AF865768

INFANCY IN UGANDA

Infancy in Uganda: Infant Care and the Growth of Love by Mary D. Salter Ainsworth, a pioneering study on early childhood attachment returns in this special reprint edition, complete with a new introduction that situates Ainsworth's work amid contemporary debates and critiques. It explores the dynamics of mother-infant attachment within the Ganda community, analyzing how cultural caregiving practices shape early emotional bonds.

Ainsworth's meticulous observations of Ganda families in the 1950s, initially praised for their insights into maternal-infant bonds, have since become a touchpoint in discussions about the importance of cross-cultural observations, the universality of attachment patterns, and evolving caregiving norms. Through detailed case studies, Ainsworth examines the methods of infant care used by the Ganda during the first 15 months of a child's life and considers the effects of these methods on the child's psychosocial development. It delves into the evolution of attachment research, addressing how modern studies question early findings, particularly in the context of cross-cultural diversity and changing family dynamics.

This classic edition showcases Ainsworth's findings and contextualises them through the lens of current psychological research and societal changes, highlighting how attachment theory remains influential—and controversial—across disciplines. This book will be invaluable to psychologists, anthropologists, educators, and anyone interested in the development of attachment theory, as well as those examining cultural contexts in child-rearing practices.

Mary D. Salter Ainsworth (1913–1999) was Professor Emerita in the Department of Psychology at the University of Virginia. She was a pioneering developmental psychologist best known for her groundbreaking work on attachment theory. Ainsworth's most influential work emerged from her observations in Uganda, detailed in this book. Ainsworth's contributions earned her numerous awards, including the American Psychological Association's Award for Distinguished Scientific Contributions. Her work remains foundational in psychology, impacting fields as diverse as psychotherapy, social work, and education, and continues to shape attachment research and theory today.

Psychology Press and Routledge Classic Editions

The *Psychology Press and Routledge Classic Editions series* celebrates a commitment to excellence in scholarship, teaching, and learning within the field of Psychology. The books in this series are widely recognized as timeless classics, of continuing importance for both students and researchers. Each title contains a completely new introduction which explores what has changed since the books were first published, where the field might go from here, and why these books are as relevant now as ever. Written by recognized experts, and covering core areas of the subject, the *Psychology Press and Routledge Classic Editions* series presents fundamental ideas to a new generation.

What Predicts Divorce?: The Relationship Between Marital Processes and Marital Outcomes (Classic Edition)
John M. Gottman

The Thin Woman: Feminism, Post-structuralism and the Social Psychology of Anorexia Nervosa (Classic Edition)
Helen Malson

Infancy in Uganda: Infant Care and the Growth of Love (Classic Edition)
Mary D. Salter Ainsworth

For more information about this series, please visit: www.routledge.com/our-products/book-series/PPCLASSICS

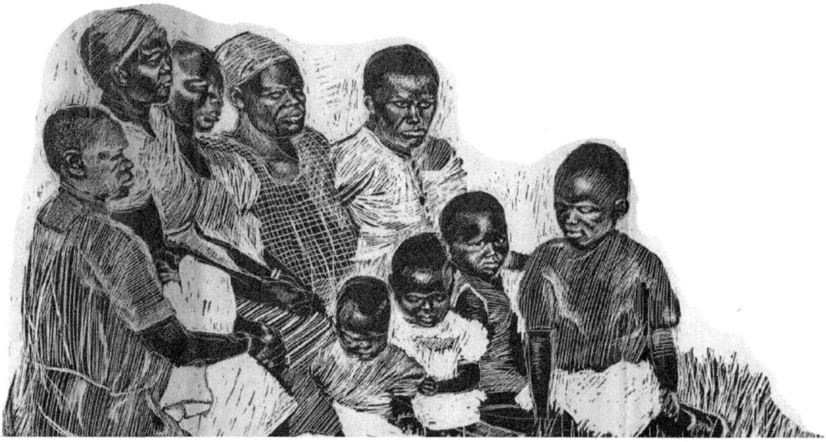

INFANCY IN UGANDA

Infant Care and the Growth of Love

Classic Edition

Mary D. Salter Ainsworth

Routledge
Taylor & Francis Group
NEW YORK AND LONDON

Designed cover image: Author supplied

Classic edition published 2027
by Routledge
605 Third Avenue, New York, NY 10158

and by Routledge
4 Park Square, Milton Park, Abingdon, Oxon, OX14 4RN

Routledge is an imprint of the Taylor & Francis Group, an informa business

First edition published by The Johns Hopkins Press 1967

Publisher's Note
References within each chapter are as they appear in the original complete work

ISBN: 9781041046615 (hbk)
ISBN: 9781041046608 (pbk)
ISBN: 9781003629337 (ebk)

DOI: 10.4324/9781003629337

Typeset in Times New Roman
by Newgen Publishing UK

CONTENTS

PREFACE TO THE CLASSIC EDITION

Everett Waters, Brian E. Vaughn, Inge Bretherton, Lenny van Rosmalen, and Robert S. Marvin

When we set out to prepare this new preface to *Infancy in Uganda*, we did what every generation of readers must eventually do: we reread it, only to be reminded that while the words remain fixed, we—and the field—necessarily read them with new eyes. Rereading it today, one wonders at the distance the discipline has traveled since 1967 and how much of what now seems foundational and innovative rests on emergent insights that Mary Ainsworth first articulated in this remarkable study.

When a long unavailable volume is reissued, a new preface can serve multiple functions. These include providing a roadmap for new readers and situating the work in relation to contemporary theory and research. Here, we also highlight the exceptional blend of openness, rigor, and insight that runs through *Infancy in Uganda*.

Context and Continuing Relevance

Infancy in Uganda provided crucial empirical grounding for John Bowlby's emerging theory of attachment. Bowlby shared early drafts of "The Nature of the Child's Tie to His Mother" (1958) with Ainsworth, and her field data from Kampala gave him rare observational support for the claim that attachment grows through signaling, responsiveness, and mutual regulation rather than simple need satisfaction. Equally, the Uganda study laid the conceptual and methodological foundation for her later Baltimore project, which produced the Strange Situation Procedure and the familiar A–B–C classifications.

Reading *Infancy in Uganda* today is an opportunity to see how much of that later system was already implicit in her design. Ainsworth traced normative sequences and individual variations in attachment formation, and she tested how maternal sensitivity—defined in terms of timing, accessibility, and cooperation—fostered infants' sense of security. Her qualitative descriptions of each infant-mother dyad's interactions anticipated the constructs that would later become central to developmental research on trust, exploration, and emotion regulation.

The book also has renewed significance in light of recent cross-cultural critiques. Because it has long been out of print, Ainsworth's fieldwork has seldom received the careful reading it deserves. Many criticisms of attachment theory's universality overlook the sophisticated cultural awareness already evident here. Contemporary readers will find *Infancy in Uganda* a far more modern, self-critical, and contextually sensitive investigator than one might expect from recent cross-cultural criticisms of attachment (see, Waters & Eagle, 2026).

Becoming Mary Ainsworth

Ainsworth's path to Uganda was both intellectual and personal (van Rosmalen, 2015; van Rosmalen et al., 2015; van Rosmalen et al., 2016). Born in 1913, she completed her Ph.D. at Toronto in 1939 and served in the Canadian Women's Army Corps during World War II, rising to the rank of Major. Returning to Toronto, she taught personality and emotion—replacing Magda Arnold who had accepted a position at Loyola University in Chicago—and in 1950 married Leonard Ainsworth. Soon thereafter, the couple moved to London, and she secured a Senior Researcher position at the Tavistock Clinic working with John Bowlby. She worked with Bowlby and James Robertson through the end of 1953, when her husband accepted an appointment in Kampala, Uganda. This gave her the opportunity to conduct the fieldwork that would set the course of her career.

Her field research from 1954 to 1956 produced the first systematic, prospective study of infant–caregiver interaction and attachment. It was, in many ways, the prototype for developmental ethnography. As she later recalled (Ainsworth, 1988), she began her Uganda study before Bowlby had published his theory; "The Nature of the Child's Tie to His Mother" appeared only in 1958. Her data thus informed his theory at least as much as the reverse.

Ainsworth's keen observational sense did not arise by chance. Bowlby, an amateur ornithologist, had cultivated a similar patience for watching behavior unfold in natural contexts. She also learned from James Robertson, whose films of children separated from parents remain classics of behavioral observation. Like Piaget, whose *Origins of Intelligence in Children* (1952/1954) she studied closely, Ainsworth combined analytic discipline with empathy for the child's point of view. As Jane Goodall (2010) observed, the ability to "see" behavior is not innate but cultivated—an amalgam of curiosity, patience, attentiveness, stamina, pattern recognition, empathic inference, and openness to observation unclouded by adult-centric or cultural bias. It also depends on trust building between observer and observed, the capacity to see subtle gestures, micro-sequences, and emotional cues that casual observers miss. Ainsworth's closeness to her participants—her willingness to sit on the floor, to share daily routines, to learn the rhythms of family life—was not merely personal warmth. It was a scientific strength that gave her data unusual depth and ecological validity.

Robert LeVine (1969) captured this in his *American Anthropologist* review, calling *Infancy in Uganda* "a landmark in cross-cultural research on infant behavior and development ... that uses naturalistic observation and systematic rating scales to discover developmental sequences and test antecedent–consequent hypotheses" (p. 123). He praised her frankness about field limitations and her "cautious and theoretically informative examination of the findings." He also noted her insight that infants form attachments even to figures who do not provide basic care—showing that attachment "does not rest on need gratification." Non-attachment, she found, reflected not hunger or deprivation but failures of responsiveness: mistimed interventions, inaccessibility, or emotional unavailability. LeVine concluded that her work "constitutes a major scientific advance that sets new standards for cross-cultural students of early development" (p. 124).

This judgment has endured. It is remarkable that *Infancy in Uganda* was her first independent naturalistic-observational project. Its combination of ethnographic richness and theoretical clarity established the empirical foundation for everything that followed.

An Inheritance from William Blatz

When Ainsworth set out for Uganda in 1954, she already possessed a theoretical framework that would shape everything she observed. Her undergraduate and graduate mentor at the University of Toronto, William E. Blatz, had developed a "security theory" that anticipated many features of attachment theory (Blatz, 1940, 1944, 1966). From Blatz, Ainsworth absorbed several enduring lessons:

- A developmental perspective; understanding phenomena by looking at them as they emerge and change over time.
- The value of prospective, longitudinal observation—to follow development rather than infer it retrospectively.
- The primacy of direct behavioral observation over verbal report.
- The significance of exploration, not as avoidance or distraction but as a natural expression of curiosity.
- Interest and mastery as intrinsic motives, countering the psychoanalytic view that emotional arousal is inherently toxic.

- The parent as a dependable base—a term she would later refine into the secure-base metaphor that became central to attachment theory.
- Security as an organizing theme, integrating affect, behavior, confidence, and social competence.

A developmental progression from dependent security, based on trusted others, to self-reliant security, based on internalized confidence—a theme Vygotsky developed in the 1920s–1934 (see Vygotsky, 1978) and later echoed by Stern (1985), Thompson (2006), and Tomasello (1999), among others.

Blatz's influence equipped her with a clear sense of what to look for and how to look. Yet she was also careful not to appropriate what was not hers. Her intellectual integrity prevented her from staking personal claims over ideas that overlapped with Bowlby's evolving synthesis. The result was a delay in full recognition of her own theoretical contributions—an imbalance that only recent historical work has begun to correct (Bretherton, 2003; van Rosmalen, 2015).

Blatz's concept of dependent security was often misconstrued. Social-learning theorists equated dependency with passivity, overlooking Blatz's broader view of dependency as adaptive social embeddedness. For Ainsworth, dependence on a trusted figure was the developmental soil from which confident independence grows. That insight animates every chapter of *Infancy in Uganda*: the mother's accessibility and responsiveness are not forms of indulgence but the conditions that allow exploration and mastery to flourish.

Observation and Theory

Ainsworth's approach also exemplified the perennial tension between observation and theory. Nineteenth-century positivists such as Ernst Mach (1886) feared that theory distorts perception; the anthropologists who followed Franz Boas inherited that caution, favoring description over inference. Among Ainsworth's contemporaries and mentors, Robert Hinde (1982) was particularly insistent that observation must precede theory. Yet Albert Einstein (1936) had influentially argued the opposite: "There is no inductive method which could lead to the fundamental concepts of physics." Facts alone, he observed, never generate concepts; theory guides attention, frames observation, and, if used wisely, sharpens perception rather than dulling it. As Marvin Harris (1969, p. 287) noted, one has merely to observe birds flying, smoke rising, or clouds drifting to realize that Galileo could not have discovered his principle of uniform acceleration without a theory, or at least a question, to focus his observations.

Ainsworth intuitively grasped this balance. Her work in Uganda was guided by theory but never constrained by it. She recorded behaviors relevant to Bowlby's hypotheses yet allowed for unanticipated findings to refine them. As she told Everett Waters, "I didn't go to Uganda to prove Bowlby's theory; I went to see whether the theory fit the data" (M. D. S. Ainsworth, personal communication, mid-1970s). This exemplifies what later methodological writers would describe as a reflexive stance, one that acknowledges the theory-ladenness of observation while treating empirical data as potentially corrective rather than merely confirmatory (e.g., Becker, 1996; Schindler, 2018). She acknowledged her theoretical commitments but treated them as part of the discovery process, not doctrines to be defended. This intellectual stance, coupled with her exceptional capacity for sustained, exacting observation, makes *Infancy in Uganda* a work of enduring value.

From Uganda to Baltimore—and Beyond

The conceptual thread linking Uganda to Baltimore is unmistakable (Ainsworth & Marvin, 1995; Bretherton, 2013). Both studies examined how infants use caregivers as a secure base—a phrase Ainsworth coined and introduced to Bowlby during their Tavistock discussions. Both traced how variations in maternal sensitivity and cooperation influence attachment security. And both revealed how a sense of safety fosters exploration and autonomy. The later Baltimore project refined her methods—introducing time-sampled home observations and, ultimately, the laboratory Strange Situation—but it did not alter her vision. It merely translated observational insights into experimental precision.

Her Uganda findings also prefigured later debates about cultural variation. She described multiple attachments, caregiving by siblings and fathers, and the ecological factors that shape infants' experiences of accessibility. Her analytic distinctions—between being attached and unattached, between the strength and security of attachment—anticipated refinements that Bowlby and subsequent researchers would formalize only years later (Bowlby, 1969).

Cross-Cultural Critique and Ainsworth's Relevance

Over the decades, attachment theory has faced a widening array of cross-cultural criticisms. Waters and Eagle (2026) catalogued nine recurrent claims: that attachment theory is monocultural; that it neglects diverse caregiving practices; that its measures are culturally biased; that universality claims are overstated; that its core postulates are narrow; that it overemphasizes mothers; that it is prescriptive across cultures; that it underestimates situational and ecological factors such as mothers' need to work; and that its evolutionary rationale is flawed.

Infancy in Uganda demonstrates, well before these criticisms were formulated, that Ainsworth fully recognized what critics claim attachment theorists ignore. She describes variability in caregiving organization as well as ecological constraints. Many infants have multiple caregivers and are attached to several of them, and most mothers necessarily devote significant time to growing food. Moreover, she treats cultural difference not as deviation from a Western norm but as a source of theoretical insight. For example, despite Bowlby's emphasis on prototypical maternal behaviors, Ainsworth contrasts hugging and kissing of and by infants, the norm in Western societies, as "largely a culture-bound behavior", learned by reinforcement or imitation, and rarely seen among the Ganda. She shows that attachment behaviors arise within cultural systems of caregiving and that secure relationships may be organized differently across contexts while serving the same adaptive functions. Far from assuming universality, she documents how universal processes take particular form in specific environments—to the point of noting in her Preface that

> The title is, of course, a misnomer. I am not concerned with infancy in Uganda but with infancy in Buganda [specifically six non-adjacent villages in the province of Buganda], and, in fact, with a relatively small sample of infants in Buganda. (p. ix)

This critical stance extended to her own role as an observer. She acknowledged misinterpretations, corrected earlier assumptions, and treated ethnographic detail not as ornament but as evidence. Perhaps if *Infancy in Uganda* had remained in print, contemporary cross-cultural critics would have been reassured by her openness, lack of dogmatism, and willingness to engage alternative worldviews on their own terms.

The Ethological Eye

Readers familiar with Ainsworth's later Baltimore studies may still be struck by how much of her mature precision was already evident in Uganda. Baltimore scales for sensitivity, cooperation, and accessibility were rooted in this field experience. She honed her eye for parsing and sequencing infant signals and maternal responses and seeing that behavior has meaning—akin to James Robertson methods—in the dusty courtyards of Kampala. LeVine's (1969) observation that her approach "derives from ethology but is nonetheless strongly environmentalist" remains apt: she shared ethology's respect for natural observation but emphasized the social and ecological matrix in which behavior is organized. Her field method combined the descriptive patience of a biologist with the interpretive curiosity of an anthropologist—a fusion rarely achieved then or since.

Ainsworth's ability to connect with her participants also shaped her science. Coming to know Ganda families, she learned their rhythms of feeding, weaning, and daily labor. She observed how infants adjusted to rotating caretakers and how small variations in maternal timing influenced trust and exploration. The intimacy of those observations produced data unmatched in texture. Her science was personal without being sentimental, empirical without being detached. That blend—an empathy disciplined by structure—would later become the signature of the attachment tradition she helped create.

Reading *Infancy in Uganda* Today

To reread *Infancy in Uganda* in the twenty-first century is to witness Mary Ainsworth, at the beginning of a storied career, discovering a new way of seeing human development.

The book is organized into four sections. The Preface and Part I provide essential orienting information about the project. They also illustrate the openness with which Ainsworth reported the background, diversity, and her relationship to the communities in which the study was conducted. Part 2 provides a mostly narrative overview of Ganda infant care practices ancient and contemporary and infants' responses to them. This is intended primarily for readers who are not expert in cultural anthropology. Part 3 consists entirely of detailed case studies of individual babies and their families. Here Ainsworth recognizes that readers have different requirements, and suggests that some, rather than exploring the details of each case study, may want to read selectively and proceed to Part 4. In particular, the four chapters that deal with attachment development and the concluding chapter, which she describes as "the book's chief contribution to the psychology of infant development" (Ainsworth, 1967, p. ix). On rereading it today, we were impressed by how precociously modern it seems, and how much more nuanced it is than many contemporary portrayals, and criticisms, of attachment theory. It is a wonder to read in a book published 60 years ago and so long out of print.

Infancy in Uganda teaches that theory and observation can and must converse, that culture and biology are intertwined, and that the everyday acts of caregiving are as worthy of rigorous study as any laboratory task. Several guideposts may help the modern reader:

- Interface of theory and observation. Both in the way insights she distilled from Blatz informed her understandings, and in adopting a posture that allowed her to benefit from Bowlby's emerging insights while remaining independent enough that her results could provide valuable guidance as attachment theory evolved.
- Expositional clarity and depth. Concepts and insights retain the richness of observed interaction, whereas Bowlby often compressed them into operational proxies, as when he equated attachment with proximity seeking and defined exploration as antithetic to attachment.

- Relatedness to the mothers, addressing them respectfully, treating them as individuals in their own individual circumstances: "… these people are my friends and know it" (Ainsworth, 1967, p. x).
- Self-awareness. She makes her reasoning transparent, acknowledges error, and trusts readers to think alongside her.
- Acuity in observing both behavior, context, and longitudinal trajectory.
- The transition from strength of attachment to attachment security.
- The emerging secure-base concept. A concept that originated with Blatz and quickly evolved toward its current meaning in her work in Uganda.
- Recognition of multiple attachments. Multiple attachments, fathers, siblings, and non-nurturing figures all find a place in her account.

Infancy in Uganda stands not merely as a historical document but as a model of how developmental science can integrate naturalistic observation, theoretical imagination, and cultural respect. Mary Ainsworth combined intellectual rigor with personal grace. Her work remains a secure base for an entire generation of researchers as they discover the wonders of behavior and explore the complexities of attachment, culture, and human growth. Routledge deserve our deep appreciation for reissuing this volume, thereby preserving its place in the history of the social and behavioral sciences and ensuring its role in the future of attachment theory and research.

Everett Waters, Brian E. Vaughn, Inge Bretherton,
Lenny van Rosmalen, and Robert S. Marvin

References

Ainsworth, M. D. S. (1967). *Infancy in Uganda: Infant care and the growth of love.* Baltimore, MD: Johns Hopkins Press.

Ainsworth, M. D. S. (1988). Security. Paper presented at the New York Attachment Consortium, Port Jefferson, NY.

Ainsworth, M. D. S., & Marvin, R. S. (1995). On the shaping of attachment theory and research: An interview with Mary D. S. Ainsworth (Fall 1994). *Monographs of the Society for Research in Child Development, 60*(2–3), 3–21. https://doi.org/10.1111/j.1540-5834.1995.tb00200.x

Becker, H. S. (1996). *The epistemology of qualitative research.* University of Chicago Press.

Blatz, W. E. (1940). *Human security.* Philadelphia, PA: Blakiston.

Blatz, W.E. (1944). *Understanding the young child.* New York, NY: William Morrow and Company.

Blatz, W. E. (1966). *Foundations of security.* Toronto, ON: University of Toronto Press.

Bowlby, J. (1958). The nature of the child's tie to his mother. *International Journal of Psycho-Analysis, 39,* 350–373.

Bowlby, J. (1969). *Attachment and loss: Vol. 1. Attachment.* Basic Books.

Bretherton, I. (2003). Mary Ainsworth: Insightful observer and courageous theoretician. In G. A. Kimble & M. Wertheimer (Eds.), *Portraits of pioneers in psychology* (Vol. 5, pp. 317–331). American Psychological Association.

Bretherton, I. (2013). Revisiting Mary Ainsworth's conceptualization and assessments of maternal sensitivity–insensitivity. *Attachment & Human Development*, *15*(5–6), 460–484. https://doi.org/10.1080/14616734.2013.835128

Einstein, A. (1936). As quoted in Miller, A. I. (1984). Imagery in scientific thought: Creating 20th-Century physics. Springer.

Goodall, J. (2010). *In the Shadow of Man (50th Anniversary ed.)*. Mariner Books Classics

Harris, M. (1969). *The rise of anthropological theory*. New York: Crowell.

Hinde, R. A. (1982). *Ethology: Its nature and relations with other sciences*. New York: Oxford University Press.

LeVine, R. A. (1969). Review of *Infancy in Uganda: Infant care and the growth of love*, by M. D. S. Ainsworth. *American Anthropologist*, *71*(1), 122–124.

Mach, E. (1886). *The analysis of sensations*. Jena: Gustav Fischer.

Piaget, J. (1952/1954). *The origins of intelligence in children* (M. Cook, Trans.). International Universities Press.

Schindler, S. (2018). *Theories and models in the social sciences: Reflexivity reconsidered*. London: Routledge.

Stern, D. N. (1985). *The interpersonal world of the infant: A view from psychoanalysis and developmental psychology*. Basic Books.

Thompson, R. A. (2006). The development of the person: Social understanding, relationships, self, conscience. In W. Damon & R. M. Lerner (Eds.), *Handbook of child psychology: Vol. 3. Social, emotional, and personality development* (6th ed., pp. 24–98). Wiley.

Tomasello, M. (1999). *The cultural origins of human cognition*. Harvard University Press.

van Rosmalen, L. (2015). From security to attachment: Mary Ainsworth's contribution to attachment theory (Doctoral dissertation, Leiden University). Document (pdf) available online via permanent link, Leiden University https://hdl.handle.net/1887/33739

van Rosmalen, L., Van der Veer, R., & Van der Horst, F. (2015). Ainsworth's strange situation procedure: The origin of an instrument. *Journal of the History of the Behavioral Sciences*, *51*(3), 261–284.

van Rosmalen, L., Van Der Horst, F. C., & Van der Veer, R. (2016). From secure dependency to attachment: Mary Ainsworth's integration of Blatz's security theory into Bowlby's attachment theory. *History of Psychology*, *19*(1), 22.

Vygotsky, L. S. (1978). *Mind in society: The development of higher psychological processes*. Cambridge, MA: Harvard University Press.

Waters, E., & Eagle, M. N. (2026). *Cross-cultural criticisms of attachment: A review and taxonomy*. Unpublished manuscript.

FOREWORD

When a baby is born he cannot tell one person from another and indeed can hardly tell person from thing. Yet, by his first birthday he is likely to have become a connoisseur of people. Not only does he come quickly to distinguish familiars from strangers but amongst his familiars he chooses one or more favorites. They are greeted with delight; they are followed when they depart; and they are sought when absent. Their loss causes anxiety and distress; their recovery, relief and a sense of security. On this foundation, it seems, the rest of his emotional life is built—without this foundation there is risk for his future happiness and health.

Despite the work of such pioneers as Mary Shirley and Charlotte Buhler, until recently our knowledge of the ways in which and the means by which a baby undergoes this dramatic transformation has been meager—and such knowledge as there was has been obscured by tenaciously held assumption and speculation. During the past decade, however, a new spirit of inquiry has been abroad, and the field has been recognized as one calling for skilled and sustained research. Among those first to embark upon such research is the author, and the study she reports here is among the first fruits of the new era.

As in any pioneer venture, Dr. Mary D. Salter Ainsworth was faced with many problems, notably those of selecting a research strategy appropriate to our state of knowledge and to her own restricted opportunities, and of deciding how best to describe her findings and to conceptualize them. In both cases, her choices, I believe, were wise. The approach she adopts is the natural history approach typical of the social anthropologist and of the ethologist; the terms she uses to present the findings are parsimonious of assumption and abstraction. As a result we are given vivid pictures of some twenty-eight babies and their mothers and the way each behaved toward the other. While the sample is small enough for each family to have been observed in some depth and the baby's social development recorded in firsthand detail, it is also large enough to give a good indication of the range of individual difference likely to be encountered.

Though in these babies, as in every other sample, the speed of development of basic social skills varied greatly, there are certain patterns of behavior and certain sequences in the development of these patterns that appeared with regularity. To have described these common patterns and sequences for a single sample of babies is an invaluable first step. The fact that it was first done for babies living in an unfamiliar culture is largely fortuitous; but Dr. Ainsworth is already applying her methods, improved in the light of experience, to a sample of babies living in the more familiar culture of middle-class American homes. This has the great advantage that in the present exposition she is able to give preliminary indication of how the two samples resemble each other and how they differ. It is already clear that resemblances far outweigh differences.

Once we have a reliable picture of common patterns of behavior and of common sequences in their development we shall be in an immeasurably better position to recognize deviant development and to explore the conditions that make for it. As a substantial start in this direction Dr. Ainsworth's book is greatly to be welcomed. On the one hand, it will provide research workers with indispensable data they will find no where else; on the other, it will provide clinicians with a few of those solid facts about early social and emotional development that have hitherto been so conspicuous by their absence.

London John Bowlby
September, 1966

PREFACE

This book is primarily a research report—a report of short-term longitudinal research into the development of a sample of Ganda infants—which I undertook while associated with the East African Institute of Social Research in Kampala, Uganda, in 1954–55. Of the various aspects of infant development observed, I paid closest attention to social development, focusing on the growth of attachment of the infant to his mother and to other members of his household.

The report is addressed to a wide variety of people interested in infant development and in the interaction of a baby with his mother. My first concern was to compile a report for those with a scientific or professional interest in child development—specifically, for developmental psychologists, child psychiatrists, psychoanalysts, and pediatricians. But parents are also interested in infant development. I have therefore tried to make this book accessible to the general reader by avoiding technical terminology and by making explicit any background theory upon which I have drawn. For the most part it was easy to write non-technically because most of the book deals with a description of people's speech and actions.

Because my investigation was of infants in an African society, the report is addressed also to the variety of persons interested in the African people and how they live. These include cultural anthropologists and others concerned with cross-cultural studies. Indeed, one of the original purposes of the investigation was to look closely at the details of Ganda methods of infant care, since these methods had not been described fully by anthropologists who had previously studied Ganda life. I was not wholly successful in achieving this aim because, despite an inquiry into ancient customs, the families whose practices I observed were more acculturated than the average Ganda family and hence were not representative of the whole society. Nevertheless, I anticipate that my findings will be of use in an anthropological context.

Finally, this is a field study—a study of babies and mothers in their natural habitat. Therefore, I can believe that behavioral scientists interested in field studies of other species—especially other primate species—will find common ground here. Certainly I myself have been much stimulated by the work of ethologists and comparative psychologists, especially as it impinges on mother-infant interaction and on care of the young. I trust that I can reciprocate by offering students of animal behavior a report of data relevant to their interests.

The book is divided into four parts. Part I, which deals chiefly with purposes and procedures, is intended for all classes of reader, but especially for the scientific reader, who always seeks to be informed of the methodological details. Field studies are becoming increasingly popular among psychologists and other behavioral scientists who have no tradition "in the field." I hope that this report will be of help to greenhorns who are contemplating field studies, whether at home or abroad. May I draw particular attention to the discussion of the problem of eliciting and sustaining cooperation from participants. Also I recommend to investigators in strange societies the blend of longitudinal and cross-sectional methods; I adopted this blend from necessity but believe that it is an excellent approach for the developmental study that must be accomplished in a relatively short timespan.

I should say a word about Chapter 2. It is intended for readers whose competence and range of information lie outside the realm of cultural anthropology and will be a disappointment to cultural anthropologists. It is a very sketchy account of Ganda life, including only what seemed essential as a background for the rest of the book. I focused my observations on methods of infant care. In regard to all other aspects of Ganda life I was a casual observer; any more adequate account that I could give of the Ganda would have to be a scholarly review of other workers' observations, and I eschewed this as peripheral to the chief purposes of this book.

Part II deals with a description of Ganda methods of infant care, contemporary and ancient, and with the babies' responses to them. It is this part which ought to be of most interest to cultural anthropologists and to others interested in cross-cultural studies. As a background for the rest of the book this part is essential for the student of infant development, for it deals with the environment in which that development took place. The general reader, also, is curious about how the people of another society manage the everyday details of family life.

Part III consists entirely of case studies—descriptions of the individual babies and their families. These descriptions are, of course, condensations of the detailed reports of each visit made to each family, but they give the reader a more intimate glimpse into the life of the families in the sample than is possible in the organized accounts given in Parts II and IV. The general reader may find his main focus of interest in this section, although he may find that his interest wanes after reading several of the case studies, and he may wish to skip on to Part IV. It is rarely possible for a clinical research psychologist to publish case studies; it is even rarer for him to publish all of them and not just an illustrative few. Yet I believe that this practice should be encouraged. Since intensive longitudinal studies are so time consuming, any one investigator can observe but a few cases. But several investigators, publishing details of the cases they have studied, can together provide a much larger sample than any single investigation encompasses. To be sure, information gathered by one investigator for his own particular scientific purposes may not be wholly relevant to the interests of others with different purposes. Nevertheless, it is my hope that my observations will be of use to other investigators, and therefore I have included for each case a fair amount of detail—more than would be required merely to give the reader the feel of how Ganda babies live and how they develop.

Part IV constitutes the book's chief contribution to the psychology of infant development, especially the four chapters that deal with the development of attachment and the concluding chapter. It was Part IV that delayed the preparation of this book for eleven years after the data upon which it is based were collected. The full significance of what I observed and recorded in my field reports emerged only gradually, not merely in the process of analyzing my observations, but also in the course of reading, discussions with others interested in mother-infant interaction, and further research into the early development of attachment. The first three parts were easy to prepare, and indeed were in advanced draft some years ago. Part IV was more difficult, but, I believe, it is the best part. In this section of the book I occasionally came to points which had to be included for the developmental scientist but which I could expect to be outside the scope of the general reader; this occurred especially in the final chapter. I dealt with the more technical points in footnotes as much as possible, in the hope that the reader, whose interest and competence did not extend to the point under discussion, could skip it without losing the main thread of the report, whereas the reader who was indeed particularly concerned with the issue in question could at least be referred to sources in the literature.

The title is, of course, a misnomer. I am not concerned with infancy in Uganda, but with infancy in Buganda, and, in fact, with a relatively small sample of infants in Buganda. But the name of the country is familiar to the Western reader whereas the name of the province is not.

The tables are included for the use of the scientific reader who values the comprehensive summary of details that they provide. The general reader can skip them as well as the footnotes without loss of essential information. The list of references at the end is limited to the works which were actually cited in the text and is given for convenience, not as a comprehensive list of relevant works.

Despite the fact that the investigation here reported was an individual rather than a team enterprise, it was dependent at one stage or another upon the help of many people, whom it is now my pleasure to thank. My deepest gratitude goes to the families of the babies themselves, and especially to the mothers, whose participation made the project possible, and whose friendship transformed a scientific investigation into a happy and unforgettable experience. It was a great privilege for me to come to know the participant families as well as I did, and to learn that cultural differences do not separate us in regard to the most deeply cherished of human values. I have not named these families, and indeed have given the infants pseudonyms, in order to spare them any embarrassment which they might conceivably experience as a result of the details I have recorded about them. To be sure, I have included some photographs to illustrate behaviors that are highly relevant to the main content of my argument. Photographs play havoc with anonymity, but since it is extremely unlikely that any embarrassment will accrue I have gone ahead, buoyed up by the knowledge that these people are my friends and know it.

I wish to express warmest appreciation to Mrs. Katie Kibuka, who was an essential and highly valued partner in the research. She served as interpreter, research assistant, and friend. Without her sensitivity and insight it would have been much more difficult to gain the confidence and cooperation of the participating families. Also essential to the project were the chiefs and leaders who helped me gather a sample in the initial stages of the project: Omwami Lwanga, the *ggombolola* chief; Abaami Kulazikulabe and Ignatio Zigudde, the *miruka* chiefs; and Omwami Sematimba, a leader by reason of tradition and ability.

Dr. Hebe Welbourn gave invaluable assistance to the project. Transportation to her child welfare clinic was the chief benefit we offered to the participants in the research; she gave them prompt and expert help with sympathy and understanding and thus benefitted them and the project greatly. Furthermore, I wish to thank her for sharing with me her insights and knowledge of Ganda ways, which are based on long and close experience with the Ganda; this helped me in planning the research, in carrying it through, and, finally, in preparing this report. Specifically, I wish to thank her for allowing me access to her manuscript on *Baganda Childhood* and for granting me permission to quote parts of it. Special thanks are also due to Dr. Marcelle Géber, who administered the Gesell Developmental Schedules to a portion of my sample, and who has kindly given me permission to quote her findings.

I wish to thank my colleagues in the East African Institute of Social Research for their expert advice, and especially Dr. Audrey Richards, who was at that time director of the Institute, and whose help has extended from the preparatory stages of the study to the present.

I must also single out Dr. John Bowlby for special thanks, both for the stimulation he has given to my thinking over the past sixteen years and for the specific help and encouragement he has lent through' out the preparation of this book. Not the least of his contributions was the convening and directing of the four Tavistock Seminars on Mother-Infant Interaction. It was of immeasurable help to meet with the members of the study group and to exchange findings and ideas. The indirect contributions of these colleagues are reflected in my frequent references to their seminar papers, which have been ably edited by Brian Foss and published in the series entitled *Determinants of Infant Behavior.*

May I express specific thanks also to the following people for reading earlier drafts of the manuscript and offering helpful suggestions, or for special encouragement when it was much needed, or both: Margaret Bullowa, Bettye Caldwell, Ellin Deese, James Deese, Leonard Doob, Wendell Garner, Harry Harlow, Jerome Hartz, Christoph Heinicke, James Robertson, Mollie Smart, L. J. Stone, and J. W. M. Whiting.

During the period of collection of the data I was supported by the East African Institute of Social Research. U.S.P.H.S. Grant M4644 was given specifically to aid me in the period of data analysis —although the task extended beyond the limits of the grant itself. During the period of preparation of the book itself I received support, specifically intended for another related project, from Grant 62–244 of the Foundations' Fund for Research in Psychiatry and from U.S.P.H.S. Grant 1 RO1 HD 01712–01. I acknowledge with gratitude these sources of support.

I acknowledge with thanks the permission from Methuen to reproduce material previously published in *Determinants of Infant Behaviour, II,* albeit in greatly expanded form.

Finally, I much appreciate the help and encouragement of the editors of The Johns Hopkins Press. The book has been long in preparation, and without their unwavering support I might never have managed to complete it.

Baltimore, 1966 Mary D. Salter Ainsworth

ILLUSTRATIONS

PART I

Purposes and Procedures

1

PURPOSES AND PLANS

The first fifteen months of the life of the Ganda infant is the subject matter of this book. A small sample of twenty-eight babies was observed as they developed over a period of several months. Their mothers told us about the methods of infant care that they employed, and indeed we could observe many of these practices ourselves. In regard to some practices there was a high degree of uniformity; in others there were substantial differences from one family to another. We were particularly interested in the course of development of early interpersonal relations and especially in the development of the baby's attachment to his mother and to others. We were also interested in variations in this development that might be attributed to differences in the infant-care practices of the mothers.

Not infrequently a research project that sets out to explore one problem becomes transformed into an investigation of a related problem. Such was the case with this project. I consider it very fortunate that the project took an unexpected turn, for it led me into a line of profitable investigation which I have pursued ever since. I would not burden the reader with an account of my original purposes and plans were it not for the fact that some knowledge of these is necessary if he is to comprehend my approach and choice of sample.

As an "experiment of opportunity," the project was originally intended to investigate the responses of very young children to separation from their mothers under conditions in which this response was not confounded by the effects either of a depriving institution or of traumatic influences such as illness or the breakup of the family. Since the Ganda were reputed customarily to separate infants from their mothers at the time of weaning and to send them to be reared by grandmothers or other relatives, this society appeared to be a good setting for such a natural experiment. Furthermore, it was generally understood that weaning

DOI: 10.4324/9781003629337-2

was, by ancient custom, sudden and traumatic among the Ganda. Therefore, it seemed likely that this society would also provide a good opportunity to contrast the effects of customarily abrupt weaning with the effects of gradual weaning practiced by those who had abandoned old customs.

My original plan was to select a sample of unweaned babies who could be expected to undergo the process within a few months and to observe them in their relations to their mothers and to other members of their families; my hope was to establish a base line of behavior before the disruption that weaning might be expected to bring. It was anticipated that some would be weaned abruptly according to ancient custom whereas others would be weaned gradually, and the responses of the two groups were to be compared. Furthermore, it was thought that some would be separated from their families at weaning according to old custom whereas others would not be, and the comparison of the separated and non-separated groups could possibly throw light on the breach of ties implicit in "pure" separation unconfounded by other traumatic or depriving conditions.

I therefore sought a sample of unweaned babies. Much preliminary work was required before I could persuade any families to cooperate in the project; this phase is described in Chapter 3. The sample itself is described in Chapter 4. For our present purposes, however, it must be said only that the sample grew gradually as we won the confidence of the first participants, and that from the outset it was more heterogeneous in age than had originally been intended.

Long before the sample was complete, information obtained from our first participants suggested that an insufficient number of babies were likely to be separated from their families for mother-child separation to remain the focus of the research. It became apparent that the "experiment of opportunity" was not going to materialize. Furthermore, inquiries about weaning plans yielded the information that abrupt weaning was *not* customary among the Ganda, contrary to the impression that Europeans commonly had gained, and thus we could not expect to make a comparison between abrupt and gradual weaning.

Meanwhile, we had been observing the development of infant-mother interaction, and were obtaining information about the development of attachment that had not previously been reported in the scientific literature. What had been conceived of as a mere base line, against which postweaning and separation responses could be evaluated, was emerging as the major focus of interest. As this shift in emphasis took place, we had the opportunity to enlarge the sample by including babies both younger and older than the age originally conceived as a criterion for selection. Since we were curious to observe the characteristic attachment behavior of these younger and older babies, the sample became even more heterogenous in age.

In retrospect, I believe that I stumbled onto a methodology that is very useful in field studies of development that must be completed within a limited time span. Ideally, a study of development begins at the beginning—or at some specified point—and proceeds by a systematic, longitudinal follow-through of all cases. Under such circumstances the collection of data is extremely time-consuming. If one wishes to study even as short a span of development as the first year of life, eighteen months or more are needed to allow for time to make arrangements, gain cooperation, and find a sample. Most investigators who have only a short time for a developmental study choose cross-sectional methods. A sample is selected from children of different ages, and through a comparison of one age level with another, a picture of the developmental process may be inferred. There are, however, two serious disadvantages to the cross-sectional study. First, the inferences derived are not an entirely satisfactory substitute for a direct study of the developmental process. Secondly, it is much more difficult to establish rapport and to gain reliable information in the relatively brief period of contact dictated by the design of a cross-sectional study than it is to do so in a longitudinal study.

The heterogeneity of the Ganda sample made it possible for me to derive benefit from both kinds of studies. Since all babies were observed over a span of time, even though it was a short span in some cases, I could observe developmental changes. Furthermore, all mothers were visited several times, and most were visited frequently. The repeated visits yielded a reliability of information which is quite impossible to achieve in a strictly cross-sectional approach. On the other hand, the inclusion of babies of different ages enabled me to deal with a much longer developmental period than would have been possible had all subjects been of uniform age at the beginning of the project.

Even though the focus of interest shifted from weaning and separation to the development of attachment, our interest in infant care practices was constant. From the beginning we attempted to gather as much information as we could on Ganda methods of infant care. We found out as much as we could about customs of weaning and separation, and these are reported in Chapters 24 and 25. We also inquired about specific details pertaining to the whole of the infancy period; we obtained information from informants who remembered traditional customs, and we observed current practices.

Thus, in retrospect, the purposes of this study may be summarized as follows:

1. To describe Ganda customs of infant care as they pertain to the first fifteen months of life, including both traditional customs and current practices.
2. To observe and record the course of development during the first fifteen months of life, with particular reference to the development of interpersonal relations, and most specifically with reference to the development of attachment behavior.
3. To ascertain the effect of variations in infant-care practices upon the course of development, particularly upon the growth of attachment.

2

THE GANDA AND HOW THEY LIVE

The Ganda[1] constitute the largest and most dominant of the societies in Uganda.[2] Buganda is the province in which they are concentrated. Uganda gained her independence in 1962, but at the time of my study it was a British Protectorate.

During the era of the early British explorers who searched for the source of the Nile in the nineteenth century, Buganda was an independent and powerful kingdom. The present *Kabaka*, or king, of the Ganda is directly descended from the *Kabakas* of the ancient kingdom, who made such a profound impression upon Speke and Grant, the first Europeans to reach Buganda, in 1862, and upon others who followed them—Stanley, Mackay, Ashe, Lugard, and Johnston.

As Richards[3] points out, these early European visitors showed remarkable unanimity in their descriptions of the Ganda, mentioning their good manners,

1 According to standard ethnographic usage, the word *Ganda* will be used as a noun to refer to the people of the society in question, and as an adjective to apply to those things pertaining to this society. The Ganda call themselves *Baganda*, however, and an individual member of their society a *Muganda;* they use the word *Kiganda* to refer to things pertaining to them. Their language is *Luganda.*

2 Uganda is in East Africa. It is bounded by the Sudan to the north, Kenya to the east, Tanzania to the south, and the Congo to the west. It has an area of 93,981 square miles, of which 8,320 are water. Its population is now 6,500,000, but in 1952 it was estimated to consist of about five million Africans, 48,000 Asians (mostly of Indian origin), and 5,600 Europeans (most of whom were British). The province of Buganda has an area of about 25,000 square miles, of which one-third is water. The Ganda themselves number some 1,500,000. Kampala is the principal city and traditional capital of Buganda; it has a metropolitan population of 123,000.

3 Audrey I. Richards, "Traditional Values and Current Political Behavior," in L. A. Fallers (ed.), *The King's Men: Leadership and Status in Modern Buganda* (London: Oxford University Press, 1964), pp. 297–300.

DOI: 10.4324/9781003629337-3

politeness, and charm, their cleanliness, neatness, modesty, and orderliness, their dignity and intelligence, shrewdness in negotiations, efficiency in the administration of their own affairs, and their centralized organization. On the less favorable side, the Europeans complained that the Ganda were touchy, competitive, legalistic, capable of surprising cruelty, reticent, difficult to know well, and fickle in their ingrained practice of shifting loyalties with shifting patterns of power. In both the characteristics that were admired by Europeans and those that were criticized, the Ganda showed from first acquaintance that they were no simple, "primitive", uncomplicated people.

Buganda, on the northwestern shore of Lake Victoria, is a land of green hills, fertile soil, and lush vegetation, much of which has given way to groves of banana-like plantain trees which yield the staple food. The climate is tropical but surprisingly moderate despite Uganda's equatorial location. At Kampala the mean maximum temperature is about 80 degrees.

The people speak Luganda, a Bantu language. Some degree of Europeanized education is characteristic of most present-day Ganda, but, since Luganda is the language used at the elementary school levels, the less educated do not speak English as a general rule. The higher the educational level, the more likely it is that English is spoken, and the quality of English spoken by the most highly educated is excellent indeed. Some have studied abroad, most usually in England, but more have attended Makerere College, in Kampala, which is now the University of East Africa. Education of women has lagged behind education of men. Relatively few Ganda women have any facility in English, despite having attended school for a few years and being able to read and write Luganda.

The babies whom I studied lived in six villages—not all immediately adjacent to each other—about fifteen miles from Kampala. Considering that it is rural, this is a thickly populated area, with one "village" melting into another without any clear boundaries between them, much as one suburban development follows another on the fringes of a large American city. The villages do not resemble the popular stereotype of an African village. There is no cluster of houses around some central focus where one could post oneself in order to observe village life. The houses are usually close to roads or paths, but each is surrounded by an acre or so of land. It would usually be difficult to make oneself heard if one shouted from one house to another. Each house has its own garden (*lusuku*) in which the staple plantain (*matooke*) and other fruits and vegetables are grown. If the family depends on farming for its livelihood, the acreage adjoining the house is more extensive than if there is only a garden. Although few of the families I visited were farm families, Buganda—and, indeed, Uganda as a whole—is primarily agricultural, and cotton is the chief cash crop.

The households that I visited tended to consist of the primary family living together in one house, with no close relatives living nearby. But some households consisted of two or more separate houses or huts, say, with husband, wife, and children living in one and the father's mother and her sister living in another.

The houses are no longer the circular, one-roomed huts that the early explorers found but are rectangular and divided into several rooms, although the partitions between the rooms are usually not complete and leave space for air (and sound) to circulate under the roof. Most of the houses are made of wattle and daub, with earthen floors and thatched roofs. The houses of the poorer people are small, crudely finished, and bare; those of the more affluent are large, well-finished, well-appointed, and comfortable, and some of the most affluent live in houses of cement block, with red tile roofs and cement floors. Increasing numbers of the wattle-and-daub houses have roofs of corrugated iron or aluminum, which are valued because they reduce the hazard of fire, even though they make for a hotter house than does a thatched roof.

Although the Europeans[4] in Kampala—and a few of the most fortunate Africans—had electricity and running water, these village houses did not. Water had to be fetched from a well, which was often some distance from the house. Most of the houses this close to Kampala had a latrine with a deep pit—dug according to health regulations —surrounded by a small house made of reeds; there might also be a a reed enclosure as a bathhouse. Usually there was a separate building for the kitchen, behind the house. Cooking was done on an open wood fire in the kitchen, although water for tea could be heated on a Primus stove which could be taken into the house itself. The houses were characteristically dark, with few or no windows. If there were windows, they were usually unglazed and had solid wooden shutters that could, like the doors of the house, be secured at night to prevent thieves from entering.

All of the houses that I visited had a few pieces of European-type furniture—at the very least a table, perhaps with a cross-stitched linen cover. Usually there were pictures on the walls—sometimes a picture of Queen Elizabeth, sometimes religious pictures, sometimes a wedding photograph, perhaps most often a calendar. The men seemed to like to sit on chairs, and most houses had at least one or two folding wooden chairs for their use—or for the use of a European visitor such as I. The women and children, however, nearly all sat on mats on the floor. The mats were handwoven, with decorative colored patterns; they were kept rolled up when not in use so as to keep them clean. When a woman sits on the floor she must sit with her legs tucked up close to one side, preferably covered with her skirts, without even her toes showing. To sit cross-legged or with her legs stuck straight out would be a breach of etiquette. When they are

4 In Uganda, white-skinned persons are called Europeans (in Luganda, *Bazungu)* regardless of their country of origin. For convenience I follow this usage.

very young, children are taught to sit properly. Similar rules apply to men when they sit on the floor.

I was not shown the bedrooms of the houses that I visited. I am under the impression, however, that most adults have beds made of wooden supports with some kind of woven substitute for springs. I know from written accounts of traditional customs that husband and wife do not necessarily share the same bedroom, let alone the same bed. I inquired about the baby's bed. Some babies slept with their mothers, and some had beds of their own but in the mother's room. Some of the babies' beds were cribs with high sides, some of which were adjustable and could be raised and lowered.

The first European explorers were soon followed by Christian missionaries, who had to compete, especially at first, with Islamic rivals. Both religions gained converts and established themselves. In 1954 it was estimated that there were one and a half million Christian Africans in Uganda and several hundred thousand Muslims, the remainder being pagan. In Buganda, especially in the countryside around Kampala, the proportion of pagans is much smaller. All the families in my sample claimed either a Christian or a Muslim affiliation.

Traditionally, the Ganda were polygynous. One of the influences of Christianity was to reduce the number of polygynous marriages. All the women with whom I discussed the matter felt that the status of women had been raised as a consequence. Some of the Christian mothers in my sample stated with pride that theirs was a "legal" union; this obviously gave them some feeling of prestige and security. A less fortunate consequence of the introduction of monogamy was to make marriages more frequently unstable than had been the case in the traditional polygynous union. If a man now wants a second wife he *may,* especially if he is Muslim, include her in his household without breaking it up, but he is more likely to leave his first wife and go off to live with the new one, even though this new union has no legal status. Usually the children, especially the young ones, remain with the mother, and all too frequently the father makes no provision for their needs. Traditionally, however, the children belong to the father—to his family and clan[5]—and he has the right to claim them and take them away at any time.

One of the chief tasks of the woman of the household is to cultivate the garden to provide food for the family. These gardens are usually, but not always, adjoining the house. The staple food—plantain—is relatively easy to grow, but nevertheless the woman characteristically spends most of every morning digging

5 Each Ganda baby traditionally was initiated into his father's clan in a special *okwalula* ceremony. Clan membership was rich in custom and ritual. Although the traditions associated with clan membership are still influential, despite changes introduced through acculturation, even a brief account is inappropriate here, for this is neither my field of competence nor an aspect of Ganda life into which I inquired.

in her garden. Just how much time she must spend depends upon how new or well-established the garden is, and upon how many mouths there are to feed. The woman may, as a side line, raise a little cotton or coffee to bring in a small cash income, and she may help her husband if he is a farmer, but for the most part she devotes herself to growing only what is needed for her family's food. She is also responsible for preparing family meals and rearing the children. Traditionally it was a man's job to make barkcloth for clothes, but now that most clothes are made of cotton fabric some women, especially those who have been taught in church schools, make clothes for their children. My impression is, however, that most men and women rely on tailors with sewing machines to make their clothing, especially if it is of the traditional type, or they buy European-type clothes ready-made.

The husband in present-day Buganda is the cash-earner. Cash is needed for clothing, animal foods such as meat, milk (for few of these families raise livestock, except, perhaps, a few chickens), household implements and furniture, school fees for the children, luxuries such as manually cranked record players, and transportation for the wage-earner—bus fares, bicycle, motorcycle, or even automobile. Some of the men are farmers raising cash crops, especially cotton. Others are employed, either commuting daily to their work, or with their jobs so far away that they can get home only on weekends or perhaps only three or four times a year. Since the families we visited were close to Kampala, they included a much larger proportion of commuters than is characteristic of the rest of Buganda.

In this part of Buganda nearly all children of school age attend school. Many of them attend local schools and return home each afternoon. Some of them, if they are bright enough and industrious enough to be able to meet the entrance requirements, and if their families can afford the fees, attend boarding schools, most of which are Church of England or Roman Catholic mission schools. Consequently, except during school holidays, the children at home during the day are under six years of age. Traditionally, babies could be left with older children, especially girls, but now mothers complain that they have no one with whom to leave their babies and very young children if they want or need to go anywhere that would exclude taking the children along.

Nevertheless, in the afternoons the Ganda housewife characteristically goes to visit friends who live nearby, taking along her babies and young children, or she receives visits from her neighbors. The ladies sit chatting on mats on the floor. The youngest babies are held on laps and are passed around from one lap to another, for it is considered a pleasure and an honor to be given someone else's baby to hold for a while. Babies who are old enough crawl about, exploring the room and the people in it, and often make excursions outside if they are permitted to do so. The children over two years of age (or thereabouts) sit politely, with their feet tucked under them out of sight, listening to the talk of their elders and speaking only when spoken to. If any young child becomes rambunctious and draws attention to himself, he is told to sit properly (*tuula bulungi*) or to be silent (*siriika*).

Ganda women clothe themselves in a modest but graceful garment called a *busuuti,* which has a square neck, short sleeves, a skirt sweeping to the floor, and a Greek-style peplum that is girdled by a bright-colored silken sash. The fabrics used for this standard garment are good quality, bright-colored, printed cottons. I understand that a similar garment was traditionally made of barkcloth; it resembled the present one except that it had no sleeves or square-necked yoke and was either held up by the pressure of one arm tucked close to the side or allowed to fall to the waist, exposing the breasts. But nowadays the breast is exposed only for breast feeding. The *busuuti* is convenient for breast feeding, for the mother is able to offer the left breast to her baby through the folds of her garment without really baring herself. To offer the right breast she has to expose herself more and must undo two buttons of the yoke of her dress. Most Ganda women feel free to suckle their babies in public, but a few (and I understand this is unusual) showed reluctance to expose themselves to me. The *busuuti* is also a very effective maternity dress; it is not until the last month or so of a pregnancy that the state of affairs is obvious at a glance. Since many Ganda housewives have babies every two years or so, it is of obvious advantage to be able to adjust the same clothing to increasing or decreasing girth merely by adjusting the folds and the sash.

The *busuuti* when new is used for visits, receiving visitors, and special occasions; when it is old it is used for household chores and gardening and may become faded and tattered before it is finally discarded. Although one may catch a housewife in an old dress if one visits unexpectedly, it is one of her new, bright dresses that she wears when she goes out. One of my best memories of Uganda is of people walking along the roadside on a Sunday afternoon—a beautiful, well-dressed group, with the women enhancing the clothes that they wear by their slow gait and dignified and graceful carriage.

Ganda men have two common garbs. For work they tend to wear the same khaki shirt and shorts that are the working uniform of the European male in Uganda, although they are perhaps less hesitant than the European to wear a bright-colored shirt rather than a khaki one. But for special occasions they resort to the garment that has been traditional since the first Arabs came in the 1840's—a long, white, cotton garment, with long sleeves, called a *kanzu.* When I was in Uganda, Europeanized Africans on special occasions, such as the Queen's visit, wore a European-type suit coat over their *kanzu*, with the trousers of the suit underneath it. I am told,[6] however, that in recent years *kanzus* have been less

6 Welbourn (personal communication).

frequently worn and that Ganda men now tend to wear long trousers rather than shorts.

Children of school age wore the uniforms of their schools, which differed in color from one school to another. The girls' uniform was a simple dress; the boys', shirt and shorts. Little boys wore European-type clothes, short trousers and shirts. Little girls wore European-type dresses.

Even babies were often clothed, although midday temperatures did not require clothing for warmth. Very young infants were sometimes merely wrapped in cloths, rather than being clothed, but some of them had dainty dresses and elaborate machine-knit shawls that would be admired in any Western country. Very few babies wore diapers, however, and then only on special occasions. When the baby was old enough to crawl, clothes were the general rule—at least in our sample. Most of our sample of babies were usually clothed when we saw them, even when we dropped in unexpectedly. Only six—all from Muslim families—were usually naked, and even they were put into clothes for special occasions, or for warmth when the sun got low in the sky in the late afternoon—and always when we suggested taking pictures.

During the first year of life both boys and girls most commonly wear dresses without underclothing. Some boys wear a shirt instead of a dress, but very few wear trousers, although a few babies—girls as well as boys—were sometimes seen in sunsuits of European style. The dresses, including those worn by boys, are often very attractive, made of bright-colored or pastel cotton, often of good quality, and sometimes beautifully handmade with tiny gathers or smocking. Sometimes these dresses match the mothers' *busuutis.* And sometimes babies are dressed in synthetic silk fabrics, which seem much too dressy and become singularly bedraggled when the baby gets grubby from crawling about on the earthen floor.

Often the dress was worn quite long, so that the walking child looked quaintly old-fashioned and the crawling baby was hampered by the skirt. Sometimes the dress was tied into a knot in the back, either to keep it clean or to free the baby from hindrance, but much at the expense of the modesty that is demanded of the older child. It was my impression that there was no clear-cut differentiation between boys' and girls' clothing in infancy.

Many babies wear strings of shiny, opaque, glass beads, usually colored blue, around their wrists, ankles, or waists, or perhaps in all three locations. Traditionally it was believed that these decorations made for slenderness, but nowadays they are worn for purely decorative purposes. Some babies—and all that we saw were Muslim children—wear little strings of cloth instead of, or to supplement, the beads, and especially a string like a bandolier over one shoulder and under the other arm, or across the back supported by strings tied around the upper arms; in either case the string crossing the back had three little bags attached to it. These bags are said to contain "medicine" to protect the baby from disease; one mother said that they were just like Daraprim, which the European doctor gives to protect the baby from malaria.

After a baby is able to walk he is usually given tight anklets of little brass bells—like Christmas jingle-bells—which ring as he walks, and which are believed to encourage the baby to walk because he is pleased with the sound. Some baby girls also wear bangles or strings of cowrie shells around their ankles, sometimes in addition to the bells. These ornaments are taken off when the child is about two years old and strong enough to break the strings.

3

PRELIMINARIES

Obviously the most important preliminary undertaking in any study of a society other than one's own is to gain a reasonable familiarity with what is already known about its customs and to find some solution to the difficulty presented by an unfamiliar langauge. Two important preliminary undertakings in any longitudinal study of child development are to locate a sample and to discover ways of gaining and sustaining the cooperation of the participants. It is hoped that an account of the way in which these three preliminaries were handled will be of interest and help to other psychologists who plan field studies in unfamiliar societies and to those who plan studies in their own society that will require sustained cooperation from the participants.

I was fortunate in having expert help from the beginning in learning the customs of the Ganda. The East African Institute of Social Research was situated in Buganda itself, and a substantial proportion of its personnel[1] were themselves engaged in studies of Ganda society. From them I gleaned much information, including suggestions about what to read of what was already published on the Ganda. It was also customary at the Institute for the newcomer, regardless of the branch of social science he represented, to be sent to live for a month or so in a village, isolated from his colleagues, to make an intensive effort to learn the local language and customs. According to this practice, I spent a month in a Ganda village about fifteen miles from Kampala. The experience was valuable in its introduction to Ganda customs and also in the establishment of contacts that

1 I wish particularly to express my appreciation of the help given me by Dr. Audrey I. Richards, who at that time was Director of the EAISR.

DOI: 10.4324/9781003629337-4

subsequently proved useful in the research project, for this village was one in which I later worked, and some of the families who participated in the research were families that I had first met during that month.

In regard to learning Luganda, however, my month in the village was not an unqualified success. Although I persisted in my efforts to learn Luganda, it was evident from the beginning that I would not be able to understand the language well enough to do without an interpreter when interviewing Ganda mothers. Some of the considerations in the selection of an interpreter may be of interest. In view of the nature of my proposed research, the interpreter would need to be a woman—and there were very few Ganda women whose English was fluent enough to play the interpreter's role. There were such women in the highest socio-economic level of Ganda society, but the danger was pointed out to me that women from this stratum of society would have been isolated from knowledge of, or interaction with, women in the villages who had been less privileged. I was warned that such a woman, acting as an interpreter, might well antagonize village women through a condescending or interfering attitude.

Very early in the search for an interpreter these problems were solved by my finding *Omukyala* Katie Kibuka, whose linguistic and personal attributes made her ideal for the job. She had a good secondary school education, but perhaps more important, she had toured the United States for a year with a group of African women under the auspices of the Y.W.C.A., and this had added both to her fluency in English and to a recognition of the differences between Western and Ganda customs. To her personal qualities of charm and tact was added the sensitivity of a "natural-born" fieldworker. She already had a genuine interest in the welfare of her fellow countrymen, particularly in regard to child-rearing, and had no difficulty in identifying herself with the purposes of the research. Furthermore, she herself was the mother of four children and had experience, particularly in ways of adapting European nutritional and hygienic principles to Ganda life, that was invaluable in meeting the demand of the women in our sample for help of precisely this sort.

Mrs. Kibuka's role in the research was much more important than that of mere mouthpiece. Her role during our joint visits to families will be described in Chapter 5. Here I will merely state that she became a valued assistant who could take my place when the need arose. Indeed, during a long illness of mine, she not only maintained contact with the families but also undertook interviews and recorded observations which prevented an otherwise irremediable gap from appearing in our longitudinal data.

The finding of a good interpreter did not lead me to desist from trying to learn Luganda myself. Fortunately for one with my academic bent, a Luganda grammar book and dictionary had recently been published and I studied them, Moreover, I enrolled in a class in Luganda provided for civil servants. With these academic supplements to my month in the village, I had learned a smattering of

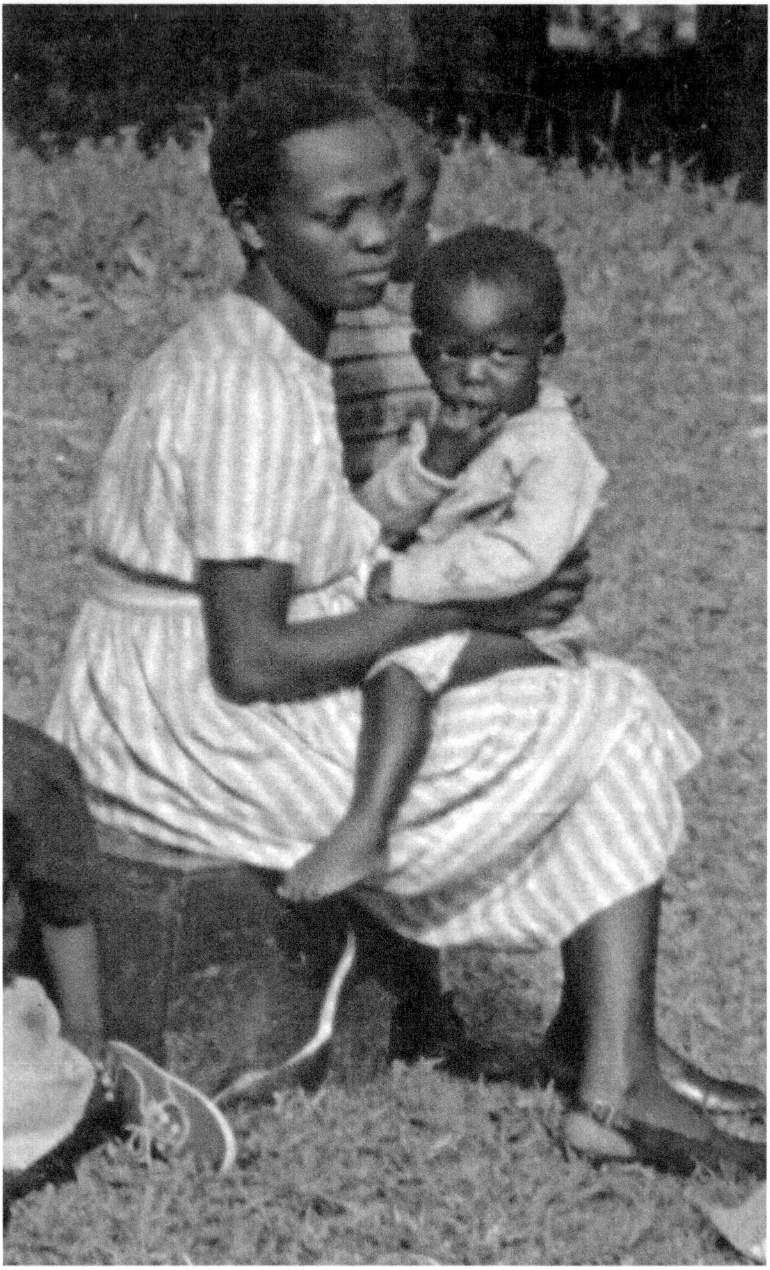

FIGURE 1 Mrs. Kibuka holding her son Robin. (Courtesy of Hebe Welbourn.)

Luganda by the time I began my research. I had learned to give the customary greetings, together with many of the elaborations of the basic greetings that facilitate polite social interaction. I had learned to ask simple questions and to understand simple replies. I had learned that most useful of all phrases for one interested in infant development— *Omwana mulungi nnyo nnyo*—"Oh! What a *beautiful* child!" I could make appointments without help. I could catch the general drift of an extensive answer to a question, even though I could not understand all the details. I prepared a speech in Luganda, which I could deliver in order to explain my purposes, but I could not carry on a question and answer period without help.

My efforts to learn Luganda were well worthwhile. The Ganda with whom I worked appreciated the compliment paid them in my efforts to learn their language, perhaps especially because so few Europeans spoke Luganda. There was, however, a more significant consequence. The language, the greetings, and the rules of good manners that regulate Ganda interaction are inextricably linked. Even a rudimentary knowledge of Luganda made it possible for me to observe the proper forms of social interaction. My linguistic efforts made by Ganda friends feel that I respected these forms—and they also made me appear less gauche in their eyes than I otherwise would have seemed. Moreover, being able to follow the general drift of conversation made it possible to interact with Ganda families more sensitively than I could have otherwise, and it was satisfying to know the participants in the project a little more intimately than would have been possible had all my contacts with them been through an interpreter.

One accident of my instruction in Luganda turned out to be valuable. The teacher of the class for civil servants taught us to address men as *Ssebo* (Sir) and women as *Nnyabo* (Madam), and to refer to a man as *Omwami* and to a woman as *Omukyala.* He did not point out that these polite modes of address and reference are used by the Ganda themselves with superiors or, at least, social equals, and not with those of inferior social status. As a consequence, I, with all gravity, addressed the villagers with whom I worked with these signs of deference. It was some months before my interpreter enlightened me; but she, with her usual tact and sensitivity, said: "I did not tell you before, because I knew that people like you to talk in this way; it shows that you respect them as individuals." Needless to say, I continued to show my respect by interjecting *Nnyabo* or *Ssebo* into my conversations.

The month in the village was useful in crystallizing my plans for carrying out the research. It was evident that there was little to be gained from basing myself in one of the villages. There were not enough babies of suitable age in any one village, even assuming that cooperation could be obtained from all parents. There was no central vantage point from which the life of an entire village could be viewed. The Ganda women themselves made it clear that they would welcome me only in the afternoon, after they had finished most of their daily chores in the garden and household. I planned, therefore, to conduct the study using Kampala as a home base, driving out every afternoon to a village to pay visits and undertake observations.

The next question was that of how to elicit and sustain cooperation since any longitudinal research of child development requires thorough-going cooperation from the families of the children and especially from the mothers. Cooperation was necessary if reliable information was to be obtained about how babies are treated and how they respond to this treatment. In any society, parent-child interaction has such deep emotional significance that, when questioned about it, parents are likely to feel defensive, especially if they interpret the questions to imply either criticism or a desire to interfere. An approach was needed that would induce parents to relax their defensive reactions—at least those defenses that they consciously adopt toward the stranger who seems too inquisitive.

In longitudinal research, once initial cooperation is elicited, time is on the side of the sensitive investigator. Through repeated visits over an extended period of time, confidence in the investigator grows and defenses are relaxed. Yet, sustained cooperation throughout a series of visits places great demands upon participants. They are asked to give many hours of their time. A potential participant could be expected to ask: "What am *I* going to get out of this?" The problem of how to gain the cooperation of the parents of babies evolved into two main questions. How can the research plan be most favorably presented in order to gain initial cooperation? What can these families be given in return for their cooperation that will make it seem worthwhile to them to sustain contacts?

The presentation of the research plan was one that had to appeal not only to the mothers of babies but also to the chiefs through whom initial contact with the families was to be made. It would have to appeal also to the babies' fathers, without whose approval the mothers would scarcely dare to cooperate. I hit upon the following general answer to the question of what I wanted to do. "As you know, your own customs differ in many respects from European customs. I am especially interested in different customs about caring for infants. I do not believe that European methods of infant care are better than your customs just because they are European, or because they are the methods used in my own country. I believe that some of our customs are probably better than yours, but I also believe that some of your customs are better than ours. But we cannot know which of your customs are better and which of ours are better until we have studied them both. I would like to learn what are *your* customs of infant care, so that we can find out which of your customs seem better than European customs." I did not add that it was unlikely that a single study of the sort that I proposed, covering only a small segment of the child's life span, could be expected to answer the questions I raised. Nevertheless, this simple formula, despite its over-statement, made enough sense to the chiefs, to whom I first presented it, and to my prospective participants to gain the toe-hold of initial cooperation that I sought. My statement put across the essential points that I was not prejudging their customs, that I wanted neither to teach nor to interfere, and that I believed I had something valuable to learn from them. Moreover, I implied that the research had a potential practical usefulness—it might be expected to help in the significant matter of rearing infants in ways that are better than those that any of us now use.

Finally, the research was presented as having a broad interest in child development and methods of infant care. When information is sought it is necessary to give the informants some general notion of the scope of the information wanted. If an investigator asks questions without making it clear why he is asking them, he is likely to evoke a suspicious and defensive attitude in his informants. Yet, there are two dangers in specifying the precise scope of one's inquiry. First, there is the danger of limiting the scope of the inquiry, since questions that stray outside the agreed area do not seem justified to the informant. In this research, for example, we could not inquire about marital status of the parents, or about some other matters that seemed relevant to us but did not seem relevant to our informants. Secondly, there is the danger of distorting the very practices in which one is most interested by focusing attention on them too specifically. In this research, for example, although the initial focus of interest was on mother-infant separation, to have specified this as the purpose of the study might well have distorted people's actions. I neither wanted infants separated from their mothers because I was interested in observing their response to separation, nor did I want them not be to separated because my disapproval of this custom could be sensed behind my interest. Even to have stated that I was especially interested in the relationship between mother and infant might have been expected to make a mother self-conscious in her relationship with her infant. Therefore, since I was in any event interested in general customs of infant care, it seemed wise to define the scope of the inquiry in broad, general terms.

My attention then turned to the question of what the cooperating families could be given in return for their time and efforts.[2] To find a satisfactory solution to this problem seemed essential, both to ensure sustained cooperation and to encourage participants to give reliable information. Clinicians know well that information gained from a patient in a therapeutic situation tends to be more revealing and more reliable than information gained from a subject in a non-therapeutic interview or survey. In the therapeutic situation the patient is motivated to give information because he believes that he will be helped thereby. In the survey kind of interview situation the subject not only may feel that he has nothing to gain from cooperating but he may feel resentful that something

2 While associated with the Tavistock Clinic in London I had been favorably impressed with the Clinic's policy of "no research without therapy." My effort to find a suitable basis for sustaining cooperation was inspired by this policy.

is being taken from him which will not be used to benefit him and, indeed, which may somehow be used against him. It seems important that the voluntary participant in a research be made to feel that he has something to gain in return for what he is giving, especially if he must invest considerable time and effort and suffer an invasion of his privacy.

In some kinds of research it has seemed reasonable to pay a wage to the participant for his time and effort. Although a wage rewards him for his time, it does not necessarily motivate him to cooperate in any but a perfunctory way. A wage is inappropriate in many kinds of research and it seemed inappropriate in this one, even had the financial resources available been adequate, which they were not. Nor did it seem appropriate to provide advice, training, or some other equivalent of therapy as a reward for cooperation. Such services would distort the very things that were to be observed. Even if I had had confidence that I could show the mothers of the babies better ways to care for their infants, such instruction, if heeded, would change their methods, and, if unheeded, would disrupt my relationship with them. From the outset, I disclaimed the role of instructor. When a mother asked for my opinion or advice, I attempted to turn the request back as a request for her opinion. Nearly always this tactic both yielded useful information and satisfied the mother that she really knew the answer to her own question. (In only one regard did Mrs. Kibuka and I find it impossible to withhold advice and that was in response to questions about infant nutrition. Nutrition was obviously an area in which European knowledge was known to be of benefit to a baby; to withhold help might have harmed the baby and would have been judged in this light.)

The most appropriate service that I could give in return for cooperation, it seemed to me, was to facilitate the provision of medical services for the baby, and indeed for other children in the family. To promote the welfare of the children—and especially the welfare of the baby, whose health was the most vulnerable—seemed to be the most likely reason for a family to cooperate with us. Medical service was the most obvious and urgently needed aspect of welfare, and it was one in regard to which there would be minimal distortion of customary methods of infant care. The Ganda in this region of the country were acculturated enough to be convinced of the value of European medicine so that to offer such a service would not seem critical or interfering.

The most generally useful medical facility available was the traveling child welfare clinic operated by Dr. Hebe Welbourn of the Uganda Medical Service and a staff of nurses and nursing aides whom she had, for the most part, trained herself. Convinced of the need for making medical service as available as possible to those who needed it, rather than relying upon a more elaborate central facility, she traveled in a van, accompanied by her staff and a basic minimum of equipment and medical supplies, going to a different center every weekday for a fortnight. In all there were ten such centers, each visited once every two weeks on a regular schedule.

This clinic provided a general pediatric service. Sick babies were treated on the spot, although hospitalization was advised when it seemed needed. Samples were taken for laboratory tests when indicated. The clinic served also as a well-baby clinic. Routine measurements of height and weight were made to provide a check on physical development. One of the duties of the nursing aides was to give instruction in basic procedures for nutrition and hygiene. Some mothers brought their babies regularly; others came only when the baby was ill, or when his failure to develop was a cause for concern.

Although the fortnightly clinic was much closer to most of the areas served than were the several hospitals in Kampala, it was still too far away from home to be readily available to many mothers. The mother would have to go on foot, carrying her baby. If she had other young children, either they had to be taken along or she had to find someone with whom to leave them—which was often difficult because the older, more responsible children attended school. Unless she lived close to the clinic center, a mother usually attended the clinic only when her baby was ill enough to cause real concern.

I offered participants in the project transportation to the nearest clinic center every fortnight, with the offer including not only the mother and baby but also other young children. No pressure was placed upon the mothers to avail themselves of this service, yet all but two did so. At first it was easy to take all who wished to go in one trip in a large Chevrolet carry-all. As our sample expanded, however, several trips were needed, and later there were so many that a driver from the Institute provided shuttle service with the carry-all, and I did also with my own car. At first it was possible to mingle with the women and babies at the clinic, observing their behavior and witnessing the medical examination of the babies in our sample and the advice and treatment that were given. Later, our time was completely occupied with bringing people to the clinic and taking them home again.

This transportation service to the clinic was the chief return for cooperation, but there were several other services we performed. I made it known that anytime I was in a village I would provide transportation to a hospital in Kampala for anyone who needed to go—immediately if the need was urgent. This service was not needed frequently, but it was used and appreciated. Dried skim milk was sold to families who needed it for a baby or young child. I originally intended to make a gift of the milk, but Dr. Welbourn strongly advised that we follow the same procedure as the clinic followed, buying the milk in large quantities wholesale and selling it at cost. She pointed out that the protein deficiency problem in this region was severe enough that the use of dried skim milk as a dietary supplement for young children, as well as for babies who needed it, should become routine. If the milk were dispensed free, people would rely upon the gift passively and would cease using it when later it was no longer available as a free service. If, however, they could become accustomed to purchasing it, a demand would be established that might persist, regardless of the original service supplying it. In a few cases where it was obvious that the milk was needed and the family did not have even the small sum available that was needed to buy it, it was provided as a repeated service and not as an occasional gift. A further small service was to provide copies of any photographs taken of the baby or his family, and this was very much appreciated.

At the outset, it was intended to limit our services to the few mentioned above. They all seemed appropriate, and served the needs of the research as well as the needs of the babies and their families. Soon, however, the need for a further type of return emerged. Ganda custom requires that food be offered to each visitor to the house, regardless of inconvenience or poverty. It was hoped that we could waive this obligation by a preliminary firm request that we be not served food. Some women nevertheless felt impelled to serve tea, if not a full dinner, and even those who had been convinced that they should not feel obliged to do so could not bear to send us away without food. At the end of a visit they made gifts of delicacies from their gardens: papaws, pineapple, sugar-cane, avocados, passion fruit, mangoes—or even eggs, which were precious sources of protein that should have been saved for the needs of their own families. It seemed necessary to reciprocate appropriately, so I brought small gifts suitable to Ganda tastes and needs—especially tea or sugar, which the villagers used regularly but which were expensive for them with their small cash incomes. Thus did we comply with the reciprocal demands of hospitality.

Before these plans for eliciting and sustaining cooperation could be put into practice or even proposed as an inducement, it was first essential to meet some of the parents of young babies. It was necessary to choose an area in which to work and then to seek the cooperation of the chief under whose jurisdiction the area fell.

The area tentatively chosen was about fifteen miles from Kampala, close enough to commute to "the field," yet not a part of the metropolitan area. This area had been covered in a survey of women's fertility undertaken a year before by the East African Institute of Social Research, and it was expected that the records of the survey might be useful. Moreover, the village in which I had spent a month was in this region; it was hoped that some of the contacts I had made there might be of use in gaining initial cooperation for the project.

It was a foregone conclusion that I had no chance of being accepted as an investigator without the approval and support of the chiefs responsible for the administration of the chosen area. The *ggombolola* chief[3] was approached first.

3 Long before the days of European administration, Buganda was a centralized kingdom, with a complex hierarchy of chiefs and little local autonomy. During the day of British overrule, the same

His support having been promised, the birth registry of the *ggombolola* was examined to estimate in how many *miruka* I would need to work to find enough babies of the right age for my sample, assuming that some parents would not be willing to cooperate. Two *miruka* were judged to be sufficient, and the judgment was correct. (Examination of the birth registry had been a useless step, however. It included none of the babies born in hospitals, and was an incomplete record even of the babies born at home.) The *ggombolola* chief chose two *miruka* chiefs whom he expected to be cooperative in the enterprise and approached them on my behalf. Since I wanted to work in the village in which I had lived, it was further decided that I should seek the support of a third leader, who, although not in the official hierarchy of chiefs, nonetheless held, by reason of family background, education, and inherent abilities, a leadership role in that village. The *ggombolola* chief, *Omwami* Lwanga, suggested that I first meet each of these three leaders to explain my purposes to them, and then, subject to their approval, ask each to call a meeting of the people in his locality so that a direct appeal could be made to the prospective participants. This plan was followed and the meetings were held.[4]

In each of the meetings I explained my purposes in a short speech, answered questions with the help of my interpreter, and asked for volunteers. In no case did volunteers declare themselves at the meetings, but, with further inquiries on the part of the chiefs, some families declared themselves willing to receive me so that I could explain to them individually and in greater detail what I wished to do. A series of visits to homes was then arranged, with the chief introducing us to each family. I again explained my purposes, and this resulted in all but one of the families visited agreeing to participate. (Those who initially agreed to participate formed only the nucleus of the group. The sample was filled out chiefly by volunteers from among the friends and neighbors of the original participants.)

Difficulties in gaining the cooperation of parents has been implied in the foregoing account. Similar difficulties could be expected in any society. It is understandable that parents resist requests to volunteer in research that will take time and invade privacy. In Buganda in 1954–55, however, there were special problems. Late in 1953 the *Kabaka* of the Ganda was deported on the order of

hierarchy of chiefs was used for administrative purposes. Buganda is divided first, according to *ssaza* or county. Under each *ssaza* chief are several *ggombolola* chiefs, each in charge of a portion of the county. Each *ggombolola* is divided into *miruka,* the chiefs of which are responsible to the *ggombolola* chief.

4 The plan for the meetings did not work out smoothly because of an illness of mine (the fieldworker in an "underdeveloped" country is indeed fortunate if his work is not interrupted by illness) and a political crisis. The meetings had to be canceled. Unfortunately, the messages regarding the cancellations were not delivered promptly—another kind of mishap that can be expected in field work of this sort. It is a tribute to the cooperation of the chiefs that they were able to persuade people to reassemble at a later date—but persuade them they did.

the Governor of Uganda.[5] The Governor's action was resented by the Ganda with increasing unanimity and intensity as the months passed. By the time my research began, about ten months later, the Ganda felt that they had been robbed of a revered figure who was the very embodiment of their national existence. Having been previously well-disposed to the Europeans living or visiting in Buganda, the Ganda were in conflict in this critical situation. Their response seemed to be a formal opposition to the British in particular and to the European in general. It was as though they said: "We have liked and trusted you in the past; we have learned much from you and we appreciate what you have taught us; you have, however, robbed us of our *Kabaka* and we protest this action; therefore we reject you whom otherwise we might have welcomed." I emphasize the formal nature of this opposition, for at no time did I encounter any violence, threat of violence, or indeed any real unpleasantness at the hands of the Ganda. Those who did not cooperate with me were either polite or invisible; those who did cooperate were very friendly, kind, and obliging.

Fortunately for the sake of the research, some Ganda could reconcile with their patriotic consciences their desire to obtain the help for their babies that the research plan offered. There is no doubt, however, that the political crisis made it more difficult to launch the research than it would have been before the crisis occurred. As it turned out, the preliminaries following my month in the village engaged the better part of two months, leaving little more than seven months for the actual collection of data.[6]

5 The events leading to this action and also the gradual resolution of the ensuing crisis are described by R. C. Pratt, "The Crisis of 1953–55," in D. A. Low and R. C. Pratt, *Buganda and British Overrule, 1900–1955* (London: Oxford University Press, 1960), pp. 317–49.

6 In Table 1 the span of observation of two cases is listed as longer than thirty-two weeks— the maximum span for most of the cases which formed the original nucleus of the sample. These two babies—Senvuma and Lusiya—were observed during the preliminary month I spent in the village, and these observations were included in the data.

4

THE SAMPLE

The sample consisted of twenty-eight babies—fifteen boys and thirteen girls. There were two sets of twins, and hence only twenty-six mothers in the sample. Only twenty-three households were visited, however, since two polygynous households included two mother-child pairs, and in one household the sister of one baby's father had a child out of wedlock.[1]

The original nucleus of the sample consisted of eight babies, seven acquired through the efforts of one *muluka* chief, and one through the efforts of another. We asked the chiefs to introduce us to mothers of babies who had not yet been weaned but who were likely to be weaned within five months or so. Since several of the original families were found to be highly acculturated in their methods of infant care, one of the chiefs at my request persuaded three less acculturated mothers to participate. Thus, through the direct efforts of the chiefs, eleven subjects were obtained. I myself took the initiative in seeking the cooperation of families in the village in which I had lived previously for a month, and thus added eight babies to the sample. One baby was born into the sample—a child in a polygynous household which we were already visiting. Eight babies joined the sample at their parents' request. Indeed, as the work continued, the requests to join in the research increased until finally offers to cooperate had to be declined because regular visits to any larger number of babies could not be sustained.

1 Samwendi's mother is Lusiya's father's sister. Still another sister, originally in the same household, had a child out of wedlock—Senvuma—but since he was separated from his mother and sent to live with relatives, a separate household was visited for him.

DOI: 10.4324/9781003629337-5

Age

At the time observations began, the babies ranged in age from two days to eighty weeks, with a median age of twenty-four weeks. At the time observations ended, the babies ranged in age from fifteen weeks to two years of age, with a median age of approximately forty-six weeks. The span of the observations ranged from seven weeks to thirty-eight weeks, with a median span of twenty-seven weeks (see Table 1).

Since the infants were of differing ages when observations began and were observed for differing lengths of time, the total age period covered by the study is longer than the duration of the study itself—from two days to two years of age. The first quarter-year of life was represented by seven babies, although the observations of six of these were limited to the third month of life. The second quarter-year was studied more satisfactorily with sixteen babies available for observation at some time during this period. The third quarter-year was represented by twenty babies and the fourth by fifteen. The fifth quarter-year was represented by a sample of ten. The number of the sample in each quarter-year includes all of those who were observed in that quarter-year regardless of the brevity of observation. Moreover, observations at the beginning were for each child less satisfactory than observations later on because of the time required to establish a relationship with the mother and to gain her cooperation. This drawback was mitigated somewhat by the fact that once cooperation had been established, information could be gained about the immediately preceding weeks which seemed to be little distorted by faults of memory. All in all, the age range spanned by the study could be most fairly stated as being from two to fifteen months, with the most adequate data in the range from three to thirteen months.

Religious affiliation

Three religious affiliations were represented in the sample—Church of England, Roman Catholic, and Muslim (see Table 1). Fifteen babies came from Church of England homes, seven from Muslim, and six from Roman Catholic. None of the families were avowedly pagan. The Muslims were clearly the least acculturated of the three groups, which is not surprising when acculturation is defined in terms of adoption of European customs and values, but they also seemed closest to old Ganda customs.

Marital status of parents

A few mothers in the sample volunteered the information that theirs was a legal union, and the situation of some others led them to confess the contrary. Apart

TABLE 1 Background facts about the sample

Name	*Sex*	*Age at Beginning (weeks)*	*Age at End (weeks)*	*Span of Observation (weeks)*	*Quarters Covered*	*Religion*	*Marital Status of Parents*
SECURE - ATTACHED							
1. Paulo	M	29	58	29	3, 4, 5	RC	monog.
2. Sembajwe	M	80	105	25	6 plus	C of E	monog.
3. Juko	M	18	35	17	2, 3	Muslim	monog.
4. Petero	M	9	36	27	1, 2, 3	RC	monog.
5. Senvuma	M	35	64	29	3, 4, 5	RC	mother unmarried
6. Mutebe	M	39	52	13	3, 4	RC	separated
7. Nakiku	F	28	60	32	3, 4, 5	C of E	monog.
8. Alima	F	7	26	19	1, 2	Muslim	polyg.
9. Aida	F	9	36	27	1, 2, 3	Muslim	monog.?
10. William	M	14	45	31	2, 3, 4	C of E	monog.
11. Senkumba	M	8	40	32	1, 2, 3	C of E	polyg., separated
12. Kyimba	M	37	43	6	3, 4	C of E	monog.
13. Samwendi	M	9	25	16	1, 2	RC	mother unmarried
14. Maryamu	F	33	60	27	3, 4, 5	C of E	monog.
15. Lusiya	F	29	67	38	3, 4, 5	RC	monog.
16. Nabatanzi	F	30	61	31	3, 4, 5	C of E	mother unmarried
INSECURE - ATTACHED							
17. Muhamidi	M	9	36	27	1, 2, 3	Muslim	polyg., separated
18. Magalita	F	42	57	15	4, 5	C of E	monog.
19. Kasozi	M	48	66	18	4, 5	C of E	father deserted
20. Sulaimani	M	25	42	17	2, 3, 4	Muslim	polyg.
21. Nakalema	F	24	39	15	2, 3, 4	Muslim	monog.?
22. Waswa (1)	M	59	91	32	5 plus	C of E	father deserted
23. Nakato (1)	F	59	91	32	5 plus	C of E	father deserted
NON - ATTACHED							
24. Nora	F	20	52	32	2, 3, 4	C of E	polyg.
25. Kulistina	F	16	47	31	2, 3, 4	C of E	polyg.
26. Waswa (2)	M	13	37	24	2, 3	C of E	monog.
27. Nakato (2)	F	13	37	24	2, 3	C of E	monog.
28. Namitala	F	0	15	15	1, 2	Muslim	polyg.

TABLE 2 More background facts about the sample

Name	*Father at Home*	*Father's Occupation*	*Other Siblings at Home* [a]
SECURE – ATTACHED			
1. Paulo	occasionally	surveyor	2
2. Sembajwe	weekends	merchant	0
3. Juko	evenings	Health Department	0
4. Petero	weekends	surveyor	4
5. Senvuma	never		0
6. Mutebe	occasionally		1
7. Nakiku	evenings	shoemaker	0
8. Alima	always	Muslim school teacher	2
9. Aida	occasionally		2
10. William	occasionally	veterinary officer	8
11. Senkumba	evenings		1
12. Kyimba	evenings	clerk	0
13. Samwendi	never	clerk	0
14. Maryamu	evenings	mechanic	1
15. Lusiya	always	farmer	0
16. Nabatanzi	never	driver	0
INSECURE – ATTACHED			
17. Muhamidi	always to never	farmer	2
18. Magalita	evenings	Electricity Board	4
19. Kasozi	never		1
20. Sulaimani	always	farmer	0
21. Nakalema	always	farmer	4
22. Waswa (1)	never	chief	4
23. Nakato (1)	never	chief	4
NON – ATTACHED			
24. Nora	weekends	surveyor	7
25. Kulistina	weekends	surveyor	7
26. Waswa (2)	always	merchant	2
27. Nakato (2)	always	merchant	2
28. Namitala	always	Muslim school teacher	2

[a] Includes both half- and full-siblings.

[b] Includes full-siblings separated, dead, or grown up and moved away. Half-siblings are not included here because other children of the father were generally not known to us unless they lived in the household. It may be noted that this excludes also other children of the mother known to be separated as in the case of Nakiku and the younger twins.

[c] Includes children other than half- and full-siblings.

Other Siblings Not at Home [b]	*Other Children in the Home* [c]	*Total Children in the Home* [d]	*Other Adults in the Home* [e]
0	0	3	1 (MU)
0	2	3	0
0	0	1	0
0	0	5	0
0	2	3	3 (MU, 2 MA)
0	0	2	3 (MGGM, MGM, MGF)
0	1	2	0
0	2	5	3 (0/wife, PU, PGM [f])
4	0	3	0 —> 1 (fem.)
1	1	10	0
0	0	2	1 (0/wife) to many
0	0	1	1 (PGM)
0	2	3	2 (MU & his wife)
0	1	3	0
1	3	4	2 (PAs)
0	2	3	2 (MGM [f], MGA)
2	0 to many	3 to many	1 (0/wife) to many
0	0	5	3 (PGM, 2 half-bros.)
0	0	2	1 (MU)
2	0	1	1 (0/wife)
0	0	5	1 (PU)
0	1	6	3 (fem.[f])
0	1	6	3 (fem.[f])
0	1	9	1 (0/wife)
0	1	9	1 (0/wife)
0	2	5	0
0	2	5	0
4	2	5	3 (0/wife, PU, PGM [f])

[d] Includes the subject and those siblings and other children who live in the household.

[e] Excluding father and/or mother.

[f] Includes grandmother and/or other elderly relatives who live in separate huts but who are truly part of the same household.

from these, we have no firm information about the formal marital status of the parents of the babies in the sample. Consequently, the classification of the families regarding marital status had to be based on our own impressions of the situation, supplemented by some direct information from informants (see Table 1).

Fourteen of the babies lived in households either known to be monogamous or assumed to be so because no other wives were present or mentioned. Seven babies lived in obviously polygynous households; three of the households in question were Muslim, two Church of England. Of the babies from polygynous households, two accompanied the mother to her parents' home when a domestic crisis arose. Three babies had unmarried mothers; three were deserted by their fathers, and one had parents who were separated (without implications of paternal desertion). It is not known how representative of Ganda families this small sample is in regard to marital instability. It is noteworthy, however, that one-third of the babies either had unmarried mothers or came from households disrupted by unstable marriages. Welbourn[2] and Richards[3] also report a high incidence of marital instability in present-day Buganda.

Fathers

Six fathers (of eight babies) were at home or close to home most of the time: four cash-crop farmers, one shopkeeper, and one teacher in a local Muslim school. Six fathers had jobs close enough to their homes to be able to commute, returning home every evening and staying at home on weekends; these were clerks and tradesmen working in Kampala or its environs. Three fathers—a merchant and two surveyors—were able to return home every weekend and sometimes during the week. Four had jobs so far away that they could get home only occasionally—two to four times a year: one surveyor, one veterinary officer, and two with occupations unknown to me. Five fathers never lived at home with the current baby—three who were not married to the mothers, and two who had deserted. The whole range is thus represented in this sample—fathers who were home so much that they were very familiar figures and fathers who were entirely absent and quite unknown to their babies (see Table 2).

Siblings and other children in the household

Three of the babies—Juko, Kyimba, and Sulaimani—were the only children in their households. Juko and Kyimba were their mothers' firstborn; Sulaimani was

2 Hebe F. Welbourn, *Baganda Childhood* (in preparation).

3 Audrey I. Richards, "Authority Patterns," in L. A. Fallers (ed.), *The King's Men: Leadership and Status in Modern Buganda*, p. 258.

his mother's third baby, but the other two had died. Five other babies were their mothers' firstborn infants, but had either half-siblings or cousins living in the same household. Seven babies lived in households with very few children, either only the baby himself or at most one other child. Twelve lived in households that included four or more other children, and three of them—William, Nora, and Kulistina—lived in households that swarmed with children. For the most part, even the babies of mothers who were unmarried or deserted were not the only children in their households (see Table 2).

Other adults in the household

Eight babies lived in households in which the parents were the only adults; four of these saw their fathers on a regular day-to-day basis, but four saw their fathers only on weekends or even less frequently. Three babies had an uncle living in the household in addition to the mother (or mother and father), and all the rest had other adult women, with or without additional adult males. These women included other wives in the family, aunts, and grandmothers, and occasionally other relatives. Thus, although few, if any, of these households were truly "extended," most of them included more adults than does the typical family nucleus of Western society (see Table 2).

None of the babies lived alone with their mothers; even those with no fathers had at least one other adult or child in the household. Few babies lived in households lacking adult males—Nabatanzi and the older set of twins, and perhaps William and Aida whose fathers were so rarely home. Most of the babies without fathers had a father surrogate in the household—either a grandfather or maternal uncle.

Unweaned versus weaned babies

It had been intended to have the whole sample consist of breast-fed babies still unweaned. Indeed, all but one of the babies had been breast-fed; Kulistina, however, was bottle-fed from the fourth day of life. Three other babies—Kyimba, Maryamu, and Senvuma—who had been breast-fed were weaned from the breast so early in the research that preweaning observations were inadequate. Data from these four babies[4] could have been excluded altogether. It was decided, however, to exclude these babies only in regard to points where information about them was inadequate and to include them in the points about which information was reasonably complete and reliable.

4 The circumstances of including each of these four babies in the sample will be presented in the case summary of each. They illustrate some of the difficulties to be encountered in field work of this sort.

Degree of acculturation

The finding that led to the judgment that the original nucleus of the sample was highly acculturated in methods of infant care was that six of the seven original babies were fed according to a schedule—a finding that is in striking contrast to the stereotype of the African baby stemming from anthropological accounts. Scheduled feeding is but one criterion of acculturation. Several of the families could be classed as relatively highly acculturated on other grounds. Two of the participating mothers had for some years attended the child welfare clinic, and one of these had much influenced a third mother. Two other women, who were friends, had sought to learn as much as they could about child nutrition and had used a book written in Luganda by Dr. Welbourn, the director of the clinic, even though their homes had a minimum of European appurtenances and they otherwise did not appear especially acculturated. One of the polygynous households was highly acculturated; the father was a college graduate who had provided a European-type house with many European amenities; the mothers had also adopted Europeanized methods of infant care, although their selection of methods differed in important respects from those recommended in the child welfare clinic. Yet two other families who were relatively well-to-do did not seem especially Europeanized in methods of child rearing.

The Muslim families in the sample seemed significantly less acculturated than most of the Christian families, and yet it was chiefly in these households that nursing bottles were used for supplementary feedings.

There seems to be no clear-cut single criterion of degree of acculturation available. We had no systematic information about the level of education of father or mother. Visible evidence of acculturation, such as European house construction, furniture, and equipment, clothing, and the like, seemed irrelevant to us, for it bore no apparent relationship to acculturation in regard to infant care. Even the visible evidence of nursing bottles and waterproof panties seemed somewhat irrelevant, since these items did not bear any apparent relationship to acculturated attitudes. The overwhelming impression was that these families had selected those aspects of European culture which suited their needs and their incomes, and it was fruitless to seek a criterion or a combination of criteria that might classify them in regard to degree of acculturation in ways that were pertinent to our interests.

It was clear that friends, neighbors, and relatives influenced each other. Each person who had attended the child welfare clinic or a mission school was at least potentially a center from which acculturation diffused.

How representative is this sample?

For several reasons it was impossible even to attempt to assemble a sample that could be considered representative of the Ganda as a whole. First, the kind of census information that is necessary for the selection of a stratified sample is lacking in Buganda. Second, a sample small enough and localized enough to be feasible for longitudinal research could not, in any event, be representative. Finally, volunteer participants are necessary to ensure the sustained cooperation required in a longitudinal research, and the very fact that they are volunteers makes them non-representative of the population as a whole.

It is obvious, however, that this sample is not representative of families throughout Buganda, for surely families such as these who live close to Kampala are more acculturated, by and large, than those who live upcountry. Moreover, Richards[5] assures me that this sample is too highly acculturated to be representative of families living within a fifteen mile radius of Kampala.

The chief corollary of the fact that the families of this sample are relatively highly acculturated is that the methods of infant care used by them cannot be assumed to be characteristic of present-day Ganda as a whole. Nevertheless, certain customs are so nearly universal in the sample and so closely in line with ancient customs that it seems likely that they are widespread. Wide individual differences were found in regard to other aspects of infant care; these differences probably highlight areas in which old customs are breaking down, even though we cannot generalize from this sample in regard to the range of practices that have replaced ancient customs.

Insofar as one of our interests is in discovering relationships between specified aspects of child development—and especially the development of a baby's attachment to his mother—and pertinent infant-care variables, it is of little importance whether our sample is representative or not; for this purpose, the chief concern is that the range of variables represented in the sample be wide enough to allow for an exploration of their relationship to the course of infant development.

Informants of traditional Ganda methods of infant care

Information on traditional Ganda methods of infant care was obtained from three informants. The first informant was *Omukyala* Mariamu, a very old great-grandmother, whom I met during my month's stay in the village, and who not only enjoyed the role of informant but gave detailed information that was remarkably vivid and coherent in view of her seemingly great age. The grandmother of one of the babies in the sample—Kyimba—proved to be another willing informant. The third informant was neither old nor female. *Omwami* Kyingi was one of my acquaintances during my month in the village; he had interested himself in traditional Ganda customs and presented himself as an authoritative source. As it turned out, his information coincided very closely with that provided by the two old ladies, although it was less detailed in many respects.

5 Personal communication.

5
PROCEDURE

Interview schedule

A schedule was prepared to cover the areas to be studied and was to include information obtained both through interview and direct observation. Some of the items in the schedule dealt with the mother—the methods she used and her attitudes. Other items concerned the child, his development, and his responses to special events and classes of events. Still other items dealt with the responses of the child to specific aspects of the behavior of his mother and that of other important figures in the household. Not all of these items could be covered by direct observation. The mother was interviewed about the period before the research began, and also in regard to daily events that our afternoon visits made it impossible to observe directly. In addition, the interview covered items that could be checked through direct observation—and this practice provided some check on the reliability of the mother as an informant.

The interview schedule was, of course, intended to ensure that a systematic body of information was obtained about each infant that would be comparable in regard to all points relevant to the age and situation of the child. It included all points that I could think of in advance as being possibly relevant to our interests.[1]

1 In the preparation of the interview schedule I was helped by three guides, as follows: *(a) Tentative Questionnaire for Handbook, of Psychological Leads for Ethnological Field Workers: Life Cycle*, originally formulated by Mead and Gorer, and revised by Sapir, Benedict, Bunzel, *et al.*, and issued by the Committee on Culture and Personality of the National Research Council. (Mimeographed); *(b) Field Quide for a Study of Socialization in Five Societies* by John W. M. Whiting, Irvin L. Child, William W. Lambert, Ann M. Fischer, John L. Fischer, Corinne Nydegger, William Nydegger, Hatsumi Maretski, Thomas Maretski, Leigh Minturn, Kimball Romney, and Romaine

DOI: 10.4324/9781003629337-6

The schedule proved to be adequate except in a few minor respects and was later modified to include the points that had initially been overlooked. It served as a guide to the collection of data about each baby in the sample; it also served as a guide to collecting information about siblings and their development and as a guide to interviewing the informants of traditional customs.

The major areas of information covered by the schedule were as follows:

Facts about the household: names of those living in the household and their relationship to the baby; ages of all children in the household and of siblings not living at home; occupation of the father and the amount of time he spent with the family; religious affiliation of the family.

Birth: date, place, and particulars.

Feeding: particulars about early lactation and suckling; method of breast feeding (i.e., schedule versus self-demand); attitude of the mother; response of the child; substitutes for breast feeding, if any; supplementary feedings, if any, when begun, consisting of what foods, how administered; feeding problems and how handled; thumb-sucking or other sucking habits.

Elimination: methods of dealing with urine and feces; attitudes expressed by adults; use of cloths, diapers, waterproofs; smearing, incidence and attitudes; problems; training, nature of methods and when begun; when bladder and bowel control were established or were expected to be established.

Cleanliness: baths, when, what kind, response of child; attitude toward general cleanliness; treatment of nasal discharges, etc.

Sleeping: in what kind of bed, where, when; how soundly; protection from noise.

Motor Development: age at which achievements (i.e., sitting, crawling, standing, walking) are expected; age at which they are achieved; training, if any; ceremonies, if any.

Vocalization: how much; what type; when, usually.

Crying: how much; how interpreted usually; how dealt with.

Distribution of Mothering Duties: who helps care for the baby; what each does for the baby; what does only the mother do; attitude and responsibility of older children in the family; proportion of time baby is left alone in a room or in the house; is baby taken to the garden by his mother or left behind; how is baby carried (i.e., on the back, on the hip, in the arms) and by whom; amount and type of attention (cuddling, rocking, crooning, playing, etc.), when given and by whom.

Interpersonal Relations: differential response of baby to mother, to other familiar women, to father, to other familiar men, to older children in the household, to

Romney. (Mimeographed); (c) *Lactation Enquiry* of the Medical Research Council Infantile Malnutrition Group. (Mimeographed.)

siblings nearest own age, to strangers (men, women, Europeans); response of baby to being left by the mother (alone, with strangers, with familiar figures); changes in these responses from visit to visit.

Sexual Behavior: reported incidence of infantile sexual behavior; attitudes of mother toward this and how dealt with.

Aggression: type of behavior considered to be aggressive; what the causes of this behavior are believed to be; how it is dealt with.

Punishment: methods of punishment used; when initiated; kind of behavior punished; response of baby to punishment. (This item of the schedule was not included at the beginning but was added when our attention was directed toward punishment of babies.)

Dangers and Concerns: aspects of the environment believed to be sources of danger; features of the baby's development that cause mother's concern.

Play: play behavior manifested by the baby; toys and playthings.

Health and Medical Care: illnesses and age of occurrence: visits to hospital; visits to clinic, how frequent; weight gain; diagnoses and treatment.

Weaning: age at weaning; method of weaning; reason for weaning at this time; response of child to weaning; sucking substitutes, if any; response of mother to child's demands.

Separation: age at each separation from the mother; length of separation; place where child was cared for during separation; substitute mother, who, and how familiar to the child; reason for separation; visits of parents; response of child to separation, to parent surrogates and caretakers, and to visits of parents.

The visits

The visits perhaps bore more resemblance to social visits than to scientific interviews. Although the interview schedule was prepared in mimeographed form, it was never brought to a visit; it served as a cumulative summary of the data already collected. After each visit I noted which items had been covered and formulated plans regarding what I hoped to cover during the next visit.

My interpreter and I knew what kinds of information we wished to obtain, but we hoped to gain it informally and with a minimum of direct questions. We chatted with the mother, with any other members of the family who were present, and with any neighbors or other guests who were simultaneous visitors. We tried to stimulate spontaneous conversation about topics relevant to our interests. We hoped that an open-ended question would bring a flood of information with little subsequent intervention. We intended to ask direct questions only when necessary—to initiate conversational interaction, or as a last resort, to gain information that could not be obtained by less obvious means.

As we came to be on increasingly friendly terms with our informants, these hopes were fulfilled to some extent but not with all mothers and not in regard to all points of inquiry. The open-ended question or comment was less successful in stimulating communication in this setting than I have found it to be in comparable situations in the United States. First, the need to use an interpreter tended to give the interview situation more structure than it would have had if I had been able to exchange information freely in Luganda (or in English). Moreover, the presence of a European probably tended to make some informants less spontaneous than they otherwise might have been. The Ganda are very polite; they are accustomed to defer to people whom they consider to be superior in status, regardless of how they feel about them privately. We consider it a tribute to the friendship and good feeling that gradually developed between us that most of the informants eventually felt free to talk spontaneously and to offer information without being asked.

The growth of comfortable rapport was in no small measure due to Mrs. Kibuka's interpretation of her role. She could not remain in the role of mere interpreter. She was actively interested in these families and established her own relationships with them. Although she had not realized how different the village way of life was from her own, she did not betray this in her words and actions. She became a friend and confidante of most of the mothers in the sample, and to the extent that she became these things, so did I, for I was drawn into her relationships rather than excluded from them.

Mrs. Kibuka's departure from the traditional role of interpreter had some disadvantages. At times she gave me the mere gist of a conversation rather than a literal translation when she judged it desirable to keep the flow of communication going without interruption. But she was conscientious in keeping me informed of what she was doing and why she was doing it, and many of the details could be filled in after the visit. Her sensitivity and her intelligent grasp of the purposes of the research enabled her to depart from the traditional interpreter's role without damaging the fact-finding purposes of the interview. Moreover, it is believed that the departures she took on her own initiative added to the reliability of the information garnered rather than detracted from it, if only because she helped our informants communicate more freely than they would have been able to do had every exchange been translated literally.

I took continuous notes throughout each visit—on answers to questions, spontaneous conversational interchange, and behavior. The delays before translation gave me time to make notes on behavior as well as on information elicited in the interview, with the result that there were minimal interruptions of the interview.

Upon returning home after each visit, the rough notes were typed up and somewhat expanded on the basis of immediate recall. These typed field notes constitute the raw data for the study.

Not all visits were equally fruitful in their yield of information. Typically, for the first few visits, while we were still a novelty, guests were invited, and neighbors dropped in to meet us. There was little opportunity for intimate interchange. We were usually asked again to explain our purposes and the services we intended to give. If there were urgent problems that the mother hoped we would help with, these were given first attention, whether other people were present or not. Occasionally it took several visits to clear away this backlog of anxieties, problems, or misgivings before we could begin gathering the information we sought.

After the early visits the pattern of a visit became fairly predictable. In most families, once the formal greetings had been exchanged, the baby was brought out, if indeed he had not been present from the beginning. He was immediately given to a visitor to hold and then was passed from lap to lap. After the ritual lap-sitting, and if he could sit alone, he was placed on the floor beside his mother. If he could crawl he was free to initiate his own social interactions or to withdraw from them at will. Much of what we wanted to know about the nature of the interaction between the infant and his mother, other familiar figures, and strangers, took place spontaneously, without any necessity for intervention. Moreover, the setting of the visit was so similar from one household to another that it provided a fairly standard situation in which we could observe individual differences in behavior.

Reliability of information

I had originally hoped to build into the study a check on reliability. I wanted my interpreter to take notes independently, which later could be checked with the notes I took. This was attempted, but abandoned, for it was impossible for her to take notes complete enough to be of use as a reliability check. Nonetheless, I checked with her after each visit to ascertain her impressions and to obtain from her the details that she had not been able to translate during the visit itself. Moreover, Mrs. Kibuka checked a carbon copy of my field notes for errors or omissions. She seemed to feel free to correct me on matters of fact. The fact that she made these amendments infrequently I take to be an indication of the reliability of my records.

The agreement of two observers is the classic criterion of reliability of observation. This criterion, however, is irrelevant to the reliability of the information given by an informant in interview. Distortions and omissions—whether deliberate or intentional—were expected in the information we were given. The chief safeguards here were that interview and direct observation overlapped at least in regard to current practices and behavior, and that the repeated visits and the services we gave facilitated the growth of rapport and confidence that tended to minimize deliberate distortions and omissions.

By the end of the study, however, it was apparent that the mothers differed in regard to the completeness of the information they had given and hence in regard to reliability. Differences in the excellence of the mothers as informants will be discussed later in this chapter.

Schedule of visits

The research plan called for a two-hour visit to each family every two weeks. There were, however, many irregularities in the schedule of visits. Although these mothers, for the most part, had calendars and clocks, appointments were sometimes forgotten, and at times emergencies arose which made the scheduled visit impossible. Illnesses and other circumstances sometimes prevented us from meeting our obligations. Although the two-hour visits were therefore less consistent than planned, we fell into the pattern of visiting briefly at more frequent intervals—to make or confirm appointments, to inquire about the health of an ailing child, to deliver medicines, or to render some other service. These frequent brief visits served to preserve good working relations, and during them some additional information was gained.

The number of contacts with each family ranged from seven to fifty-one, with a median number of twenty-three (see Table 3). This total is composed of (1) "long" visits, which were visits lasting for two hours or more, and including both a detailed interview with the mother and direct observation of the infant in interaction with his mother and with any other members of the household who were present; and (2) "short" visits, which included initial rapport-building visits, later appointment-confirming or service-rendering visits, visits that were cut short because of emergencies in the family, contacts in connection with transporting the mother and children to the clinic, final farewells, and the like. The number of long visits ranged from 0 (in the case of Senvuma with whose foster parents we never did achieve enough rapport for us to be able to conduct an adequate interview) to 9, with a median of 4.5. The number of short visits ranged from 3 to 45 with a median of 16.5. It is believed that the number of total contacts provides the best single criterion of the adequacy of our contact with the family concerned. In some cases it was felt that reliable and fairly comprehensive data were obtained despite the fact that the number of long visits was four or fewer.

Regardless of the number and length of contacts, the completion of the interview schedule provides a criterion of the adequacy of the contact. In nearly all instances the schedule was completed, although there were a few in which gaps in information were evident. Although in two[2] cases the gaps were in part

2 The worst gaps existed in the case of Senvuma. My first contacts with him and his mother took place during my preliminary month in the village, where I had an excellent opportunity to observe

TABLE 3 Number of visits and excellence of informants

Name	*Number of Visits*			*Mother's Excellence as Informant*
	Long	*Short*	*Total*	
SECURE – ATTACHED				
1. Paulo	7	20	27	7
2. Sembajwe	3	11	14	7
3. Juko	2	8	10	4
4. Petero	5	19	24	7
5. Senvuma	0	15	15 [a]	–
6. Mutebe	5	5	10	6
7. Nakiku	6	33	39	5
8. Alima	5	11	16	5
9. Aida	5	25	30	7
10. William	7	17	24 [a]	7
11. Senkumba	4	25	29	7
12. Kyimba	4	3	7	6
13. Samwendi	4	7	11 [a]	5
14. Maryamu	4	14	18	4
15. Lusiya	9	15	24 [a]	4
16. Nabatanzi	7	15	22	7
INSECURE – ATTACHED				
17. Muhamidi	4	19	23	4
18. Magalita	4	16	20	7
19. Kasozi	5	18	23	6
20. Sulaimani	4	12	16	5
21. Nakalema	3	5	8	2
22. Waswa (1)	6	45	51	5
23. Nakato (1)	6	45	51	5
NON – ATTACHED				
24. Nora	7	33	40	4
25. Kulistina	7	33	40	3
26. Waswa (2)	4	19	23	1
27. Nakato (2)	4	19	23	1
28. Namitala	4	7	11	3

[a] Not including informal visits before research began.

them in interaction, although the lack of an interpreter made interviews impossible. At the very beginning of the research proper, Senvuma was separated from his mother. It proved very difficult to establish a cooperative relationship with his foster parents, and consequently interview data are sparse. Enough information was gained through direct observation, however, to justify retaining him in the sample.

Nakalema was seen only eight times, partly because the family moved about and was difficult to trace for a while, and partly because the mother seemed less enthusiastic about cooperating with us than did any of the other mothers.

attributable to reluctance to cooperate, in four[3] cases the mothers had been highly cooperative and had been visited often enough that it seemed unbelievable that data could be incomplete.

The mother's excellence as an informant

The phenomenon of finding incomplete data, despite numerous visits, highlighted the fact that these mothers differed in their excellence as informants. This important variable was obscured by the fact that some mothers were very pleasant, welcoming, and cooperative while still being relatively poor informants. In each of these instances it seemed that the mother was eager to be a gracious hostess and to establish a relationship with her visitors but much more interested in talking to us about things other than the baby.

These women were in striking contrast to some others, who were equally hospitable and proved to be excellent informants. Although these others seemed to appreciate our visits, they did not attach more importance to chatting with us than to talking about the baby. When led to answer questions about the baby, they responded readily, volunteering relevant information and giving much spontaneous detail about the baby's behavior.

A seven-point scale was devised to rate each mother's proficiency as an informant. Although attention had first been directed to this variable by incompleteness of information obtained, the scale itself (except for rating 7) was based on other criteria: readiness and detail in responding to questions, spontaneity and detail in volunteering information, relevance of conversation to the current topic, patience in enduring a long interview, and concern with entertaining the visitor instead of giving information about the baby. The rating scale was as follows:

7 *The mother was an excellent informant. She stuck to the topic, volunteered information, gave much spontaneous detail about the baby, and never seemed impatient in interview.* The mothers of eight babies received this rating (see Table 3).
6 *The mother was a good informant. She talked readily and stuck to the topic.* The mothers of three babies received this rating.
5 *The mother was a good informant. She answered questions readily but did not volunteer much information.* The mothers of six babies received this rating.
4 *The mother answered questions briefly, volunteering little, but was cooperative, with her attention focused on talking about the baby.* The mothers of five babies were rated thus.

3 Kulistina, Namitala, and the younger set of twins.

3 *The mother was a good informant at times but seemed more concerned with her relationship with the visitor than with talking about the baby.* The mothers of two babies—Kulistina and Namitala—were rated thus.
2 *The mother was a fair informant at times, but it was difficult to keep her conversation focused on the baby for any length of time.* Only one—Nakalema's mother—was given this rating.
1 *The mother was a poor informant; little information was obtained about the baby despite at least an average number of visits.* The mother of the younger set of twins received this rating.

Special difficulties

Certain gaps in our information are due to special difficulties encountered in this particular society, and perhaps they could not have been avoided even had we known in advance that we would encounter them. First, it proved to be difficult to gain information about the composition of the household. I discovered that it was not customary for people to be introduced, as they are in this country, in recognition of the implicit question "Where does this person fit into the family picture?" The Ganda mother did not introduce a child by saying "This is my son" or "This is my sister's boy who is visiting us for a month." Nor did she introduce a man by saying "This is my brother-in-law" or "This is my next-door neighbor." On the contrary, each person present went through the traditional greetings with each other person, whether they had met before or not, and if anything was said in introduction of strangers it was the mere mention of a name. Indeed, it was considered impolite to offer identifications of relationships. Consequently, it took some weeks to differentiate between members of a household and visitors or neighbors. Even then it was difficult to distinguish between children who were the actual offspring of the householders and children who had been entrusted to them for upbringing. It was considered to be a humiliating rejection to a child to say in his presence that he was not a member of the family by reason of birth. It was therefore only gradually, and from general conversation, that one could sort out householders from visitors and children from foster children.

Another difficulty was of my own making. In presenting my plan to prospective participants I emphasized that my interest was in babies prior to weaning and shortly afterward. This emphasis was interpreted to mean that we were not interested in things that did not pertain to babies—and, indeed, that other things were none of my business. On the whole this emphasis facilitated rather than limited the research, but there were limiting features. We could not, for example, inquire routinely about the mother's education, about details of the parents' marriage, or about the composition and dispersion of the household. Moreover, I sensed that it would be considered rude for me to ask to see the behind-the-scenes living arrangements of the family or, indeed, to penetrate into family relationships except as I was invited to do so.

Still another difficulty was introduced by the high degree of mobility in Ganda life and the instability in Ganda marriages. Four of the twenty-eight babies moved during the period of research—one without his mother, two with their mothers only, and one with the entire family. Although contact was renewed to some extent after the move, it proved difficult in each case to re-establish it promptly and to continue the schedule of visits at the previous level of frequency and intensity.

PART II

Methods of Infant Care and the Infants' Responses to Them

6

FEEDING

Traditionally, all Ganda babies were breast-fed throughout the first two or three years of life, and even today most Ganda babies are breast-fed for the greater part of the first year of life or longer. In our own sample there was only one baby who was not breast-fed— Kasalina. Most babies are weaned directly from the breast to an adult type of diet, without an intervening period of bottle feeding. Final weaning from the breast now takes place most commonly between twelve and fourteen months of age. Before weaning, however, mother's milk is by no means the only source of nourishment; supplementary solid foods and fruit juices are introduced when the baby is still only a few months old, and although it is rare for a child to be fed entirely by bottle rather than by breast, in a substantial minority of cases supplementary feedings of milk are given by bottle or cup. Despite these supplementary sources of nourishment, most babies in our sample, including some whose mothers' milk supply had dwindled to an inadequate level, continued to suckle the breast until they had reached the age that the Ganda consider normal for weaning.

In view of the importance of breast feeding, we inquired what measures, if any, were taken during the first few days of a baby's life to ensure a successful feeding relationship and what was done either before or after delivery to encourage adequate lactation.

Early lactation and sucking

Potential difficulty in establishing suckling was acknowledged tacitly in ancient customs. According to our three informants, the newborn infant was customarily given food "for the purpose of clearing the throat"; this food contained *amafuta*

DOI: 10.4324/9781003629337-8

(butter or other fat) as an essential ingredient. Next, he was given unspecified "medicine" (*eddagala*). Only after these two preliminary precautions were taken was the baby put to the breast—but ordinarily this occurred within two hours after birth. All three informants recognized that the colostrum secretion was not milk, for they specified that it was two days before the milk came, even though the baby was expected to suckle from the beginning, if only momentarily at first. They recognized that suckling was sometimes established only with difficulty, if at all. They agreed that if the baby boy did not suck well at the beginning, a spear belonging to his father was laid beside him as a specific remedy. The baby girl, under similar circumstances, was given a knife (*akambe*) such as her mother customarily used to peel *matooke* when preparing it for cooking.

Only five of the mothers in our sample were aware of the existence of any traditional method for ensuring successful suckling, and none of these had faith in the efficacy of traditional methods. Only one had a vague and uncertain recollection of the ancient custom of giving a baby a spear (or knife). One said that the remedy was to put on the baby's tongue the dried and powdered leaf of the kyangwe plant or, in the case of an older child who failed to eat well, to mix it in his porridge.

We inquired of all the mothers in our sample about the circumstances of childbirth and early suckling (see Table 4). Eighteen babies were born in hospital and only nine at home.[1] Of the latter, only one bore her child without assistance; the rest received help either from a midwife or from a relative, usually one of the baby's grandmothers. Most (five of nine) of those who were delivered at home were Muslim, and even one of these had intended to have her baby in hospital; she arrived too early and was turned away, and later, when labor began in earnest, she had no time to get back to hospital. One of the non-Muslim mothers who had her baby at home had intended to go to hospital, but could not find transportation when her time came. The fact that most of the mothers in our sample wanted to have their babies in hospital is an indication that they are more acculturated than the average Ganda mother. Welbourn[2] reports that only 30 per cent of the babies attending child welfare clinics were born in hospital; the estimate is that between 20 and 30 per cent in Buganda as a whole are born in hospitals or rural maternity units.[3]

1 In this, as in many subsequent statements, we refer to twenty-seven rather than twenty-eight babies because one (Senvuma) had to be omitted; his mother had not been interviewed adequately before their separation, and subsequently it was very difficult to obtain information from his foster family.

2 Annual reports for Child Welfare Unit, 1955–61, Uganda Ministry of Health.

3 Billington, W. R., Welbourn, H. F., Wandera, K. C. N., and Sengendo, S. "Custom, child health, pregnancy and childbirth," *Trop. Geogr. Med.*, 1963, *15*: 124–33.

TABLE 4 Birth and early sucking

Name	*Where Born*	*Midwife*	*Day Breast First Offered*	*Day First Sucked Well*
SECURE – ATTACHED				
1. Paulo	hospital		1	1
2. Sembajwe	hospital			
3. Juko	hospital		1	2
4. Petero	hospital		2	3
5. Senvuma				
6. Mutebe	hospital		3	3
7. Nakiku	hospital		2	2
8. Alima	hospital		1	4
9. Aida	home	?	1	"not at first"
10. William	hospital		2	3
11. Senkumba	home	midwife	1	1
12. Kyimba	hospital		3	5
13. Samwendi	hospital		1	2
14. Maryamu	hospital			
15. Lusiya	home	PA	2	
16. Nabatanzi	home	MGM	2	2
INSECURE – ATTACHED				
17. Muhamidi	home	mother alone	1	"not at first"
18. Magalita	hospital		2	2
19. Kasozi	home	midwife	2	2
20. Sulaimani	home	relatives	2	2
21. Nakalema	home	PGM	1	
22. Waswa (1)	hospital		3	3
23. Nakato (1)	hospital		3	3
NON – ATTACHED				
24. Nora	hospital			
25. Kulistina	hospital		2	
26. Waswa (2)	hospital		2	
27. Nakato (2)	hospital		2	
28. Namitala	home	MGM	1	2

Of the nine babies born at home, six were given the breast shortly after birth and the rest on the second day of life. There was delay in the case of more of the hospital-born babies. Only six were put to the breast on the first day, but only four were delayed as long as the third day.

The success of initial feeding was reported in the case of nineteen infants. Of these, nine had some initial difficulties, and most of them had been offered the breast on the first or second day of life. By the third day, difficulties had cleared up in most instances, and by the fifth day all were reported to suck well.[4] None of the mothers seemed concerned about initial difficulties in suckling (except for Kasalina's mother, who claimed lactation failure). Three mothers, whose babies did not suck well at first, seemed content in the belief that the baby "was tired when he was born."

We asked all the mothers in our sample how initial difficulties in suckling might be overcome, if indeed they did occur. Apart from the five mentioned above, who had some awareness of ancient customs, these mothers seemed at a loss in replying to our question. Five had only tentative suggestions, with no apparent feeling of conviction. Two seemed to reflect hospital practices when they suggested that glucose be given or that water must be boiled. The others suggested that warm water might be given "to clear the throat" or that one should be persistent but patient in offering the nipple. The question about overcoming early difficulties in suckling was an academic question for these mothers. By the time we observed the babies, all were sucking well.

We inquired also what measures could be taken during pregnancy to ensure adequate lactation. All of our informants about ancient customs agreed that nothing was customarily done during pregnancy itself to encourage subsequent lactation, but that soon after the birth of the infant the mother received specific medicine—the name of which was not divulged, although salt was said to be added as an important ingredient. (Magalita's mother later said that the specific was the juice of the *kitembe* plant.) If lactation continued to be scanty, the mother was encouraged to eat plenty of vegetables, especially if prepared in soups.

We asked the mothers of our own sample how lactation might be established and maintained. The two who had had least success with lactation said that they had tried traditional "medicine," presumably as a last resort, but without success. Three mothers believed that adequate nutrition during pregnancy facilitated lactation, but the rest stressed an adequate diet for the mother during the period of breast feeding. They gave emphasis to corn meal porridge and liquids, particularly tea and orange juice, and some believed hot foods had special efficacy. None of them said anything that suggested that they recognized the importance of emptying the breasts of milk and hence of the stimulating function of frequent and adequate suckling by the infant.

Later lactation

These Ganda mothers did not conform to the stereotype of the "primitive" mother whose milk supply is so abundant that it can serve as the sole (or at least the

4 Gunther's observations of British babies suggest that if successful suckling is not established before the fifth day, it cannot be established. (Mavis Gunther, "Instinct and the nursing couple," *Lancet*, 1955, *1*: 575.)

chief) source of nourishment for a baby during his first two or three years of life (sec Table 5). Only eleven mothers seemed satisfied that they had an adequate milk supply throughout the entire period of breast feeding (or as long as we were in touch with them), and one of these suckled her baby until he was twenty-two months old. Two more lactated well until a new pregnancy intervened. All the rest reported difficulty in maintaining adequate lactation.

Three mothers reported difficulty from the beginning. Kulistina's mother claimed that she had had no milk at all and had had none for two of five previous babies.[5] The mother of the older set of twins had too little milk for two babies, and Magalita's mother felt that her supply was scanty from the beginning. Kulistina and the twins were, in fact, markedly malnourished when our study began and were not only well below age norms for height and weight but also obviously retarded in motor development. Indeed, concern over the babies' malnutrition was probably the chief reason for their mothers' cooperation in the research. Magalita was also somewhat below average for her age in height and weight although she was not obviously retarded otherwise. Her mother had had clinic help and advice about supplementary feeding all along, but, nevertheless, Magalita did not thrive—proabably because of recurrent diarrhea.

Twelve other mothers reported difficulty in lactation, claiming that their milk supply was adequate at first but dwindled later. It is by no means clear in which cases the insufficiency of lactation was real and in which cases it was imagined; but even if the original "insufficiency" were a figment of the mother's insecurity, it could well lead to a real insufficiency. When a mother suspected her milk supply was inadequate she immediately introduced supplementary feedings—of milk by bottle or of solids, or both. These supplementary feedings usually were given in lieu of the breast or at least before the breast feeding. Thus, the breast was suckled less frequently or after the baby's hunger had been satiated; it may be assumed that this led to less stimulation of milk secretion and to a true insufficiency, if indeed the insufficiency had not been real in the beginning.

Welbourn[6] comments that "failure of breast milk" may mean several things: the mother thinks her baby is not satisfied; the baby is observed not to gain weight or to lose weight; the mother wants to bottle feed, for whatever reason; the mother is anxious and externalizes the tension between her and the baby as a feeding problem. She goes on to say that after the baby is five or six months old the mother's judgment of insufficiency of breast milk for the nutritional needs of the baby is probably realistic, for he now needs other foods

5 Welbourn, in a personal communication, says that the statement "I have no breast milk" is often made by a mother at the child welfare clinic, although she is seen suckling her baby at the clinic. "She may say it in order to appear refined and educated—or, more likely, as an expression of her feeling of confusion and uncertainty."

6 Personal communication.

TABLE 5 Breast feeding

Name	*Mother's Milk Supply* [a]	*Mother's Enjoyment of Breast Feeding*	*Method of Feeding*	*Number of Night Feedings*	*Baby's Sucking Reponse*	*Baby's Initiative in Seeking & Managing Breast*
SECURE – ATTACHED						
1. Paulo	good	much enjoys	demand comfort [e]	3–4	good	actively seeks (30)
2. Sembajwe	good	enjoys	demand comfort	3	eager	seeks & manages (80)
3. Juko	failing (30) [b]	enjoys	demand comfort	1	good	actively seeks (32)
4. Petero	failing (30)	enjoys	demand comfort	2–3	eager	reaches for breast (9)
5. Senvuma	good	enjoys	demand comfort		eager	does not seek [j]
6. Mutebe	good	enjoyed at first	demand comfort [e]	3–4	good	passive
7. Nakiku	good	enjoys	schedule flexible	2	good [h]	
8. Alima	failing (10)	enjoys	demand	3	greedy	angry when removed (12)
9. Aida	failing (14)	enjoys	demand	1–3	eager	actively seeks (33)
10. William	good	enjoys [c]	schedule flexible	2[g]	eager	does not seek
11. Senkumba	failing (30)	duty	schedule flexible	2	eager [i]	does not seek
12. Kyimba	failed (32)	enjoyed at first	demand comfort [e]	2–3	eager [h]	
13. Samwendi	failing (13)	enjoys	demand comfort	3	good [h]	hits breast when hungry (19)
14. Maryamu	failed (37)	enjoys	schedule rigid	1–2	good [h]	does not seek
15. Lusiya	good	enjoys	demand comfort [e]	3	good	actively seeks (38)
16. Nabatanzi	good	enjoys	demand	2	greedy	actively seeks (46)

TABLE 5 (Continued)

Name	*Mother's Milk Supply* [a]	*Mother's Enjoyment of Breast Feeding*	*Method of Feeding*	*Number of Night Feedings*	*Baby's Sucking Reponse*	*Baby's Initiative in Seeking & Managing Breast*
INSECURE – ATTACHED						
17. Muhamidi	failing (31)	enjoyed at first	demand comfort	5	eager	actively seeks (32)
18. Magalita	insufficient	duty	demand	2	good [h]	
19. Kasozi	good	enjoys [c]	demand comfort [e]	2–3	good	actively seeks (48)
20. Sulaimani	good	duty	demand	often	greedy	hits breast when hungry (35)
21. Nakalema	failing (24)	enjoys	demand comfort	2–3	good	actively seeks (35)
22. Waswa (1)	insufficient	enjoyed at first	schedule flexible	2	greedy	actively seeks (59)
23. Nakato (1)	insufficient	enjoyed at first	schedule flexible	2	greedy	actively seeks (59)
NON – ATTACHED						
24. Nora	good	duty	schedule flexible	0–1	greedy	does not seek
25. Kulistina	none	enjoyed at first [d]	sch. flex, (bottle)	1		bottle-fed
26. Waswa (2)	failing (21)	no reply	demand [f]	0		
27. Nakato (2)	failing (21)	no reply	demand [f]	0		
28. Namitala	failing (8)	enjoys	demand comfort	1–2	good	does not seek (15)

[a] The adequacy of the mother's milk supply is based on her own report. The reports of "failing," "failed," or "none" may be inaccurate (see text).

[b] Age of baby in weeks throughout the tables.

[c] These mothers implied that breast feeding was a duty made pleasant by affection for the child.

[d] This is based on mother's statement about her enjoyment of breast feeding in the case of other children for whom she had milk.

[e] These mothers gave the breast for comfort sometimes, but not under all circumstances.

[f] This mother stated that she fed her babies on demand but observation suggests that it was at her own convenience.

[g] William was schedule-fed at night also, whereas the others who were schedule-fed during the day were fed on demand at night.

[h] In these cases feeding was not observed during our visits; the response of the baby is based on the mother's report.

[i] For a while, at about twenty-one weeks of age, this baby interrupted his breast feeding to cry.

[j] The mother offered the breast so readily and in response to such minimal cues that a seeking response was not observed.

as well. Nevertheless, four of the mothers in our sample judged their milk supply to be insufficient before the baby was more than about three months old and without any objective evidence of failure to gain.

Five Muslim mothers attributed a dwindling milk supply to the month-long Ramadan fast, during which they could not eat or drink between sunrise and sunset. In one of these Muslim mothers the effect of the fasting was complicated by illness, but in none did lactation return to normal when the fasting period was over. Indeed, only one Muslim mother in the sample was able to maintain an adequate milk supply during and after Ramadan. It is not clear how the fasting affected lactation. The total intake of food probably was not much less than usual, for after sundown one could eat well—and the main meal of the day for the Ganda comes after sundown. Perhaps regular meals are required to maintain lactation—or, more likely, regular intake of fluids. Perhaps the tension and irritation induced by fasting had an adverse effect on lactation—or made the mother believe that lactation was affected. In any event some effect communicated itself to the babies because they were fussy and irritable during visits made in the Ramadan period—both the babies of the sample and the babies belonging to women who were visiting the household simultaneously. It was easy to interpret their fussy crying as an indication of hunger. The Muslim mothers dealt with the problem by introducing supplementary bottle feedings. The babies seemed to bounce back to normal, despite the fact that their mothers' milk supply did not.

Since the whole issue of dwindling lactation is so closely related to supplementary bottle feeding, further discussion of it will be continued later in this chapter.

Enjoyment of breast feeding

Without expecting anything reliable or significant to come of it, we asked the mothers whether they enjoyed the process of breast feeding (see Table 5). One, Paulo's mother, said that she enjoyed it so much that she was reluctant to wean him, although he was already a year old and walking sturdily. Three implied sensuous pleasure in breast feeding, two by the Luganda word they used to describe it, and one by the embarrassed way she laughed when admitting that she enjoyed the experience. In all, fourteen mothers stated without qualification that they enjoyed breast feeding. Two more qualified their statements—one saying "I like it because it is good for him," and William's mother (who throughout seemed a very perceptive and competent mother) saying "I like it because I like the person I feed." The mothers of six babies said that they had enjoyed breast feeding at first, but that it had become burdensome after some months, while the mothers of four confessed that they had not enjoyed it at all but had undertaken it only out of a sense of duty. One—the mother of the younger twins—simply evaded our question, although she was asked on several occasions.

As it turns out, the answers to this question must have been reasonably reliable because reported enjoyment of breast feeding emerges as one of the few variables that, for this sample, is significantly related to outcome (see p. 362).

Method of breast feeding

The popular stereotype of African infant feeding is that the mother's breast is perpetually accessible and the infant feeds ideally according to his own desire. There is some question as to whether even ancient practice approximated this stereotype. Two of the informants of old customs among the Ganda said that the baby was fed whenever he was hungry or indeed whenever he cried—by "self-demand." But the third informant, old Mariamu, who always gave most realistic detail, scoffed at this interpretation of the facts. She said that the mother fed her baby early in the morning, but that for a long time after this she was much too busy digging in her garden and preparing food to take time to feed the child. Finally, after the fire had been lighted and the mid-day meal had been put on to cook, she could sit down. Then she would call to the child: "Now come, and I can feed you." Obviously Mariamu was thinking of an older baby, who could walk and understand language; she did not elucidate what was done with the tiny infant. She said, however, that only women who were weak or who wanted to avoid working used breast feeding as an excuse for not doing the work expected of them.

All informants of old customs agreed, however, that at night the ideal "demand" situation pertained. The baby slept with his mother and had free access to her breast whenever he woke and wished to suckle. Although most mothers fed infants while lying down during the night, Mariamu—the realist as always—pointed out that women have breasts that are differently shaped, and some mothers must sit to give the breast, even at night.

My own preconception of African feeding relationships was certainly that the baby would be fed according to "self demand." To my astonishment I found that eight of the babies in the sample (including Kulistina, the bottle-fed baby) were fed according to schedule (see Table 5). The schedules were not followed rigidly—except by one mother who said she fed "by the clock"[7]—for sleeping

7 A good many present-day Ganda families possess clocks, but even those who do not can tell time with reasonable accuracy. This close to the Equator, sunrise and sunset vary little from season to season, so that it is fairly easy to get a sense of time even without consciously noticing where the sun is in the sky. Moreover, the Ganda distinguish a twenty-four hour day, although the numbering varies by six hours from ours—so that noon is the sixth hour after sunrise. This six-hour discrepancy can cause embarrassing misunderstandings if the two people making an appointment do not agree whether they are going by Ganda time nomenclature or by European.

babies were not awakened to be fed, and seemingly hungry babies were not made to wait for the appointed hour. A four-hour schedule was usual, but one mother used a three-hour schedule during the first few months, and the mother of the older set of twins used a two-hour schedule—well into the second year of life. None of these mothers, however, attempted to adhere to scheduled feedings at night; if the babies woke, they were fed.[8]

How was schedule feeding learned in the middle of Africa? Two mothers said they had learned about it at school, and one specified that she had been taught that babies who are not fed on schedule cry more that those who are. One mother was introduced to the practice at the child welfare clinic, and she adopted it with alacrity for she found it helped her to be more efficient in planning her day's work. (On the other hand, two of the mothers had rejected schedule feeding as impractical, one saying that she was "too busy," the other that she had too many children to care for to manage it.) The other women who used a schedule had learned about this method from neighbors.

Twenty babies in the sample were fed "on demand." "On demand," however, does not mean the same thing from case to case. Eight mothers offered the breast whenever the baby seemed either hungry or to need comfort, and, indeed, four of them were observed to do so at the slightest signal from the child (often imperceptible to the observer), sometimes as often as four or five times in the course of a two-hour visit. Five mothers said that at times they offered the breast for comfort, but by no means always, and usually only if the baby was upset enough to cry hard. Five other mothers also described their feeding methods as "on demand," but they made it clear that "demand" was always interpreted as hunger and that under no circumstances was the breast offered for comfort or to alleviate distress. In other words, they said they fed a baby "when he was hungry" and the mother was the judge of whether or not he was hungry. One mother —the mother of the younger set of twins—claimed that she fed the babies on demand, but it seems likely that she met her own convenience rather than their needs, for she was not prompted to attend to them if they cried persistently during our visits.

In most instances, especially in the case of babies fed "on demand," firsthand observation during our visits enabled us to check on the information gathered in interview. Some women, however, seemed reluctant to bare the breast, despite the relative degree of modesty made possible by the *busuuti*\ they yielded to the baby's demand only if he were very insistent. Six babies were not observed while suckling during any visit. This figure includes Kulistina, who had been bottlefed from the beginning, and two babies who were weaned at the outset of

8 Except for the younger twins, whose mother discontinued night feedings when the twins were a few months old.

the study or soon thereafter. It includes also one schedule-fed baby. This leaves only two babies—Samwendi and Magalita—who were perhaps not fed in my presence because of the mothers' reluctance.[9]

Mothers' reports indicated that nighttime feedings tended to be more frequent with babies fed on demand than with those fed according to schedule. Four were said to be fed "often"—which was sometimes specified to mean as many as four or even five times during the night, while nine had three feedings on at least some nights. Four of the babies fed on demand awoke only once or twice in the course of the night whereas none of the schedule-fed babies woke more frequently than twice. Two babies—the younger set of twins—were not fed at all during the night; when they were ten weeks old their mother decided to ignore their cries at night, and soon they slept through without waking. With this one exception, no mother seemed to make an effort to train her baby to sleep through the night so as not to interrupt her sleep for a feeding. I could detect no note of triumphant accomplishment in the voices of mothers who reported that their babies sometimes slept through until morning; nor did I hear exasperation in the voices of mothers who said that their babies woke often for feeding.

The frequency of nighttime feedings seemed to have little or no relationship to age. Some of the youngest babies were fed only once or twice, while several of the oldest were fed three or more times. On the other hand, the babies who slept in their mothers' beds were all fed at least twice at night, and only those who slept in their own beds woke only once to be fed or slept through without feeding. Nevertheless, three of the babies who slept in their own beds roused their mothers four or more times for nighttime feedings.

We made no systematic note of the length of time taken for a feeding, but our impression was that these were generally relaxed and unhurried, often terminated by a tiny baby falling asleep at the breast or by an older baby initiating social interaction with his mother. The times when we visited were in the afternoon hours, which are usually filled with leisure in any event; it may be that at other times of day a mother might be more perfunctory in feeding. Nevertheless, I did not observe any Ganda mother terminating the feeding because the baby was not really sucking but only mouthing the nipple, nor did I observe one who put her baby aside impatiently, saying, in effect: "There! That's over with, and now I can get on with more important things."

For daytime feedings, including bottle feeding, the mother typically held the baby in a cradled position, supporting the baby's head with one arm loosely circled about him. No exceptions to this characteristic posture were observed in the case of very young babies, but when babies became old enough to take some

9 Nevertheless, the facts that some babies were not fed in my presence in the course of repeated visits, and that their mothers showed reluctance to breast feed, further indicate that my sample included a large proportion of relatively highly acculturated women.

initiative in seeking and managing the breast the mother did not always give the cradled support that they no longer needed. At night some of the mothers fed their babies while lying down—all but one of the mothers who shared their beds with the baby and eight of the mothers whose babies had their own beds. The others assumed the same sitting position that they took during the day.

"Burping" or patting "for wind" after feeding occurred in fifteen cases. Most of the mothers who did not pat for wind had never heard of such a practice. Most mothers—all but eight—said that they held the baby or played with him for a while after feeding him and before putting him down to sleep, except, of course, when the baby fell asleep at the breast; however, this after-feeding interaction tended to occur only after daytime feedings.

Response of the baby to breast feeding

All of the babies were said to suck well, and indeed, most of those who were observed while they suckled could be described as sucking actively and vigorously, if not greedily (see Table 5). Only once was a baby observed to fuss at the breast.[10] If a baby had been crying before the breast was offered, he accepted the nipple readily and stopped crying.

We did not ask the mothers about the initiative their babies took in seeking the breast, but our observations suggested that this was considerable, especially with babies fed on demand. Nine children, all six months of age or older, amazed me by the initiative they showed in seeking the breast, fumbling in the folds of the mother's dress, and often succeeding in gaining the breast by themselves, or at least in prompting the mother to help them. Sembajwe, who was over nineteen months of age when first observed, managed the whole business by himself. Standing beside his mother, who was seated in a chair, he pushed the folds of her dress aside, exposed the breast, lifted it up, and started to suck. Only one of the babies fed on demand appeared somewhat passive when feeding. One baby, who first signaled hunger by crying, soon needed only to whimper, and then only to "make a special sound" to inform her mother that she wanted to be fed. Two babies made it clear that their cries were hunger cries by hitting the breast while crying—a type of signal that could be specific only when the baby was being held by the mother. One nine-week-old baby had only to reach for the breast and his mother would respond appropriately to his signal. On the whole, the babies fed on demand, particularly those over six months old, were strikingly active in initiating suckling. The schedule-fed babies were usually passive—crying

10 This absence of fussing during feeding seems noteworthy in contrast with the fairly high incidence of impatient or frustrated fussing during feeding (both breast feeding and bottle feeding) in a sample of American babies currently under observation.

when hungry and accepting the breast when it was offered, but not directing an efficient, specific demand or search for the breast.

Supplementary feeding

Mair[11] seated that solid food was begun among the Ganda when the infant was but a few months old. That breast feeding was traditionally supplemented by solid food was confirmed by Mariamu, although she believed that this did not occur until the child was old enough to walk. The most usual foods offered to the very young child were said to be *matooke* (the staple plantain), *amenvu* (sweet bananas), and soup. Meat was not given because it was scarce and was usually served only when guests came. If the child learned to like meat, he might cry for it when guests came, and "this would not be right." By the time of weaning, the child was eating nearly everything in the adult diet, except meat, but in smaller portions. There was a standard amount that was considered appropriate for a young child, and he was given no more. Breast feeding was supplemented with solids before the age of walking only if the mother's milk supply was insufficient—according to Mariamu. In this case the most usual supplement was very ripe, sweet banana steamed in a banana leaf wrapping. Our other female informant recalled that supplementary solids were never given before weaning except when the mother's milk supply was inadequate, and even then not before the infant was two months old. She agreed that sweet bananas were the most usual supplement but mentioned also *ensujju* (a type of squash that the Americans call summer squash and the English vegetable marrow). Our male informant had no information to offer regarding supplementary feeding.

Present-day Ganda babies tend to begin to eat solid foods about the middle of the first year of life, according to both Welbourn[12] and the reports of the mothers in our own sample. The sufficiency or insufficiency of the mother's milk supply did not appear to influence the time of beginning solid supplements to breast feeding. The variety of foods available and given to the infant is greater than in the old days and reflects acculturation.

No other aspect of infant care was of more concern to the mothers in our sample than supplementary feeding, and nearly all of them asked repeatedly for information and advice. So great was their concern and so well-grounded in reality that it was quite impossible to refuse the advice they sought. Moreover, principles of infant nutrition were a major aspect of the instruction given by the child welfare clinic to which we offered to take mothers and babies, and this instruction emphasized early introduction of supplementary foods, stressing

11 Lucy B. Mair, *An African People, in the Twentieth Century* (London: Routledge, 1934), p. 56.

12 Hebe F. Welbourn, "Bottle Feeding: A Problem of Modern Civilization," *J. trop. Pediat.*, 1958, *3*: 165.

particularly vegetable proteins, which were more readily available than animal proteins. The clinic staff hoped to train their clients to become accustomed to serving these proteins since even the adult diet was deficient in this respect, and kwashiorkor—a serious disease in which protein deficiency is an etiological factor—was all too common among young children after weaning.

Because of the obvious danger of contaminating our information by our own advice and clinic instruction, we were careful to inquire about supplementary feeding on our first visit and before such advice or instruction had been given—at least before that given by us or through our services. The following information is based entirely upon feeding practices independent of our influence, unless otherwise specifically noted (see Table 6).

One of the first supplements added to the diet of the breast-fed baby was orange juice,[13] usually at about three months, of age, although two infants received it from the beginning. At some time between three and seven months solid foods were added, although one infant received some solids even earlier. Only two children—Kyimba, who was weaned before nine months of age, and Namitala, who was only four months old when the study ended—received no solid supplements. The most popular supplements were papaw, sweet bananas, *matooke,* squash (*ensujju*), sweet potatoes, and porridge made of corn meal (*kasooli*) mixed with a little milk. More rarely, bean soup, potatoes, beans, rice, bread, or avocados were given. It may be noted that, except for beans, these foods are very deficient in protein. Some infants received eggs, peanut soup, or pea flour mixed with water or milk, but these foods were almost invariably added as a result of clinic advice. The supplementary foods were introduced gradually in each case, and there seemed no outstanding preference for beginning with one food rather than another. Most mothers said they were careful to mash lumpy or fibrous foods before offering them to the baby.

A few mothers fed supplementary solids—especially papaw—by spoon.[14] More frequently the child fed himself with his fingers, although sometimes the mother used her own fingers to feed him. The mother of the younger set of twins began feeding corn meal porridge to her babies when they were but three months of age; she used a spoon at first but found this so tiresome that she made the porridge thinner and fed it by cup.

13 Welbourn reports: ". . . A previous generation of health educators had encouraged the planting of citrus trees and the use of orange juice for babies. This had become so firmly accepted as a rule of health that after ten years of trying to teach about the vital importance of beans and other protein foods I found that most conscientious parents regarded orange juice as the only essential supplement needed in a child's diet." Welbourn, *Baganda Childhood.*

14 The use of the spoon is another indication of a high degree of acculturation. Audrey I. Richards reports (personal communication) that spoons are not used even by adults in remote Ganda villages.

It was not uncommon for a baby to refuse a new food when it was first offered, but apart from this, little difficulty was encountered in feeding these supplementary foods. Indeed, the only persistent refusals were reported of Mutebe, who disliked orange juice, and Petero, who was reluctant to accept solid foods, although his refusal was neither consistent nor adamant.

During the first three months, supplementary foods (except orange juice) were rarely given unless the mother believed her milk supply to be insufficient. Except for one baby, supplementary feeding before three months of age consisted entirely of milk given by means of a nursing bottle and excluded solid foods. Bottle feeding of very young babies was observed in even the least acculturated families in our sample and was independent of advice from us or the clinic. Fresh cow's milk was difficult to obtain and hence was rarely used. More often the mother bought an expensive imported brand of powdered whole milk. There seemed to be prestige associated with the use of these imported preparations, but even for the more affluent families of our sample the cost was out of proportion to the family income. Perhaps because of this the tendency was to use a very dilute solution. Most of the mothers in our sample were, however, easily persuaded to substitute dried skim milk, which both we and the clinic bought wholesale and sold at cost. The supplementary bottle feeding often consisted of weak tea mixed with powdered milk and sugar. When a mother was asked what she gave the baby, she might reply: "Tea"—a reply that horrified Europeans who did not realize how weak it was. Indeed, this "tea" was perhaps preferable to a simple milk and water mixture, for everyone knew that water had to be boiled to make tea whereas only the best informed knew that milk or water given to an infant should be boiled.

Four infants in our sample received supplementary milk feedings during the first quarter-year of life, and one was entirely bottle-fed. Thirteen babies began to receive supplementary feedings in the second quarter-year—six because the mother's milk supply was dwindling and the rest because the mother thought it was a good thing. Indeed, all but three infants received supplementary milk feedings of some kind (see Table 6).

Bottle feeding was favored over cup feeding by the mothers of infants under six months of age, although two changed to cup feeding because they had such difficulty in keeping the bottle nipples clean and in good condition. Cup feeding was nearly always preferred to bottle feeding for infants whose supplementary feeding began after six months of age. Only Muhamidi's mother, who always did things the hard way, fed milk by spoon.

There seemed to be no common pattern regarding times for supplementary feeding, especially in the case of supplementary milk, although only one baby received it on demand. Supplementary solids were usually given at noon, if at no other time, and were sometimes followed immediately by breast feeding. Some babies received their solid food three times a day, at the time of family meals,

TABLE 6 Supplementary feeding and weaning

Name	*Supplementary Milk Begun (Weeks)*	*Supplementary Milk Given by*	*Supplementary Solids Begun (Weeks)*	*Feeding Problems: Dislikes or Refuses*
SECURE – ATTACHED				
1. Paulo	24	cup	24 [b]	none
2. Sembajwe	none	—	19	none
3. Juko	30?	cup	30?	None
4. Petero	30	bottle	30	milk, solids
5. Senvuma	—	—	—	—
6. Mutebe	22	cup	22	orange juice
7. Nakiku	28	cup	28	none
8. Alima	10	bottle	15	none
9. Aida	14	bottle	22 [a]	none
10. William	24 [a]	cup	24 [a, b]	new foods
11. Senkumba	20	cup	21	none
12. Kyimba	none	—	none	none
13. Samwendi	13	cup	15	none
14. Maryamu	22	cup	22	none
15. Lusiya	50 [c]	cup	17	none
16. Nabatanzi	48	cup	22 [a]	none
INSECURE – ATTACHED				
17. Muhamidi	31	spoon	22	none
18. Magalita	13 [a]	bottle [d]	13 [a]	milk
19. Kasozi	24	cup	24	none
20. Sulaimani	25	bottle	25 [b]	none
21. Nakalema	24	bottle	24	greedy, cries at the sight of food
22. Waswa (1)	16	bottle [d]	26	milk [e]
23. Nakato (1)	16	bottle [d]	26	milk [e]
NON – ATTACHED				
24. Nora	refused	(cup)	26 [a]	milk
25. Kulistina	1	bottle	27 [a, b]	new foods
26. Waswa (2)	18 [a]	cup	17 [b]	none
27. Nakato (2)	18 [a]	cup	17 [b]	none
28. Namitala	8	bottle	none	none

[a] Advised to begin supplements either at the clinic or by us on request.
[b] Orange juice begun earlier than solid supplements.
[c] Not begun until first phase of weaning was started.
[d] Changed later to cup feeding because of difficulty in keeping bottles and nipples clean.
[e] For a while, after illness.
[f] During the Ramadan fast only.
[g] After weaning only.

Malnutrition or Persistent Hunger	*Weaning Begun*	*Weaning Completed*	*Non-Nutritive Sucking*
no	—	—	no
no	21 mos.	22 mos.	habitual
no	—	—	occasional
slow gain	—	—	occasional
no	10 mos.	10 mos.	no
no	—		no
no	51 wks.	53 wks.	occasional [g]
hunger [f]	—	—	habitual
no	—	—	habitual
no	—	—	habitual
slow gain	—	—	occasional
no	—	34 wks.	no
no	—	—	habitual
no	36 wks.	37 wks.	habitual
no	50 wks.	52 wks.	no
no	49 wks.	56 wks.	no
hunger [f]	—	—	occasional
undernourished	—	55 wks.	habitual
no	57 wks.	59 wks.	occasional [g]
hunger [f]	—	—	no
hunger [f]	—	—	no
malnutrition & hunger	—	—	no
malnutrition & hunger	—	—	no
no	43 wks.	48 wks.	no
malnutrition	3 days	3 days	occasional
slow gain	—	—	occasional
slow gain	—	—	no
hunger [f]	—	—	occasional

but there were many idiosyncratic patterns, usually seeming to be determined by the mother's own convenience.

Although some babies accepted supplementary bottle feedings readily, none preferred a bottle to the breast, and five babies tended to refuse supplementary bottles. Nora and Magalita were persistent in their refusal of supplementary bottle feedings—which was unfortunate for Magalita especially, because her mother's milk supply was inadequate from the beginning. The older set of twins also went through a phase of refusing supplementary feedings of milk after a period of illness which occurred at eighteen months of age; this was also unfortunate for them since they were very undernourished. Petero preferred the breast to the supplementary bottle and was reluctant to accept solid foods.

Welbourn[15] reports that bottle feeding is on the increase among the Ganda, especially as a supplement to, rather than a substitute for, breast feeding. She notes three main causes: (1) physical, especially illness of mother or baby; (2) failure of lactation, which she believes to result from underfeeding at the breast; and (3) personal reasons, especially the mother's loss of confidence that she can adequately nourish her baby by breast feeding alone. Since Luo mothers living in Kampala lactated more abundantly than Ganda mothers living in the same town, Welbourn concedes the possibility that genetic factors may influence the abundance of milk supply, although she emphasizes personal psychological factors—alone or in interaction with genetic factors. If a mother believes that her baby is "not growing well"—whether this is true or not—she is likely to introduce supplementary feedings. If the baby cries excessively, especially at night, she may believe he is hungry and malnourished. Welbourn judged that supplementary bottle feeding was unnecessary in over half of her sample seen in child welfare clinics. Moreover, she implies that supplementary bottle feeding is undesirable when not truly necessary. Babies who receive supplementary bottles gain less satisfactorily than those who do not, probably because the mothers, through ignorance or economy, use too dilute a solution for the artificial feeding. Bottle-fed babies had a higher incidence of diarrhea, vomiting, and acute respiratory infections than babies who were entirely breast-fed. Moreover, babies fed supplementary bottles are weaned earlier—at a mean age of 6.6 months—than babies who are fully breast-fed, who are weaned at a mean age of 12.7 months. Welbourn implies that supplementary bottle feedings tend, especially when they are unnecessary, to diminish lactation and hence lead to early weaning and its hazards.

Our own data are by no means in opposition to Welbourn's findings. Supplementary bottle feedings were used more commonly by mothers with an inadequate milk supply than by those who had enough, but it is difficult to

15 Welbourn, "Bottle Feeding: A Problem of Modern Civilization," pp. 157–66.

distinguish cause from effect. Were the supplementary feedings begun because there was too little mother's milk, or did they themselves cause the milk supply to dwindle? Careful examination of our records confirmed the fact that in every case of a dwindling or insufficient milk supply the mother had complained of this before beginning supplementary feedings of milk. It may well have been, however, that she merely believed her supply to be inadequate because the baby cried or was not growing as quickly as expected, or that she, as Welbourn suggests, had lost confidence in her adequacy as a nurturer. In any event, once supplementary bottle feedings were begun they were used in such a way as to cause mother's milk to decrease. Rather than offering the bottle only if the baby still seemed hungry after exhausting the possibilities of the breast, these mothers tended to give the bottle instead of the breast at certain times, reserving the breast for what might be termed a between-meal snack. One woman—Samwendi's mother—often gave only one breast at a feeding (despite the fact that she believed she did not have enough milk) and began supplementary bottle feeding when her baby was only three months old. Although two women continued to have abundant lactation for at least twelve months, despite giving a bottle as a substitute for, rather than a supplement to, some breast feedings, it seemed likely that other mother-infant pairs were caught in a vicious spiral in which bottle feeding, introduced because of a real or imagined deficiency in milk supply, served to further diminish the milk supply, until finally some "unweaned" babies were suckled at a dry or nearly dry breast.

In our sample—apart from the four malnourished children mentioned earlier, Kulistina, Magalita, and the older twins—failure of the mother's milk supply (real or imagined) did not seem to have any strikingly adverse effects on development, presumably because supplementary feedings were provided, accepted, and utilized. (The general health of the babies of our sample is discussed in Chapter 11.)

Thumb sucking

In view of the hypothesis derived from psychoanalytic theory that one cause of thumb sucking is the failure to satisfy the need to suck in nutritive sucking at the breast (or bottle),[16] it is of interest that sixteen babies in our sample sucked their thumbs or fingers. In nine instances the sucking was said to be occasional, but in seven cases thumb sucking was habitual. The mothers of four of the seven claimed they had an insufficient milk supply and provided supplementary

16 A good discussion of this hypothesis and a review of the research literature relevant to it are given by Bettye M. Caldwell in her chapter entitled "The Effects of Infant Care," in M. L. Hoffman and L. W. Hoffman (eds.), *Review of Child Development Research* (New York: Russell Sage Foundation, 1964), I, 33–41.

feedings; the mothers of two fed by schedule. Thus, it could be said that six of the seven habitual thumb suckers had not experienced an ideal, natural suckling with an abundance of milk. The seventh was Sembajwe. He was a confirmed thumb sucker, despite the fact that his mother had a plentiful supply of milk, and despite the fact that he was fed on demand and, indeed, managed the breast by himself. He was not weaned until he was nearly two years of age, and therefore, as far as one could judge, he should on all counts have had his sucking needs gratified at the breast; nevertheless, he sucked his thumb.

7

CLEANLINESS

Personal cleanliness and tidiness is stressed in Buganda. Although water must be carried from wells, which are often distant, a daily bath, be it only a sponge bath, is customary for an adult. Hands are washed before eating. Laundry may often be seen drying on bushes in the hot sun. Old clothes, earth-stained and faded from many washings, may be worn for working in the banana garden, and babies and young children may get grubby as they play on the impacted earth of the floor of the house or the yard outside, but in the afternoons when it is time for visitors or for going visiting, everyone is cleaned up and the clothes are bright, clean, and freshly ironed. Perhaps less emphasis is placed on house cleaning than on washing bodies and clothing, and the folding chair that is brought for the European visitor may have to be dusted off before it is offered, but the houses, although tending to be bare and sparsely furnished, are tidy and free from litter.

Baths

The daily bath is routine for everyone, but babies are bathed even more frequently. After mouth-rinsing, a bath was traditionally the first experience of the newborn child. According to Mair[1] the newborn child used to be washed in warm water mixed with crushed herbs. "Medicines" were rubbed on his navel; he was massaged; and if he seemed ill, medicines were dropped into his mouth. Only then was he handed to his mother to be put to the breast. Our informants of old customs said that the herbs used for this first bath were *ekiirikiti* and

1 *An African People*, p. 42.

DOI: 10.4324/9781003629337-9

omulova, which were believed to prevent skin rashes. The traditional herb bath had been given, however, to only one of the babies in our sample, and it was delayed until after mother and baby had returned from hospital where the baby had been born.

Both Roscoe[2] and Mair[3] reported that infants used to be given baths daily in hot water. Mair said that medicinal herbs were mixed in the water during a baby's first four or five months, and that at about that age a midday bath in cold water, which was believed to increase a baby's appetite, was added. Until about three or four years of age all but the midday baths used to be given in warm water, but after that, unheated water was used. The child was not dried with a cloth but was allowed to drip dry.

Our informants of old customs elaborated on the accounts given by Roscoe and Mair. They all said that a baby was usually given *three* baths a day—in the morning, at noon, and before being put to bed in the evening. One informant said that the midday bath used to be optional (was usually given only when the weather was hot) but that that the other two were compulsory. They agreed that warm water was customarily used, although unheated water could be substituted at midday. Each baby in the household used to be bathed in his own special vessel, which in the old days was made of pottery, but which more recently has been of European metalware. There was no soap in the old days, but with the influx of Europeans, soap came into common use, and each child had his own piece. As the child grew older, it was customary to give him only two baths a day—at midday and at bedtime. The same type of herbal infusion that was used for newborn babies was customarily used from time to time throughout the early months, especially during the first two months. Other herb baths were considered to be specific treatments for illnesses of various kinds and were used especially for fever.

Present-day practices of the families in our sample closely resemble the traditional customs, except for a tendency for herb baths to be used less commonly (see Table 7). All but three babies in our sample had baths two or three times a day, and oddly enough it was this influence of European instruction that accounted for less frequent bathing. William's mother learned from the child welfare clinic that a single morning bath was standard European practice and welcomed the modification since she was busy with so many children. The mother of the older set of twins adopted the single daily bath as one of her several ways of easing the burden of twins. Fifteen infants received two baths a day, one in the morning, usually after the mother returned from the garden, and the other in the evening; with these a third bath was often added if the weather was

2 John Roscoe, *The Baganda* (London: Macmillan, 1911), pp. 58–59.
3 *An African People*, p. 54.

very hot or if the child had become particularly dirty. Nine babies received the traditional three baths a day, and these tended to be the youngest in the sample. Some were always bathed in warm water, but quite often water was not heated at midday or in very hot weather. The mothers agreed that older babies might need only one bath a day, and the shift was placed at some time between eighteen and thirty months. No mother expressed a belief that baths aided appetite, but Aida's mother believed that a baby would not sleep well unless he had been bathed just previously.

Our afternoon visits came at a bath-free time, but one afternoon Aida was given a bath in our presence—in preparation for a nap. She was held standing in a large basin of unheated water, outside in the sunshine, with the mother supporting her at the shoulders. Using her hands, with no cloth, the mother soaped her all over, and then rinsed her off. The mother gave careful attention to her nose, cleaning it with her fingers. She was then brought into the house in her mother's arms, still dripping, and dried with a cloth of thin unbleached cotton (*amerikani*). This was not a proper bath, the mother insisted; in a real bath she would have been seated in the tub, and her head would have been lathered too. Indeed, all the mothers agreed that bathing should include the hair, even three times a day.

Although herb baths were not used routinely for very young babies in this sample, fourteen had received them as specific treatment for illnesses. One mother said that an herb called *mululuga* was specific for fever (presumably malaria), while *bombo* was good for measles. The mothers who did not employ medicinal baths tended to be the more acculturated mothers; they believed them to be ineffective or even harmful.

Nearly all the babies enjoyed their baths; some liked particularly to play in the water and splash it about. Only two babies protested when the water was unheated and another two began to fight against bathing after they had been weaned.

As can be imagined with this amount of bathing, these Ganda babies appeared clean and tidy. Sixteen of the mothers kept themselves, their babies, their other children, and what we could see of the house and its environs especially clean and neat. The other families were less meticulous, but in only five cases was the baby more usually unkempt than clean and tidy, and in two of these cases—Senvuma and Lusiya—the child was usually being cared for by a nursemaid when we arrived to visit. In most households we found everything in order, even on a surprise visit, although we might find the mother in an old *busuuti* that she used for work. On a few occasions we were surprised to find a usually clean and well-groomed family of children looking grubby and unkempt, only to be informed that the mother was away—in hospital or at a funeral—and the children were being cared for temporarily by someone else.

TABLE 7 Cleanliness

Name	*Number of Baths per Day*	*Herb Baths*	*General Cleanliness*	*Elimination Training Begun*
SECURE – ATTACHED				
1. Paulo	2–3	yes	marked	4 mos. [a]
2. Sembajwe	2	no	fair	not trained
3. Juko	2 (prev. 3)	yes	marked	5 mos. [a]
4. Petero	3	no	marked	5 mos.
5. Senvuma			often unkempt [b]	
6. Mutebe	2	yes	marked	4 mos. [a]
7. Nakiku	2	no	marked	6 mos. [a]
8. Alima	3	yes	marked	2 mos.
9. Aida	3–4	yes	fair	2 mos.
10. William	1	no	marked	3 mos. (pot)
11. Senkumba	3	no	fair	3 mos.
12. Kyimba	3	once	marked	5 mos. [a]
13. Samwendi	3	no	marked	2 mos.
14. Maryamu	2	no	marked	6 mos. [a] (pot)
15. Lusiya	2	no	often unkempt	4 mos. [a]
16. Nabatanzi	2	yes	fair	4 mos. [a]
INSECURE – ATTACHED				
17. Muhamidi	2	yes	fair	1 mo. [a]
18. Magalita	2 (prev. 3)	yes	marked	
19. Kasozi	3	yes	marked	1 mo. [a]
20. Sulaimani	2	yes	fair	2 mos. [a]
21. Nakalema	3	yes	often unkempt	3 mos. [a]
22. Waswa (1)	1	yes	often unkempt	2–3 mos. [a]
23. Nakato (1)	1	yes	often unkempt	2–3 mos. [a]
NON – ATTACHED				
24. Nora	2–3	no	marked	4 mos.
25. Kulistina	2	no	marked	4 mos.
26. Waswa (2)	1	no	marked	4 mos.
27. Nakato (2)	1	no	marked	4 mos.
28. Namitala	3	yes	marked	2 mos.

[a] Based on retrospective report.
[b] After weaning and separation.
[c] If heard.
[d] Reported to be very close to reliable control.
[e] If the mother manages to wake up in order to hold him down during the night.
[f] The twins were not dry at sixteen months, but were reported to be dry at night when inquiry was next made at twenty months.
[g] Smearing was said to occur when bowel movement went unnoticed.
[h] Only when "very young," e.g., before four months of age.

Elimination Control Achieved

Bowel (Bed)	*Bowel (House)*	*Wetting (Bed)*	*Wetting (House)*	*Smearing*
9 mos.	not by 13 ½ mos.	13 mos. [e]	not by 13 mos.	yes [g]
7 mos. [a]	"early" [a, c]	22 mos.	22 mos.	no
4 mos. [a]	not by 8 mos.			no
8 mos.	not by 8½ mos.			no
		not by 11 mos.		
"very young" [a]	10½ mos. [c]	not by 11½ mos.		yes [h]
8 mos.	8 mos.	10 mos.	not by 14 mos.	no
5 mos.	not by 6 mos.			no
5 mos.	not by 8½ mos.			no
7 mos.	10 mos. [c]	10 mos. [c]	10 mos. [c]	no
6 mos.	not by 9 mos.			no
8 mos.	not by 10 mos.[d]			no
not by 6 mos.				no
11 mos.	not by 14½ mos.	not by 14½ mos.		yes [g]
5 mos. [a]	not by 8½ mos.	not by 14 mos.		no
9 mos.	9½ mos.	13½ mos.	13½ mos.	Yes
5 mos.	not by 8 mos.			yes [g]
6 mos. [a]	12 mos.	12½ mos.[c]	12½ mos.	no
4 mos. [a]		9 mos. [a]	not by 15 mos.	yes [h]
5 mos.	not by 9½ mos. [d]			once
8 mos.	not by 9½ mos.			no
6 mos. [a]	not by 21 mos.	19 mos. [f]	not by 21 mos.	once
6 mos. [a]	20 mos.	19 mos. [f]	not by 21 mos.	once
not by 12 mos.				often [g]
not by 11 mos.				often [g]
not by 8½ mos.				often [g]
not by 8½ mos.				often [g]
not by 3½ mos.				no

Other cleanliness practices

The general cleanliness associated with bathing did not necessarily extend to other aspects of bodily hygiene. Sometimes the baby's runny nose was wiped with a handkerchief or clean cloth, but sometimes it was wiped on whatever was at hand—a corner of mother's dress or even a dirty rag. Similarly, discharging eyes were wiped by the mother with her fingers or with any cloth at hand. Few of these mothers had any inkling of European knowledge of preventing infection or reinfection through hygienic practices.

Some traditional customs, however, in addition to bathing, promoted good hygiene. For example, the staple food, *matooke*, as well as similar foods like sweet potatoes or cassava, were cooked by long steaming. The food was wrapped in banana leaves, tied securely, and placed over a pot of boiling water, the bundle being just large enough to rest on the rim of the pot without dipping into the water. When the bundle was opened the housewife tore off a piece of the leaf in which it had been cooked, and with it divided the food, handing it to each person without touching the food with her hands. The hands of the diners, meanwhile, had been washed as a necessary preliminary to eating. Since we had meals with only a few of our sample families, it is not known how general this method of cooking and serving is today, nor what modifications have been introduced with plates and cutlery. We often noticed, however, that cooking and eating utensils had been placed on racks to dry outside in the sunshine.

Elimination practices and training

Contemporary specialists in child training in our culture place much emphasis on the importance of delaying any serious effort towards training in elimination control until the child had matured enough to be capable of control and of understanding what is required of him. Fraiberg,[4] for example, suggests that children are not likely to be mature enough until fifteen to eighteen months of age or even older to cooperate in learning bowel control. She and many other authors stress the adverse influence of methods of training that begin too early and are enforced too rigidly or even punitively, often making the child feel anxious and guilty, delaying the acquisition of the very control he is pressed to achieve, and usually resulting in making the issue of elimination control a battleground between parent and child.

If early and rigid toilet training can be viewed as a misguided effort of civilized societies to socialize the child, the stereotype of the primitive society is

4 Selma H. Fraiberg, *The Magic Years* (New York: Charles Scribner's Sons, 1959), p. 91.

one in which natural processes are not subject to social interference, and also in which civilized standards of cleanliness are not observed. Roscoe,[5] for example, while observing the personal cleanliness of the Ganda adult, said of the baby: "It was not trained in habits of cleanliness, and it grew up more like an animal than a human being. . . ."

Arriving in Uganda with this stereotype in mind, I was astonished to find, in response to my first inquiries, that training of eliminative functions is begun when the infant is very young indeed—usually at four months of age or earlier—and is carried through consistently and conscientiously. It was perhaps even more surprising to find that the Ganda mode of training was effective in bringing about the early acquisition of control of eliminative functions without any apparent anxiety, guilt, or struggle. Moreover, it was discovered that the methods of training in elimination control are by no means a result of acculturation influences. On the contrary, our informants of old customs made it clear that traditional training began as early as two and a half or three months of age, and was identical with the methods used today by all but the most acculturated families in our sample.

The method of training consists in holding the baby down in a squatting position, his feet on the ground, with the mother's arm passing across the baby's back, supporting it, and holding him under the arm farthest away from her. The mother's other hand usually was on the baby's body also, but it was not clear to my eye whether it was used to provide support or pressure. The baby is "held down" immediately after he wakes from sleep and immediately after feeding. Indeed, as one of our old informants told us, the mother might interrupt feeding, if she sensed that he was about to have a bowel movement, and thus avoid soiling.

The Luganda word for holding the child in this manner is *okusimba*, which is the same word as the verb "to plant." Mrs. Kibuka translated it as "to hold down," and this is the term I shall use. Welbourn[6] uses the term "hold out" and has shown me a photograph of a baby being held out rather than down. The baby was supported under the armpits, with his feet touching the ground. There was no pressure downwards, and no squatting position. I myself have observed babies being held thus, after having surprised the mother by wetting on her lap, although usually under these circumstances the baby is held out with his feet dangling in the air. Otherwise I have observed holding down in a squatting position as described above. It may well be that there are two methods used. Perhaps younger infants are held out while older babies are held down.

5 *The Baganda*, p. 60.
6 Welbourn, *Baganda Childhood.*

It is not clear whether holding down is believed to facilitate the eliminative process, but it seems likely that this might be true, particularly in the case of bowel movements. In any event, it is clearly the intention of the mother to hold the child in this position at times when a bowel movement or urination are most likely to occur, and, as one mother explained, the child eventually builds up an association between being held in this manner and the process of excreting waste. Most mothers implied quite clearly that the practice of " 'holding down" was designed to catch the child at an opportune time when he was ready to excrete but had not yet done so. They all placed stress on the need for vigilance if the child was to be caught. They attached importance to the convenience of avoiding soiled or wet beds by undertaking this practice, but at the same time they believed it to be a method of training. But, perhaps because of the recognition that the practice of holding down was as much for their own convenience as for training, they showed great patience throughout the long period before the child gained control. They seemed to realize that very young infants were unable to learn control and that their own lapses of vigilance were to blame for any accidents that occurred. Consequently, the babies—at least in the age group we observed—were never scolded or punished for accidents, but rather, lapses of control were dealt with in a matter-of-fact fashion without fuss.

Although this much emerged clearly, it proved to be exceedingly difficult to obtain any precise information about the age at which training was instituted or about the ages at which control was finally established. Mothers who in other ways seemed to be reliable informants were caught in seemingly contradictory statements—for example, one moment saying that training had been begun at seven months of age and the next moment saying that the infant had stopped soiling his bed at four months of age—and inquiries often ended with both inquirers and informants looking perplexed and confused. My interpreter was just as confused as I, since she herself used European "potting" training for her children. The grandmother in one household found it hilarious that we should be interested in such matters; she could understand our interest in feeding practices, for feeding was important; but elimination training was such a trifle for Europeans to inquire about. The mothers themselves seemed to feel that this training was a legitimate field of inquiry. Only one seemed touchy on the subject—and she was touchy in many areas since she was defending her own idiosyncratic child-rearing practices. Indeed, she claimed that she used no training at all.

It gradually emerged that one difficulty was purely semantic. When the word *okusimba* was used, it was always qualified by the purpose for which the child was held down, whether for a bowel movement or for urination. So, when an unqualified question was posed as to when holding down had begun, the mother sometimes answered in regard to one function and sometimes in regard to the other. Furthermore, these mothers made a clear-cut distinction between learning not to soil the bed and learning not to defecate elsewhere in the house or yard. They made the same distinction between wetting the bed and wetting elsewhere. We gradually realized that training was thought of as having at least three stages, in regard to both soiling and wetting. The first stage in bowel training, and the one to which they attached most importance, was keeping the bed clean. Therefore, their first concern was to be alert to the baby even while he slept, so at the first sign of waking he could be taken up and held down. Holding down after feeding helped to accomplish the second purpose of avoiding defecation in the house as well. The baby was taken outside, around the corner of the house, and out of sight when he was held down for a bowel movement. The final stage of learning to use the same latrine as adults used was delayed for several years.[7]

Similarly, the first objective in control of micturition was a dry bed. It was of relatively little concern to the mother if the baby wet elsewhere in the house, for the urine was quickly absorbed by the dirt floor, leaving no trace even of odor. An effort was made, nevertheless, but considerably later, to train the child to go outdoors to urinate, and the method was the same—by holding down. Before the child was able to crawl or walk he was not necessarily taken outside to urinate. We sometimes observed a baby being held down in the house, away from the mats that covered part of the earthen floor.

There were major variations in elimination-training practices in only three cases (see Table 7). Sembajwe's mother claimed that she did not attempt to train him at all,[8] but suddenly, just after he was weaned at twenty-two months of age, he quite spontaneously acquired control and henceforward on his own initiative went outside to eliminate. William's mother, on the other hand, used a potty for training, although otherwise she followed the traditional pattern closely, and Maryamu's mother imitated the potting practice. Maryamu's mother, however, lacked the vigilance of most of these mothers, and her babies had more accidents. Two other variations were attributable to lack of vigilance; Kulistina and Nora were kept in their cribs in a bedroom most of the time, and their signals

7 Welbourn (*Baganda Childhood*) provides more detail for the older child. "As the child grew old enough to move about he would be smacked gently and put outside to teach him not to soil in the house. At first he would soil near the doorway of the house and the mother would pick up the mess in a bundle of leaves and throw it away. Later he would be taught not to soil in the compound near the house, and later still he would be taught to use the latrine if there was one. Old fashioned people sometimes had an idea that a person could be got at, by witchcraft, by means of his excreta. A baby's stools were wiped up with leaves and thrown away under his special banana-tree. It was sometimes said that it was dangerous for children's stools to mingle in the same latrine as adults'. Usually, in practice, older children ran about in the banana gardens and passed their stools wherever they felt inclined so long as they were out of sight of adults."

8 I suspect, from other things she said, that she followed the practice of holding him down, to "catch," but that she went even further than the other mothers in refusing to consider this "training."

therefore went unnoticed. Otherwise their mothers followed the usual practices in holding down.

There was some variation in the age at which holding down was begun. In the case of babies whom we visited during their first six months of life, we were told, and often observed for ourselves, that training began at three months of age, or earlier—in one case as early as one month. The retrospective reports of the mothers of the older babies suggested that training began slightly later—at a modal age of four months. It may seem unlikely to the Western reader that a baby of three months of age or younger could have enough control of his head and back musculature to be held in a squatting position for several minutes with only slight support. Ganda babies, however, were very accelerated in motor development.[9] Moreover, if motor development lagged, as it did with Kulistina and Petero, for example, training was delayed until the baby was judged strong enough to be held down.

Let us turn now from techniques of training to ways of coping with the untrained child. Ganda babies are rarely diapered. Only two of our sample—Kulistina and Lusiya—wore diapers, and these only for special occasions when they wore waterproof pants also. The diapers were made of *amerikani* cloth—which is thin, unbleached muslin, not very absorbent, and hence ineffective for the purpose. *Amerikani* cloth is much more frequently used in lieu of diapers; instead of being pinned around the baby, it is spread out on the lap of the mother (or visitor) when she holds him. Six babies in our sample had waterproof pants, which they wore only for special occasions, such as visits to the clinic. Especially when worn without diapers—as they were in four cases—the waterproof pants were absurdly ineffective. I noted one occasion when a baby in waterproof pants urinated while held on his mother's lap. His mother exclaimed and quickly held the baby away from her while the urine trickled down his legs. She then removed the pants, shook the remaining drops of urine on the floor, dried the baby with a cloth, and then dried the pants and put them back on. On the other hand, the mothers who dressed their babies without pants of any description had less difficulty with accidents, for usually clothing did not have to be removed.

The effectiveness of these training methods will be discussed later in more detail; here it is necessary to say only that they were effective enough—in "catching" the child if in no other way—that accidents were not common during our visits. Only half of our sample were observed to have an accident in the course of a visit, and most of these were observed to have only one during our entire acquaintance. Only four instances of soiling were observed. Therefore, the mothers' attitudes toward the eliminative functions of their babies must in large part be inferred from interview data in the context of our inquiries about training

9 See Chapter 19.

procedures. Their attitudes seemed, without exception, tolerant and accepting. A few could verbalize that it was in a child's nature to function in this way, and that it took a long time before he was old enough to learn control.

The closest these mothers came to any expression of disgust or displeasure was when an accident occurred while the baby was being held. We observed, almost invariably, that the mother exclaimed and quickly held the baby away from her in order to avoid getting wet or soiled. Once the initial reaction was over, she dealt with the accident with neither scolding nor fuss. The results of wetting were often ignored; the wet spot on the earthen floor or even on a mat would soon dry. Perhaps if the baby seemed likely to put his fingers in the little muddy spot, she would deter him or place a chair or other obstacle over the spot. Cement floors presented more difficulty. In one house we observed that a puddle was swept with a broom, spreading the urine so that at least it would dry more quickly.

Coping with soiling was less casual, but still very matter-of-fact. The baby was first cleaned up, and then the feces themselves were removed. In the four instances we observed, different materials seemed to have been kept at hand for this specific purpose. In one instance it was toilet paper, in one, newspaper, and in the others, leaves.[10] Some mothers even carried leaves about with them in a handbag so as to be prepared for any emergency.

Establishment of control of elimination

Our most reliable information was gained in regard to the first landmark in elimination control—not soiling the bed. The mothers' expectations, judging from their retrospective reports about their older children, seemed to be that this control should be established by the age of seven months. In the cases of the babies whom we visited before control was acquired, the range of ages at which bed-soiling ceased was from five to eleven months. In the case of babies not visited until after this control was acquired, the range of ages, reported retrospectively, was from four to eight months (see Table 7).

There were three babies who were late in achieving control—the only ones who had not done so by the age of nine months—Kulistina, Nora, and Maryamu. In none of these cases did the mother pay adequate attention to the baby's signals. In each case of the establishment of early control, the baby either evacuated very regularly and predictably so that he could always be "caught" or he began to give signals of his intentions which the mother heeded. The acquistion of early, reliable control was clearly a matter of intimate interaction between infant

10 Welbourn (personal communication) says that leaves from a particular tree—"the toilet-paper tree"—are used for this purpose; they are soft and slightly absorbent.

and mother, the child giving signals and the mother (or her deputy) being close enough and alert enough to respond to the signals promptly.

The second landmark of not soiling in the house was achieved by seven babies. One baby achieved this by eight months of age, six by twelve months of age, and one much later. Five of the seven were able to go outside on their own initiative when they wanted to move their bowels. Three babies, however, including Sembajwe at an "early" age, achieved a reputation for control because they were never alone and always managed to signal their needs in time to be taken out and "held down." Five babies did not achieve bowel control by twelve months of age. Two (the older twins) were generally retarded; Maryamu's and Nora's mothers did not heed their signals; this leaves only Paulo, who was slow for no apparent reason.

In regard to smearing—fourteen mothers said that their babies had never smeared, although thirteen admitted that theirs had. Seven of the latter explained that smearing occurred only if a bowel movement went unnoticed. Since the practice was so commonly to hold the child down immediately after waking or feeding, and for the mother or some responsible adult to be omnipresent and alert to the child's signals, smearing was a real problem only with the four children who spent considerable time unattended—Kulistina, Nora, and the younger twins.

Nine babies achieved the third landmark of not wetting the bed, six before fourteen months of age, and two as early as nine or ten months. Sembajwe, who was said to have received no training, spontaneously stopped wetting at the time of weaning at twenty-two months of age. In all instances of early control there was emphasis both on the child's recognizable signals and the mother's alertness to them, and on the mother's practice either of wakening him during the night to be held down or herself waking as soon as he awoke. The mothers themselves understood that control was contingent upon alertness and close interaction with the child. When questioned about the age at which older siblings stopped wetting the bed they placed it at about eighteen months, which is later than the times observed in this sample.

The fourth landmark—not wetting in the house—was achieved by only four children during the age span observed. Sembajwe, as mentioned above, without previous training began to manage his own eliminative processes effectively and reliably at the age of twenty-two months. Magalita and Nabatanzi were successful in managing to get outside to urinate by the time they were little more than a year old. William, who was almost never alone, could delay until placed on the potty by the time he was ten months old, but on rare occasions when his signals were not heard, he wet.

It is clear from the foregoing account that Ganda training in elimination control is at least as effective as the training methods used in our culture. It rests for its effectiveness not so much upon a schedule of holding down but upon the child's own indications of need. Before he can actually signal his needs the mother gears her practices to what she has observed of the child's rhythms, and holds him down at times when he is most likely to defecate or urinate. Soon he is able to signal his needs with special sounds that she recognizes even before he can verbalize. The extent to which control is something accepted by the child rather than imposed upon him is shown by his tendency to take the initiative himself in finding the appropriate place to excrete waste when he is old enough to get there under his own steam. All of this is contingent upon the mother's (or some other adult's or responsible child's) omnipresence and responsiveness which ensure that the baby's signals will not go unheeded.

The gradation of the purposes of training is itself interesting. It may well be that the task of learning first of all that the bed is a place *not* to be wet or soiled is an easier one than learning that elimination can take place only in one place—on a potty or toilet. Having grasped this notion it is perhaps easier to take the next step of delaying until the proper place is reached than it would be to learn that all at once without intermediate objectives.

Delay in the acquisition of elimination control was found in the case of children whose mothers were either not present enough of the time or, if present, not alert enough to signals. Delay also occurred in children whose general development was retarded presumably because of malnutrition or illness. Moreover, diarrhea, which was unfortunately common, could wreak havoc with any training program, and accounted for accidents even in children who otherwise were said to be reliable.

The success of a technique of training in elimination control must be evaluated not only in terms of its initial effectiveness but also in terms of its effect upon later characteristics of the individual, including the long-term maintenance of effective control. We have almost no information about the long-term results of Ganda training. It is clear even from our own sample that this early training, although often effective, does not prevent further difficulties, for several mothers asked for advice about handling a problem of bed-wetting in an older child. I am very much inclined to agree with Welbourn who wrote to me as follows: "I was surprised that your babies were dry at night and learned not to soil in the house so early. I think this may have been because they were still, even those who had been weaned, interacting closely with their mothers—still almost at the 'holding down' (or 'out') stage. I would be willing to bet that they regressed as they became independent of their mothers. . . . As you say, there is a lot of difference between learning by interaction with mother that you *don't* soil in the house or in bed, and being caught up in mother's obsession that you *must* use a particular time and receptacle." But regardless of its eventual degree of effectiveness, the most impressive evidence that it was effective at least in its "catching" aspects was that only half the babies were observed to wet once (or more) during our whole series of visits. Holding an undiapered baby on one's lap did not present as much of a hazard as one might suppose!

8

SLEEPING

In the old days the Ganda infant slept with his mother until he was weaned. Even weaning did not necessarily end this sleeping arrangement, according to two of my informants about old customs. The child might continue sleeping with her until he was separated from his mother and sent elsewhere to be reared. The child's father, meanwhile, slept elsewhere.

Roscoe[1] reported that the Ganda wife lived apart from her husband for three years while nursing her child, although, if she was his only wife, they continued to live together. Mair,[2] in 1934, stated that none of her informants had any recollection of prohibition of sexual intercourse during the period of breast feeding, such as Roscoe implies. Our oldest informant, Mariamu, recalled, however, that intercourse was discouraged, if not virtually prohibited. Relatives, especially the father's sister, brought pressure upon the father to desist in his demands on the mother during the suckling period. It was considered a disgrace for the mother of an unweaned baby to become pregnant, and if this happened, her husband would be abused by the mother's brother or father. Mariamu hastened to point out that the disgrace lay not in sexual relations but in the resulting pregnancy. It was expected, she said, that if sexual relations took place, the husband should practice coitus interruptus. If, despite social discouragement, the husband wished to have relations with his wife before their baby was weaned, she was obliged to go to him, leaving the baby behind in her own hut, for the

1 *The Baganda*, pp. 55–56.
2 *An African People*, p. 55.

DOI: 10.4324/9781003629337-10

child, however young, should not witness sexual relations between his parents. Mariamu said that the mother was in conflict when such demands were placed upon her, because she was also expected immediately to give the breast to the baby should he wake and cry.

Inquiries were not made about the parents' sleeping arrangements in our contemporary sample, although, except for those who were separated, they must at least have slept in the same house rather than in separate huts. The sleeping arrangements of the infants in our sample varied (see Table 8). Most of them slept in beds of their own.[3] Only eleven babies in the sample slept in their mothers' beds, and of these, three did so for no longer than the first four months of life. By and large, it was believed to be best for a baby to have his own bed—even by the mothers of three babies who did not. Kasozi's mother could not afford to buy him his own bed; Kyimba refused to sleep by himself, so he slept with his mother until he was weaned and thereafter with his grandmother; Mutebe slept with his grandmother from six months onwards at her urgent request and returned to his mother's bed only when the grandmother was away from home. Each baby who had a bed of his own nevertheless shared his mother's bedroom with her.

Sixteen babies who had their own beds, either from the beginning or later on, had European-type cribs with sides, and two of these were provided with mosquito netting. One mother placed the baby's crib tight against her own bed, with one side down so that she could reach the baby easily when he woke at night to be fed. Four babies were said to have beds with no railings. Perhaps these were low beds; but in one case, at least, the bed must have been raised from the floor for the mother was concerned because the baby fell out of bed now and then.

Most of the babies in our sample slept well at night, crying only if they woke to be fed, and settling down well afterward (although two of these, the younger twins, did so only after three months of age). Five of the eight babies who slept poorly at night were also fussy and cried a lot during the day; a sixth baby who fussed at night had done so only since weaning. Sleeping problems thus seemed to be infrequent, perhaps because even those babies who were schedule-fed during the day were fed on demand at night. Only one problem other than crying at night was even mentioned; one mother was concerned because her baby persisted in sleeping on his face, and turned again to his favored position no matter how often she turned him over onto his back.

3 Richards (personal communication) believes this to be atypical, that it is another indication of the relatively high degree of acculturation characteristic of this sample.

TABLE 8 Sleeping

Name	*Sleeps with Mother*	*Sleeps Well at Night*
SECURE – ATTACHED		
1. Paulo	no	no
2. Sembajwe	no	yes
3. Juko	no	
4. Petero	no	yes
5. Senvuma		
6. Mutebe	to 6 mos.	yes
7. Nakiku	no	yes
8. Alima	to 2 mos.	yes
9. Aida	yes	yes
10. William	no	yes
11. Senkumba	to 2 mos.	yes
12. Kyimba	till weaned	no [a]
13. Samwendi	yes	yes
14. Maryamu	no	yes
15. Lusiya	till weaned	no
16. Nabatanzi	no	yes
INSECURE – ATTACHED		
17. Muhamidi	yes	no
18. Magalita	to 4 mos.	no
19. Kasozi	till weaned	yes
20. Sulaimani	no	no
21. Nakalema	to 6 mos.	yes
22. Waswa (1)	no	no
23. Nakato (1)	no	no
NON – ATTACHED		
24. Nora	no	yes
25. Kulistina	no	yes
26. Waswa (2)	no	yes [b]
27. Nakato (2)	no	yes [b]
28. Namitala	no	yes

[a] After weaning; no information about how well he slept before weaning.
[b] But not during the first three or four months.

A tiny baby, as might be expected, slept most of the day—perhaps in bed (his own or his mother's), with his mother or some other responsible person nearby, perhaps on a heap of old cloths in a corner of the living-room, or perhaps on a mat in the garden while his mother worked. William had his naps in a wheelbarrow which served as a baby carriage, and the younger twins napped together in a gocart. Most of our sample soon settled into a routine of two naps a day, morning and afternoon, although among those over fourteen months of age there was only an afternoon nap.

All but five babies took daytime naps without difficulty. Muhamidi, however, was said to be restless and to have only one nap during the day, while Sulaimani, Juko, and the younger set of twins were said to sleep very little during the day.

9

MOTHERING PRACTICES

The term "mothering" can include everything that a mother or substitute mother does for a child or in interaction with him. At a minimal level, mothering includes only such routine care as is needed to ensure that the baby is fed, clean, warm, dry, and safe. Optimally, mothering includes much more than routine care, and the term must therefore be extended to cover many kinds of interaction between mother and child.

This chapter deals with two aspects of mothering practices: (1) the quantity and mode of physical contact between mother and child; and (2) the extent to which a mother shares her mothering duties with other people. A third important aspect—a mother's response to a baby's emotional states—will be dealt with in the next chapter.

Quantity and mode of physical contact between mother and baby

We are concerned here with handling, carrying, and holding, chiefly. And, as pointed out in the last chapter, some babies, even in this relatively highly acculturated sample, slept with their mothers; this for them is also an important aspect of physical contact.

Carrying and Handling

There are four ways in which Ganda mothers carry their babies —held cradled in the arms, held up against the shoulder, straddled across one hip, or on the back held in place by a sling of cotton cloth. Very tiny babies are usually carried

DOI: 10.4324/9781003629337-11

cradled in the mother's arms, or held up against her chest and shoulder—and even older infants are often carried thus for short distances. The stereotype is, however, of the Ganda baby being carried on his mother's back, and some observers even fancy that this implies skin-to-skin contact, despite the facts that the mother is obviously clothed, the baby is usually clothed also (especially if a journey is involved), and, moreover, that the cloth of the sling is between them. Mair[1] commented that babies were carried on their mothers' backs, implying that this was the usual practice at that time. In this sample eleven babies were said never to be carried on their mothers' backs (see Table 9). On the whole it was the more acculturated[2] mothers who never adopted this method of carrying a baby; however, both Sulaimani and Nabatanzi, whose mothers otherwise did not seem highly acculturated, were carried straddled over their mother's hips, not in a sling nor on the back. Even a mother who sometimes carried her baby slung across the back often carried him in her arms, or up over the shoulder, or straddled across the hip instead. By and large it seemed to be the distance that the baby was to be carried that dictated the method. If the distance was long, it was easier to carry a baby on the back; if the distance was short it was more convenient to use another method. Even so, there were disagreements. Lusiya's mother said that Lusiya had outgrown being carried on the back by the time she was eleven months old and that it was easier to carry her in arms or on the hip. Mutebe's mother carried him on her back when he was a year old and a very big baby at that. Sembajwe's mother said that it was more comfortable to carry him on her back than on her hip if she was going a long distance, even when he was a sturdy boy of two years.

Namitala at three months of age was the youngest baby I observed being carried on the mother's back; but my observation and inquiry on this matter were not systematic at the beginning, and it may well have begun earlier. Certainly Ganda mothers do not take care to support the heads of even newborn babies.

1 *An African People*, p. 55.

2 In personal communications both Richards and Welbourn expressed astonishment that there were this many babies in a Ganda sample who were not carried in the traditional way. Richards says the finding is "atypical" and holds it as still another piece of evidence that my sample was relatively highly acculturated. Welbourn says: "I can't believe that there *could* be eleven Baganda babies *never* carried on the back! I think they would have been carried on the back on a journey—perhaps you saved them journeys by providing car transport. I have a feeling that this is something a woman might say she never did because she did it without thinking." I doubt that a woman could carry a baby in a sling on the back without thinking, if only because of the use of the sling. I believe it is possible that, in an attempt to appear refined and acculturated, a mother might deny the practice. I have no doubt that providing car transport to the clinic made it unnecessary for babies to be carried on the back to the clinic. I suspect, however, that most of the mothers who said they did not carry their babies on their backs would be reluctant to undertake a journey with a baby if to do so made it necessary to carry the baby thus. In any event, I observed no discrepancy between what these mothers did in my presence and what they said they did.

TABLE 9 Mothering practices

Name	*Carries Baby on Back*	*Amount of Holding*	*Rating Amount of Mother's Care*	*Rating Amount of Total Care*
SECURE – ATTACHED				
1. Paulo	yes [a]	much	7	7
2. Sembajwe	yes	little [c]	7	7
3. Juko	yes	much	7	7
4. Petero	yes	much	6	6
5. Senvuma	yes	much [d]	5	7
6. Mutebe	yes	little [c]	5	7
7. Nakiku	yes	much [d]	5	7
8. Alima	yes	much	5	7
9. Aida	yes	much [d]	4	6
10. William	never	some	4	6
11. Senkumba	never	much	4	5
12. Kyimba	yes	much	4	6
13. Samwendi	never	much	4	6
14. Maryamu	never		4	5
15. Lusiya	yes till 11 mos.	some	4	5
16. Nabatanzi	never	much [d]	3	7
INSECURE – ATTACHED				
17. Muhamidi	yes [a]	much	7	7
18. Magalita	yes	much	4	6
19. Kasozi	never	some	3	4
20. Sulaimani	never	some	4	2
21. Nakalema	yes	much [e]	4	7
22. Waswa (1)	yes [b]	much	3	6
23. Nakato (1)	yes [b]	much	3	6
NON – ATTACHED				
24. Nora	never	little [f]	2	2
25. Kulistina	never	little [f]	2	2
26. Waswa (2)	never	little [f]	1	2
27. Nakato (2)	never	little [f]	1	2
28. Namitala	yes	much [e]	2	2

[a] Carries baby on back even when working in garden.

[b] Carries one twin on back, other in arms.

[c] Mother says she cuddles baby little, but was observed to hold him and interact with him a great deal.

[d] Report regarding cuddling was not obtained from mother, but she was observed to hold the baby and interact with him a great deal.

[e] Mother says she cuddles the baby much, but this seems unlikely from observations during visits and from other information given by the mother.

[f] No report regarding cuddling was obtained from the mother, but other information and observations suggest that she cuddles the baby little.

One sees a mother hurrying along the road, her baby on her back, with its head bobbing about. Ganda mothers very frequently pick up their babies by taking hold of one arm near the shoulder, swinging the baby up, taking no precautions whatsoever to support the head. The youngest baby I saw handled in this way was eleven days old. The babies themselves do not find this seemingly rough manner of handling uncomfortable, for they do not protest. It may be that the accelerated motor development of the Ganda infant (see Chapter 19) makes him able to tolerate this kind of handling better than European babies could. On the other hand, it may be that some of the precautions taken in our society to support a baby's head are unnecessary and overprotective and indeed it may be that babies develop control of head and trunk musculature more rapidly if they are not given constant support.

Holding

Before they can sit unsupported, Ganda babies spend most of their waking hours being held by someone. To be sure, if a mother had no one with whom to leave her baby while she worked, she was likely to place him on a mat nearby (only two of our mothers said they ever worked in the garden with the baby in a sling on the back). But when hours of leisure came she held the baby if he was awake (see Table 9).[3] When visitors came, each was given the baby to hold in turn, seemingly as a courtesy, for it was assumed that anyone would want to hold a baby. (I observed this in the case of male visitors also, but in each case these were relatives; I do not know whether a male stranger would have been offered a baby to hold.)

Even before the baby was able to sit unsupported, he was often held propped up on the lap, facing the assembled company, rather than lying on the lap or cradled in the arms. After he could sit alone he was often held on the lap anyway, although sometimes he was placed on the floor close to the mother or another familiar person. Another mode of handling that seemed to me more frequent among Ganda mothers than among American mothers whom I have observed was to hold the baby in a standing position, long before he was able to stand unsupported. The mother usually held him standing in her lap, while she caressed his leg with her hand, and he bounced up and down happily.

Cuddling, Play, and Affectionate Display

I am not sure what Luganda phrase Mrs. Kibuka used to translate *cuddling.*[4] When I inquired about cuddling I meant to imply holding cradled in the arms

3 There were exceptions here; Kulistina, Nora, and the younger set of twins were held relatively little.

4 Welbourn (personal communication) says that *cuddling* is not translatable in Luganda.

rather than merely holding seated on a lap, and I also meant to imply an active initiation of interaction with the baby by the mother, probably accompanied by vocalization. It was my intention to use the amount of cuddling as an index of warmth in interaction. We found it very difficult, however, to assess this variable in our sample because there was so much discrepancy between the mothers' reports and their behavior as observed in interview. I have concluded that there was a semantic difficulty, which, had I recognized it before the end of the project, might have been corrected.

I believe that the difficulty was that some mothers were responding to the implication of "interacting with and playing with," others were responding to the notion of "holding," and some were responding to the notion of "cradling in the arms." In fact we rarely observed a mother holding her baby cradled in her arms except during feeding. Sometimes a baby in need of soothing was cradled thus, but in that case the breast was usually offered as well. Babies were usually held in a sitting position, often facing out, or were held in a standing position. My notes contain only one observation of a mother holding her baby so that there was a face-to-face confrontation—Nabatanzi's mother once held her high in the air in a gesture of delight, talking to her and smiling, while the baby responded with delighted laughter. I noted no instance of a mother bending over her baby trying to coax a smile or a coo. Indeed there was only one mother—Nabatanzi's again—who could be described as playing with her baby. Except for her, we noticed no one playing games of peek-a-boo or pat-a-cake. When we inquired about such games we sometimes received the response "when he is older." All of this suggests that the information we received about "cuddling" referred merely to holding.

Holding most frequently took place after feeding. Twenty babies were, according to their mothers, held for a while after they were fed, although in three cases there was some qualification—"briefly" or "if I am not too busy." The mothers of seventeen babies specifically mentioned that they held their babies when they finished their day's work —or "after lunch," which implied the same thing. Most mothers said that they held their babies when they cried in order to comfort them or calm them. Other specific occasions for holding were after the bath and before sleep.

The kind of play that took place between mother and baby seemed to be in the context of physical contact. While holding the baby the mother gently patted or stroked him. Or the baby scrambled over his mother, touching her face, reaching for her hair or eyes, or manipulating her clothing. Or the baby bounced up and down while she held him standing. Exchanges of smiles usually took place over a distance, for close face-to-face confrontation seemed infrequent, even among the babies younger than four months of age.

If baby games were infrequent, so were hugging, nuzzling, and kissing. We saw no baby being coaxed to kiss or hug. I noted only three mothers who nuzzled and kissed their babies as they held them —the mothers of Kyimba, Nora, and Nakiku.

These Ganda mothers did not interact with their babies through toys. I noted no instance of a mother trying to elicit a response from her baby by dangling a plaything in front of him. I saw no instance of a mother attempting to direct a baby's attention to a physical object and away from herself. Their interaction was direct and not mediated by playthings.

Manufactured toys were very rare. Four babies had toys of their own—respectively, a string of celluloid beads, a toy cat, a ball, and a doll—and the younger twins liked to play with their sister's doll. The mothers of Nora and Kulistina could have afforded to buy toys, but they had none, and said that the toys which had belonged to the older children were all broken. There were playthings, however: small tins, often with stones inside of them to rattle; empty spools which had held thread or adhesive tape; household objects picked up by the baby, such as a comb, a bottle, and bottle caps; and fruits, berries, sticks, and flowers.

Sharing of mothering

Anthropologists report that babies in some non-literate societies are reared by "mothers-in-parallel" or "multiple mothers." When the child's survival depends upon breast feeding it is an easy assumption that a close relationship would be built up between the infant and the woman who suckles him. Margaret Mead[5] challenges this assumption, pointing out that dependence upon breast feeding does not necessarily lead to an exclusive mother-infant pair relationship. On the contrary, in some societies the infant is suckled by two or more women, or is at least cared for by other women or prepubertal girls during a mother's absence and given food other than breast milk if he becomes hungry. Since it is likely that the child will form a less exclusive attachment to the mother—if not a weaker one—when mothering is shared by several figures, the sharing of these duties is of interest.

The sharing of mothering by several figures is most likely to occur in a society in which extended households are common, and in which, for example, a man brings his wife to live in close juxtaposition with his parents, his brothers and their wives and families. Even where this kind of extended household is not customary, polygynous marriage may make for distribution of mothering duties because of the sheer increase in the number of women and children who are available to share the responsibility for the care of a given infant. In still other

5 "A Cultural Anthropologist's Approach to Maternal Deprivation," in "Deprivation of Maternal Care: A Reassessement of Its Effects," *Public Health Papers, No. 14* (Geneva: World Health Organization, 1962), pp. 55–58.

societies, for example, the Ngoni,[6] the mother customarily turns over a large part of the care of her infant to a young girl who becomes his own special nursemaid; thus he has virtually two mothers—his own mother and his nursemaid.

The Ganda traditionally lacked extended households. Fallers[7] reports that a young man did not customarily bring his wife to live with his parents or even close to them. On the contrary, he was more likely to go elsewhere, his choice being determined by land that was available to him or by the favor of a chief from whom he hoped for help or advancement. Polygyamy was practiced, but, as one of our informants of ancient customs pointed out, only the rich man had many wives while the common man could afford but one. This informant, Mariamu, stated that the common man lived alone with his wife and children. Perhaps in rich households there might be other women to help look after the baby, for a rich man tended to attract many relatives who came to live in his household.

Roscoe[8] stated that traditionally, each Ganda child had a girl appointed to take charge of it soon after birth and expected to be in constant attendance on the child. He noted, however, that the mother had to take care of the baby herself, even while she worked, if the father were unable to find a girl from his own clan to come to serve as nurse-maid. Mair[9] and our informants of old customs are in general agreement with each other and with Roscoe regarding the traditional mothering pattern. The mother often took her baby with her to the garden, carrying him on her back and laying him on the ground while she worked. But it was also common for a baby to be left behind in the care of an older child while his mother worked in the garden. Even a firstborn might have a nursemaid, for the young mother could call upon a younger sister to come to live with her and share her responsibilities.

It was very rare, according to our informants, for a woman other than the biological mother to suckle an infant, if the mother was alive and producing enough milk.[10] Mariamu said emphatically that a woman suckled a child not her own only if she lived in the same household with a mother who had insufficient milk and if she had more than enough milk for her own baby. Another informant insisted that the infant could be suckled by a woman other than his own mother only if the woman belonged to his own clan—usually one of the father's close relatives. Of course, should the child's mother die, an effort would be made to

6 Margaret Read, *Children of Their Fathers* (New Haven, Conn.: Yale University Press, 1960), pp. 57–58.
7 L. A. Fallers, "Social Stratification in Traditional Buganda," in L. A. Fallers (ed.), *The King's Men: Leadership and Status in Modern Buganda.*
8 *The Baganda*, p. 58.
9 *An African People*, p. 55.
10 Welbourn (personal communication) agrees that this practice is now very rare and says she has never observed it. She knows of no documented reference to wet-nursing among the Ganda, although the practice is well-documented for many other African tribes.

find a substitute mother for him, and this would preferably be one of the father's sisters.

In all of the households in our sample the child's own mother was the person primarily responsible for the care of the infant, and it was she who spent most time with him. On the other hand, only five babies were looked after exclusively by their mothers. In all other instances the mother shared her duties to some extent with other figures—other adults or older children in the household or neighbors. Indeed, in seventeen cases the mother shared the mothering duties with two or more other people—with at least one other adult and at least one child. In only one case was a child the only helper, but usually children supplemented the care provided by additional adults.

Usually, the mothering duties shared with these helpers were restricted to "baby-sitting"—looking after the baby while his mother worked in the garden, holding him, carrying him, and generally keeping an eye on him. Some helpers, however, shared also in the routine care of the baby—in giving him his baths, holding him down to defecate or urinate, or feeding him the foods that were commonly used to supplement breast feeding—but these were usually adults and very rarely children. We are not counting as "mothering" merely holding a child in his mother's presence, for all of our babies were used to being held on the laps of whomever was there—even the laps of children much too young to be baby-sitters.

Most fathers who were regularly present in the home took some share in the routine care of the baby—especially in baths and the feeding of supplementary foods—but some did not and merely held their babies and played with them after returning from work. In no family of this sample was the father the only person with whom the mother shared her mothering duties.

The children who helped look after the baby were either his older siblings or cousins being reared in the household, or both. Since nearly all children of school age in these villages did in fact attend school, their help with the baby was limited to after-school hours or holidays. Preschool children were sometimes asked to "mind the baby," but usually only if the mother was no farther away than the garden and could readily be recalled in an emergency. Boys as well as girls acted as baby-sitters, and in some families only boys were available. Only two babies were assigned to nursemaids who regularly looked after them for long periods of the day. Lusiya was regularly looked after by a nine-year-old girl, who had been sent to live in the household in order to attend a school to which she failed to gain admission. Senvuma, after weaning and separation from his own mother, was regularly cared for by one or the other of two young girls who appeared to be about eight or nine years old.

Breast feeding by a woman other than the child's own mother was observed only once, and in the only household that included two women lactating simultaneously. Namitala was left with Alima's mother while her own mother was away working in the garden. She became fretful and finally cried in earnest; her demand was answered by Alima's mother, who gave her the breast. The scene was interrupted by Namitala's mother returning from her work; she exclaimed and laughed. Both women explained that this was a very unusual occurrence. In this instance the foster mother did not have surplus milk; both women were complaining of scanty milk supplies because of the long Ramadan fast, and both babies were said to be frequently hungry and fretful.

The diversity of patterns in the sharing of mothering duties was great, even in a sample as small as this one. It seemed desirable, however, to rank the babies in accordance with some scheme that would simplify the picture. Two seven-point rating scales[11] were devised accordingly—one dealing with the amount of care given to the baby by his own mother, and the other with the total amount of care he received from all the people who shared mothering duties (see Table 9).

Amount of Care Given by Mother

Two main considerations were incorporated into this rating scale: (1) the amount of time spent by the baby with his mother rather than with other people or alone; and (2) the extent to which the baby was indeed mothered by his mother.

7 *The mother takes the baby with her everywhere she goes. When he is awake she never leaves him, except perhaps for a few moments. She gives him much motherly care.* Four babies were rated 7—Paulo, Sembajwe, Juko, and Muhamidi.

6 *The mother rarely leaves the baby, and tends not to share mothering duties with others.* Only one child was rated 6—Petero. Although the mother did not share mothering duties, she regularly left him in a room alone for short periods if she was working nearby and within earshot.

5 *The mother is chiefly responsible for the care of the child but to some small extent shares mothering duties with another adult and sometimes leaves the baby briefly in the care of another adult or child.* Four babies were rated 5—Mutebe, Nakiku, Alima, and Senvuma. The only problem in rating was presented by Senvuma, who was rated on the basis of the care he got before weaning and separation and in the absence of a formal interview with the mother. During this preweaning period she was observed always to be with him and to give him a great deal of affectionate attention, but since there were two other women in the household available to care for him—the mothers of

11 These scales have been reworded since publication elsewhere (Mary D. Ainsworth, "The Development of Infant-Mother Interaction Among the Ganda," in Brian Foss (ed.), *Determinants of Infant Behaviour, II* [London: Methuen, 1963]) in order to substitute "mothering duties" for "caretaking"; no substantial change in meaning was introduced thereby.

Samwendi and Lusiya—it seemed best to give him the conservative rating of 5 rather than a rating of 7.[12]

4 *The mother is chiefly responsible for the care of the baby but leaves him fairly regularly for short periods while she works in the garden; to some extent she shares mothering duties with others.* This was the most common rating since it was given to ten tables.

3 *The mother leaves the baby regularly for long periods but gives much mothering when she is at home and at those times does not share mothering with others.* This rating was given to four children—Kasozi, Nabatanzi, and the older set of twins, Waswa and Nakato. The only problem was presented by Kasozi. Up until seven months he could have been rated 4. Then, however, his mother began to leave him with a neighbor for most of the day while she established a new garden. Since our observations did not begin until he was eleven months old it seemed best to base our rating on the practice at that time, namely, 3.[13]

2 *The mother leaves the baby regularly for long periods and shares her mothering duties with others even when she is available to look, after him.* Three children were rated 2—Namitala, Nora, and Kulistina. Although rated the same, Namitala was held by someone for most of her waking hours while Nora and Kulistina spent most of the day alone in their cribs. It seemed best, however, not to make the distinction between the two patterns of mothering in this rating scale. An alternative would have been to rate Nora and Kulistina 1, but this seemed unsatisfactory since these babies received affectionate mothering from their own mothers for much of the time that they were out of their cribs.

1 *The mother gives the baby relatively little motherly care even when she is available to do so.* Two babies were given this rating—the younger twins, Waswa and Nakato.

Total Amount of Care

The two considerations in devising this rating scale were: (1) the amount of waking time the baby spent with other people in contrast to the time he spent alone; and (2) the total amount of motherly care he received from his mother and other adults and children who shared the mothering duties.

7 *The baby is given much mothering and is alone only when asleep.* Ten babies received this rating; indeed, this was the modal rating.

12 In an earlier publication *(ibid.*, p. 73) he was rated 7.

13 In an earlier publication *(ibid.*, p. 73) he was rated 4.

6 *The baby is given much mothering but sometimes for brief periods is alone and awake.* Nine babies received this rating.
5 *The baby is given much mothering but is quite often, although for brief periods, alone and awake.* Three infants were rated 5—Senkumba, Maryamu, and Lusiya.
4 *The baby is attended to when he demands care by crying and in addition is given a fair amount of motherly care even when he is not demanding; he is, however, alone and awake for only brief periods.* Only one baby—Kasozi—was given this rating. His busy mother, even when she was available to him, could not give him as much attention as babies received in most other households, and it is assumed that the neighbor with whom he was left for long periods gave him somewhat less mothering than most of the babies in this sample received.
3 *The baby is attended to when he demands care by crying; otherwise he is left to his own devices, although he is not left alone for long periods.* No baby received this rating.
2 *The baby is left alone for much of the time, even when awake, but is given some mothering that goes beyond routine care such as feeding, bathing, etc.* Five babies received this rating—Sulaimani, Nora, Kulistina, and the younger set of twins. There was no problem in rating the latter four, but Sulaimani presented some problem. He was often left alone in the house while his mother worked, but unlike Senkumba (who was rated 4) he did not sleep while his mother was gone. Moreover, he cried a lot for attention when his mother was present—so much so that she quite often ignored his demands. On the whole, he seemed best to fit this rating, but a rating of 3 was also a possibility for he received more total care than the other infants rated 2.
1 *The baby is left alone for much of the time, even when awake, and is given little mothering that goes beyond routine care.* No infant was given this rating.

In summary, despite the great diversity in patterns of mothering in this sample, the modal tendency was for the mother to be chiefly responsible for mothering but to share her duties with others during her relatively brief absences in the garden so that the baby was seldom if ever left alone. The total amount of motherly care given the typical baby in this sample was very considerable. Even the younger twins, who received low ratings in both scales, would not have been considered grossly neglected by Western standards. Nor would Kulistina and Nora, who were left alone in their cribs for much of the day.

10

DISTRESS, ANGER, AND DISCIPLINE

A baby's crying and his mother's response to it are of great interest to one who would understand the relationship between them. A mother's characteristic responses to her baby's distress are a significant aspect of her mothering practices. It is my belief that the ways in which a mother responds to her baby's distress have much to do with the strength and security of her baby's attachment to her. On the other hand, a baby's crying—when he cries, why he cries, and how much he cries—is by no means independent of the way his mother responds to it. Since the baby's behavior and his mother's response are interlocked, it is an arbitrary decision which should be discussed first. It is proposed, however, to deal first with the baby's behavior.

Crying

Our interest in crying was sustained throughout repeated visits. Notes were made of any episodes of crying that occurred during the visits. Inquiries were made about crying at every visit. With almost no exceptions, the reports of the mothers and direct observations coincided in regard to frequency of crying, cause of crying, and the mother's response.

The babies fell into two groups—those who cried frequently and those who did not. Since, in a later chapter this classification is combined with a classification of infant-mother attachment and is seen to be related significantly to several infant-care variables, the distinctions will be discussed here in some detail.

Seven babies were classed as frequent criers (see Table 10). The mothers of all of these babies said they cried a lot; six of the babies lived up to their

DOI: 10.4324/9781003629337-12

reputations during our visits and clearly cried more than did the babies described as infrequent criers. The seventh, Kasozi, did not seem to cry excessively during our visits, and only he and Kyimba presented any problem of classification.

Kasozi's mother said that he cried a lot but added that he had cried more in previous months than he did by the time our visits began. She explained, moreover, that he was content when sitting on her lap. Since he spent most of the time during our visits sitting either on her lap or close to her, we could not check the mother's account of his crying frequently during the greater part of the day when she was too busy to devote herself to him. On the basis of her report, however, he was classified as a frequent crier.[1]

Kyimba, on the other hand, was classed as an infrequent crier despite the fact that he was said to cry frequently and did in fact cry a great deal during our visits. Weaning, however, had taken place just before our visits began, and his mother believed weaning to be the reason for his unusual fussiness. Since in the cases of all other children we based our classification upon preweaning behavior if it differed from postweaning behavior, we did so with Kyimba.

Except for Kyimba and Kasozi, the dichotomy between frequent and infrequent criers could be established upon the basis of observations and reports relevant to the period spanned by our visits. Three babies, however, were reported to have cried frequently during an earlier period of their lives, but these three—Kulistina and the younger set of twins—were obviously infrequent criers during the period of research.

Even some babies classified as infrequent criers cried frequently during *some* of our visits. As may be seen in Chapter 24, some babies responded to weaning with much more frequent crying. Moreover, babies undergoing a temporary period of illness cried more than they usually did when they were well. We based our observations upon the preweaning period, and ignored the occasional patches of crying attributable to illness that occurred within it. If, however, the state of poor health was chronic and the baby cried frequently, he was classified as a frequent crier.

Regardless of how frequently the baby was reported to cry, we asked the mother about his reasons for crying and how she responded. Among the most commonly reported reasons was hunger (see Table 10). If crying was believed to be caused by hunger (and often when it was not), the mother offered the breast.[2] If the hunger cries signaled a baby's impatience for food that his

1 In an earlier publication, "The Development of Infant-Mother Interaction Among the Ganda," in Brian Foss (ed.) *Determinants of Inf ant Behaviour, II*, I classed Kasozi as "secure"—i.e. as an infrequent crier. It is now believed that he would be more accurately classified as a frequent crier.

2 Except, of course, in the case of schedule-fed babies, and even with these the schedule was usually not followed closely if the baby seemed hungry.

mother was in the course of preparing—after weaning, and even before weaning to a certain extent—the mother continued her preparations. The baby had no alternative but to wait. We observed babies who seemed to be crying from hunger during our visits. Usually the mother responded with an offer of the breast and the crying ceased. Persistent fussiness was observed with Muslim babies during the Ramadan fast; sometimes they hushed if breast or bottle was offered, but at other times they persisted in crying as though breast, bottle, and life in general were unsatisfactory. The most pathetic hunger cries that we observed came from the older twins. These malnourished babies strove in the most persistent manner to capture the breast, competing with each other in their striving. The mother both fed on schedule (believing that this was appropriate because of her insufficient milk) and was reluctant to feed her babies in our presence. During later visits, after the twins had reached a better state of nutrition through our gifts of dried skim milk, they were less compelled to strive for the breast, but in our early visits their striving was heart-rending both for the observers and for their mother who tried to calm them without feeding them.

The three most common reasons for crying—more common than hunger, illness, or weaning—were: (1) crying to be picked up by the mother or crying when put down by her; (2) crying when the mother left the room; and (3) crying when some activity in progress was interrupted. The first two occasions for crying are clearly related to the child's attachment to his mother; the third is the general case of frustration.

Crying when the mother leaves the room is considered to be an important feature of attachment behavior and will be discussed in more detail in Chapter 20. The youngest age at which this reaction was reported was fifteen weeks, but it commonly emerged before six months of age and continued to be common with the older babies in the sample, especially before weaning. Only five babies did not cry for this reason—Nora, Kulistina, Namitala, and the younger twins, Waswa and Nakato.

Crying to be picked up by the mother was much less common than crying when the mother left the room. Even after attachment to the mother as a special person had developed,[3] most of these babies were content to be in their mother's presence and did not insist upon actual physical contact with her; however, Nakalema, Muhamidi, and Sulaimani regularly cried when their mothers put them down after holding them or otherwise attending to them. In addition, Magalita, Sulaimani, and the older twins frequently cried and conveyed to their mothers the desire to be picked up, even though the context was not that of

3 This is discussed in Chapter 20.

TABLE 10 Distress, anger, and beating

Name	*Frequency of Crying*	*Reasons for Crying* [d]	*M's Response to Crying*
SECURE – ATTACHED			
1. Paulo	infrequent	M	holds breast [g]
2. Sembajwe	infrequent	M, I, B	breast [g]
3. Juko	infrequent	M, B	holds
4. Petero	infrequent	M, P [e], B, O	holds [h] breast [g]
5. Senvuma	infrequent	—	—
6. Mutebe	infrequent	M	holds breast [g]
7. Nakiku	infrequent	M, I, F	holds
8. Alima	infrequent	M, B, O	holds
9. Aida	infrequent	M	holds [h]
10. William	infrequent	M, O	holds [h]
11. Senkumba	infrequent	M [f], B, F	holds [h]
12. Kyimba	infrequent [a]	M	—
13. Samwendi	infrequent	M, I, B	breast
14. Maryamu	infrequent	M, F, B, O	holds
15. Lusiya	infrequent	M, I, B	holds breast [g]
16. Nabatanzi	infrequent	M, I, F, B	holds
INSECURE – ATTACHED			
17. Muhamidi	frequent	M, D, B	breast
18. Magalita	frequent	M, P, B, I	holds
19. Kasozi	frequent [c]	M, F, P	left to cry
20. Sulaimani	frequent	M, D, P, I, F	holds [i]
21. Nakalema	frequent	M, D, B, O	holds
22. Waswa (1)	frequent	M, P, B, O	holds
23. Nakato (1)	frequent	M, P, B, O	holds
NON – ATTACHED			
24. Nora	infrequent		left to cry
25. Kulistina	infrequent [b]	I, B	left to cry
26. Waswa (2)	infrequent [b]		left to cry
27. Nakato (2)	infrequent [b]	O	left to cry
28. Namitala	infrequent	P [e], B, I	holds

Frequency of anger	*Angry and Aggressive Behavior* [l]	*Reason for Anger* [m]	*M's Response to Anger*	*"Beating" (Age Reported)*
occasionally [j]	B, C, T, H	F, U	holds punishes [n]	yes—13 mos.
occasionally	H	F	comforts	—
never [j]	H	—	—	no
occasionally	C	M	breast [o]	no
—	—	—		—
occasionally	C, B, O	F, A	punishes [n]	yes—5 mos.
occasionally	C	F	holds	—
occasionally	C, T	B, F	holds	yes—5 mos.
never	—	—	—	no
occasionally	C, H, O	F, M, U	holds	yes—8 mos.
occasionally	C	F, A	holds punishes [n]	yes—8½ mos.
occasionally	C, T	B	holds	—
occasionally	C, H	B	breast	no
occasionally	C	F	holds	—
never [j, k]	H, T	F	holds	yes—14½ mos.
occasionally [k]	C, H, T, O	B, F, P, M	holds punishes [n]	yes—5½ mos.
occasionally	C, H	B, F	breast	yes—8 mos.
occasionally	C, B, T	B, F, A	holds	—
occasionally	C, T	B, F	withholds	yes—6 mos.
occasionally	C, H, T	B, F, M, P	breast punishes [n]	yes—9½ mos.
often	C, H	M, U	—	yes—8 mos.
never	—	—	—	yes—14½ mos.
occasionally	C, H, T	F, A, U	holds	yes—14 ½ mos.
often	B, C, H, T	F, P, A	ignores punishes	yes—11 ½ mos.
rarely	H	A	—	yes—11 mos.
rarely	C	B	—	—
rarely	C	B	—	—
occasionally	C	B	—	no

See Following Page for Footnotes

[a] Before weaning.
[b] But not during the first three or four months.
[c] Especially during the first twelve months.
[d] The symbols used in this column indicate the following reasons for crying:
B: for the breast or because of hunger.
D: when put down by the mother.
F: frustration or interference with activity in progress.
I: when ill or hurt.
M: when the mother leaves the room.
P: to be picked up.
O: other.
[e] Rarely.
[f] Sometimes.
[g] The mother stated specifically that she did not invariably offer the breast to the crying child.
[h] The mother stated that she picked up the baby and cuddled him when he cried, except when he had just been fed. Under these circumstances, if he cried after he had been put down to sleep, the mother did not respond to the cry, but rather hoped to train him to go to sleep without attention.
[i] This mother was very inconsistent in her response to the baby's crying, although sometimes she cuddled him.
[j] Sometimes aggressive without seeming angry.
[k] But often angry after weaning.
[l] The symbols used in this column indicate the following forms of angry or aggressive behavior:
C: crying.
T: tantrum, throwing self about.
B: biting.
H: hitting.
O: other.
[m] The symbols used in this column indicate the following reasons for angry or aggressive behavior:
B: breast or food not provided quickly enough.
F: other frustration or interference.
M: mother leaves room, or puts baby down.
U: unwelcome attention of another child or stranger.
A: aggression from another child, or presence of a sibling towards whom aggression is initiated.
P: punishment by the mother.
O: other.
[n] Punishment for anger is only occasional; usually it occurs only if child's behavior is particularly aggressive.
[o] Mother sometimes gives the breast to the angry child; sometimes leaves him to cry.

having just been put down, and so did Kasozi, although less frequently. Only two other babies—Petero and Namitala—were said to cry to be picked up, although only rarely, and Namitala did not show a differential response in this regard—she cried to be picked up but not especially to be picked up by her mother. Thus, the seven babies who often cried to be picked up by the mother or in response to being put down by her are the same seven classified as frequent criers.

Crying from frustration when the child was unable to obtain some object that he wanted or when he was stopped from doing something he was doing or wanted to do was considered by most mothers to be an expression of anger and will be discussed in that context. It did not become a common reason for crying until about the end of the first year of life, until locomotion and manipulation had become important activities. In the few instances in which babies under nine months were said to cry when they could not have something they wanted, the desired object was specified as food.

Other reasons for crying were mentioned. Crying when physically hurt seemed to these mothers so obvious as to be worth mentioning only in comments such as "He cries only when he is hungry or hurt." Crying for the breast or when refused the breast was specifically mentioned by a few without implying that hunger was the reason for crying. Senkumba, William, and Alima were said to cry when they were sleepy. Maryamu's mother said that her baby cried briefly when she woke from a nap "to let me know that she is awake." Alima cried when picked up by a child rather than by an adult, and, indeed, some other babies were said to dislike being picked up by a child. Nakalema was reported to cry when a stranger was present; other babies obviously did so too, but their mothers did not think to mention this fact when asked the reasons for the baby's crying.

In short, the answers to our question "Why does the baby cry?" did not serve to elicit a comprehensive list of the situations that could be depended upon to stimulate crying but emphasized only the ones that seemed most conspicuous to the individual mother as reasons for the crying of the individual baby.

Furthermore, lest there be misunderstanding, it should be stated clearly that the babies classified as infrequent criers cried when they were hungry[4] or hurt, and most of them at a certain stage of their development cried when their mothers left the room. The only *reason* for crying that seemed to distinguish between the frequent and infrequent criers was crying to be picked up or when put down. The criterion for distinguishing frequent from infrequent criers was not the reason for crying, however, but was the sheer frequency of crying over the *preweaning* period spanned by the research; moreover, the mother's report was given priority to our own observations, although these were in close agreement in every case but Kasozi's.

4 Except for undernourished Kulistina, who, left in her crib alone for most of the day, cried very little, although she must have been hungry.

Response of the mother to the baby's distress

The question "What do you do when the baby cries?" was asked each mother on repeated visits as a corollary to the question "What makes the baby cry?" And, of course, the mother's response to any episode of crying that occurred during a visit could be observed directly.

The mother's response to the crying of her baby obviously depends in part on her interpretation of the cause of the crying. If the crying is interpreted as a hunger cry, the mother's response is to give the breast, except in the case of the eight schedule-fed babies. This was so obvious that the mothers did not think to mention it when asked: "What do you do when the baby cries?" Most mothers, perhaps because of the context in which the question was asked, interpreted the question to refer to their practice of picking up or not picking up a baby who is crying for reasons other than hunger. The most common response of the mother was to pick the baby up to soothe him and in some cases to give the breast as well (see Table 10). There were some qualifications and exceptions. The mothers of four babies— William, Aida, Senkumba, and Petero—regularly picked them up when they cried unless the crying occurred following a feeding when the baby was put down in the hope that he would sleep; these babies usually did sleep and rarely cried when put down. The mothers of five babies— Kulistina, Nora, Kasozi, and the younger set of twins—said that they did not make a practice of picking up their babies in response to crying and that they did so only if the crying continued for a long time. One mother—Sulaimani's—was very inconsistent in her handling of crying; sometimes she picked him up and jiggled him about, sometimes she did so roughly and impatiently or only after a delay, and sometimes she just let him cry.

On the whole, these mothers comforted their crying babies in much the same way as American mothers do, either cradling them in their arms in a breast-feeding position (and these often enough gave the breast) or holding them against the shoulder and patting them on the back. One pattern of comforting, however, was new to me. The mother swung the baby up onto her back so that he was lying prone on her back, held him by one arm over her shoulder, and, leaning forward slightly while she sat on the floor, bounced him vigorously up and down. The mothers of three babies who cried frequently —Sulaimani's and the older twins'—seemed to do this as a last resort, when merely picking the baby up proved of no avail in stopping the crying. Indeed, the mother of twins sometimes bounced one twin in this manner while she held the other against her breast. This bouncing-on-the-back pattern was also observed with some babies after weaning and seemed to be used instead of cuddling in order to keep the child away from the tempting breast.

By and large these mothers seemed to believe that a baby's distress called for holding and comforting, whether with or without suckling. Only four mothers deliberately and consistently ignored all but the most persistent crying—the mothers of Kulistina, Nora, and the younger twins.

Angry behavior

The following questions were asked of each mother: "What makes the baby angry?" "What does he do when is he angry?" and "What do you do when he is angry?" There is an obvious overlap of these questions with those concerning crying because some crying can be, and indeed was, interpreted as angry crying, even in the absence of aggressive movements or verbalization. It was evident from their replies that some mothers interpreted crying in a given situation as indicative of anger while others did not. Thus, our findings, for the most part, merely reflect the mother's interpretation of the child's behavior (see Table 10).

Four children were said never to become angry—Juko, Aida, Lusiya, and the older Waswa. At twenty-four weeks of age Petero was said to be too young to get angry. On the other hand, the mothers of Namitala at fifteen weeks and of Senkumba and Samwendi at twenty-one weeks sometimes interpreted crying as an indication of anger. We observed that Lusiya did indeed have a very high tolerance for frustration and when about a year old did not protest when a plaything was taken from her; moreover, she was said to express anger after weaning, so it is likely that before weaning she was, in fact, less aggressive than many babies. Waswa at fourteen months of age was said never to get angry; we observed that his response to frustration was in sharp contrast to that of his twin sister—she usually had a tantrum and often hit out whereas Waswa only cried (see Table 10).

Three babies seemed to us, as observers, to become angry frequently during our visits, although their mothers did not volunteer any comment that they were often angry. After weaning, Nabatanzi was fussy and seemed easily aroused to angry aggression. Nora also was outstandingly aggressive during our visits; she, more than any other child, was continually interfered with in her activities. She kept crawling away from her mother toward the door of the house and was repeatedly caught by one leg and dragged back. Nakalema showed less directed aggression than either Nora or Nabatanzi but often had tantrums during our visits; she was also classified as a frequent crier.

In this sample, crying was an almost invariable component of the behavior interpreted by the mother as an expression of anger. In some babies, crying seemed to be the only expression of anger—there was no tantrum with the baby throwing himself about or hitting out or biting. These babies tended to be in the younger age range—from fifteen to thirty-seven weeks—although Maryamu at twelve months and Nakiku at thirteen months also "just cried." It seems likely that some of the mothers of young babies who "just cried" did not interpret the crying as an indication of anger. When tantrums or crying with more directed aggression occurred, however, all mothers identified the response as anger. Most of the babies who were observed or reported to have tantrums were nine months of age or older, although Alima was said to cry and throw herself about in anger as early as five months of age. Hitting was the most frequently reported directed aggressive response, occurring usually after eight months of age, although sometimes younger children (e.g., Samwendi at five months) were reported to hit the mother's breast when hungry and angry. Biting was reported in the cases of only four children—all over ten months of age; it may have been more frequent, however, for it was not the subject of systematic inquiry. Other occasional forms of directed aggression were kicking, throwing things, and fighting to keep something that was being taken away. These also tended to occur only in children of nine months or older. There were no sex differences in the incidence of these directed forms of aggression.

Five babies were observed or reported to hit or slap without crying and without obvious anger. Paulo at forty-six weeks was said to hit and bite his sisters but to do it "like a game." Juko at thirty-two weeks was observed during one of our visits to hit Aida repeatedly over the head with a corncob; he seemed to be enjoying the game, and Aida did not protest. Lusiya at thirty-nine weeks was said to hit both her mother's breast and her child nursemaid without crying and without anger. Nabatanzi at thirty-one weeks was said to slap her mother's breast when she was hungry, although her mother did not consider this anger. She was reported also to hit her mother whenever her mother "beat" her, and this was done sometimes in fun by both. During one visit at twenty-one months, the older twin Nakato was observed cheerfully to hit her twin, Waswa. Waswa cried and was comforted. Since the twins were in constant competition for their mother's breast and lap, however, it would be naive to assume that Nakato's hitting, though cheerful, was entirely free of aggression.

The most frequently reported antecedent condition for anger was frustration of, or interference with, the child's activities or desires. "He becomes angry," the mother reported, "when he is kept from something he wants," "when something is taken away from him," or "when he is stopped from doing something." Most of the sixteen babies who became angry under these circumstances were ten months of age or older, although some were eight or nine months, and one — Alima—was as young as five months (although frustration in the desire for food was the specific reason for her anger).

Hunger, wanting the breast, or wanting supplementary food together formed another class of causes of anger. Babies as young as three months of age were reported to be angry when hungry, although most of them were between five and nine months old.

Although it was common for babies over five months of age to cry when their mothers left the room, this crying was not commonly interpreted as anger. In other words, frustration of the desire to be near the mother was not interpreted as a cause for anger as frequently as were other frustrations—the desire for the breast, for food, or for locomotor or manipulative activities. Five mothers, however, did so interpret it. The presence of strangers or the unwelcome attention of even more familiar figures was reported as a cause for anger in four babies, all at least eight months of age. Punishment was said to evoke aggression in three babies—Sulaimani, Nabatanzi, and Nora. In only one case was aggressive behavior by other children stated as a stimulus to anger, although four children were said to initiate an attack on another child, and another was reported to push away the aggressor.

Response of the mother to the baby's anger

The mothers' responses to anger were much the same as their responses to crying. Fourteen mothers usually picked their babies up when they believed they were angry and tried to give them comfort. Some of these mothers also gave the breast for comfort to an angry child, even though he was not judged to be hungry. Sometimes, if the anger seemed to be prompted by impatience for food that the mother was in the course of preparing, she did nothing until the food was prepared but then fed him immediately.

Some mothers, however, did not comfort the angry child, and some punished aggression. Nora's mother was perhaps least comforting when the baby became angry: sometimes she punished her by "beating" her; more frequently she simply ignored the tantrum. Sulaimani's mother often fed him when he angrily demanded feeding, but at times also she "beat" him. Three other babies who were usually held and soothed—Senkumba, Nabatanzi, and Paulo—were sometimes punished for anger, especially if it was expressed in directed aggressive behavior such as hitting. The mother of small, sickly Petero usually cuddled him when he cried, but at times when his crying seemed angry she just let him cry. William's mother interpreted his crying as anger when she was about to leave him for a short or long period; under these circumstances she did not return to comfort him but relied on the person with whom he was left to do so. When Kasozi was thirteen months old his mother attempted to teach him that he could not have everything he wanted by angrily demanding it; when he angrily cried for something, especially food, she deliberately withheld the desired object.

On the whole these mothers, especially when their babies were quite young, seemed to sympathize with the angry baby, recognizing the frustration and helplessness and also the distress, and they looked upon comforting as a matter of course. For the most part it was only when the baby approached the end of the first year, if then, that these mothers attempted to handle the angry baby by ignoring or punishing him.

Discipline

Okukuba means "to hit," "to strike," or "to beat." It is the word used also for spanking, slapping, smacking, or whipping children as a mode of discipline. In this context it is usually translated "to beat" —which to me conjured up an image of a child being whipped hard with a stick. I knew that "beating" was a mode of discipline used for the older Ganda child, because at a preliminary meeting held in one of the villages, several fathers in the audience questioned me carefully about my opinions on beating. They believed beatings were necessary. Several women in the audience demurred. The ensuing discussion brought out the point that, while beatings might be appropriate for the older child, they were inappropriate for a baby who was too young "to understand."

It did not occur to me to include in the interview schedule a question about physical punishment. I was struck with the tender and gentle interaction between Ganda mothers and their babies; it did not cross my mind that they might "beat" their babies. In a later study, I saw American mothers slap their babies to make them keep still while having their diapers changed or to deter them from reaching toward forbidden objects, but at that time I had never seen a woman strike a small baby. But in the course of one interview a mother volunteered that she tried to teach her baby by beating him, and from then on I inquired about this point.

Fortunately I had the sense to inquire precisely how the beating was done. My first informant told me—and this was confirmed by all the others—that she cupped her hand and gently struck the baby's arm or hand. She pointed out that it was necessary to cup the hand in order to avoid the sting of a smack with the flat of the hand. The objective was not to hurt the baby or to punish him but to "teach" him.

Thirteen babies had been "beaten," seven had not, and about seven we had no information. The harassed mother of the older twins did not beat them, even though they were over fourteen months old, but all the other mothers who did not beat their babies said that they were still too young—"too small, can't walk, can't understand." It may be seen from Table 10, however, that three of those beaten—Mutebe, Alima, and Nabatanzi—were as young as five months when this mode of discipline began, while Juko was considered too young to be beaten at seven months and Aida too young at eight.

The reasons for beating varied widely. Three were smacked to prevent their reaching for something the mothers did not want them to have, either because they might spoil it or because it might hurt them—Juko, Kasozi, and Nabatanzi. Four were beaten if they cried a lot or "for nothing"; this group included Nabatanzi again, but it also included three babies whose mothers admitted that the beating was given because they themselves were angry rather than because of a desire to "teach" the child—Kulistina, Alima, and Sulaimani. Two children were disciplined for hitting or biting other children—Paulo and Mutebe— and Senkumba was beaten for angry behavior. Mutebe at five months was beaten during training for sitting; when he tried to pull away the cloths that were wrapped around him to support him, his mother tried to deter him. Three babies—Nora, William, and Lusiya—were beaten to teach them not to do something that was wrong or that the mother "did not like." To this list could be added three—Nabatanzi, Sulaimani, and Juko—who were smacked when they smeared feces. Nakalema was taught by beating not to put her hands in a puddle of her own urine, and she and Senkumba were smacked for touching their genitals.

This is perhaps as good a context as any in which to report the results of our inquiries about infantile masturbation. We obtained information about twenty-one babies. The mothers of fourteen, seven girls and seven boys, said that there was no masturbation or even touching of genitals. Some of these women looked embarassed when the inquiry was made, and some replied "no" so flatly that I wondered how much lay behind the denial. William's mother said that he did not masturbate but that some of her other children had done so. Kulistina's mother said that girls never did. The mothers of seven, five boys and two girls, reported at least one instance of manipulation of the genital region. The mothers of two boys—Juko and Muhamidi — noticed fingering of the genitals, especially after urination, and both "tried to stop" them from doing so. Kasozi's mother, noticing him handling his penis frequently, examined it and thought it looked irritated. She "stopped him" from touching it, and soon he discontinued doing so. Magalita's mother, noticing her scratching herself, investigated and found a mango worm embedded; for a while after it was removed she continued to scratch herself and her mother "tried to stop her." Nakalema's mother said that she noticed her touching her genitals just once; she "beat" her and it never happened again. Sekumba's mother, on the other hand, had not been so successful in her efforts to stop him from touching his genitals; nevertheless, she smacked him every time she noticed him doing so. There was, however, only one child who presented a persistent problem in regard to masturbation—Kyimba. His mother resorted to keeping him in pants to discourage him—and most Ganda babies do not wear pants or diapers. In summary, it was clear that Ganda mothers discourage infantile masturbation, if indeed they notice it and acknowledge its occurrence. All the mothers of babies who were reported to have masturbated took action to stop it, although only two "beat" the baby.

The response of three babies to beating interested me enormously. Although Kulistina cried harder than ever when punished for crying, and Kasozi and Senvuma tended to stop doing what was forbidden, three babies responded to aggression with aggression. Despite the fact that these Ganda mothers stressed the gentleness of their "beating" with the cupped hand and said that the objective was to teach and not to hurt or to punish, three babies retaliated by hitting the mother. This was particularly vivid with Nabatanzi; in Chapter 13 it is reported how she responded to "beating" by hitting her mother and to a threat of beating by a similar threat. Sulaimani and Nora retaliated in like manner. In each of these three cases it appeared to me that the physical intervention of the "beating," gentle though it was, was interpreted by the baby as aggression, and the baby responded in kind. In these cases the "beating," instead of teaching the baby to conform to the mother's wishes, seemed to be teaching him to strike back.

11

HEALTH AND SAFETY

From the beginning the offer of transportation to the child welfare clinic was clearly the most attractive reward for participation in the research. If the sample was biased in any direction, it was certainly biased in consisting of babies whose parents were especially concerned about their children's health. In seven cases the baby's health was already poor, and the mother hoped for help. In other instances the severe illness or death of older children made the mother overanxious about the new baby's health, even though his present state gave no objective cause for concern. In still other instances the parents were motivated to learn as much as they could from Europeans about child nutrition and health, even though there seemed no special cause for anxiety or concern.

We do not know exactly what the attitudes of the mothers in our sample were toward witch doctors and traditional "medicine." Inquires were avoided so as not to pose any direct European challenge to Ganda beliefs and customs. Even indirect and seemingly innocent inquiry could be negatively construed because churches and schools had been so outspoken in their criticism of superstition—witch doctors, witchcraft, and the "medicine" associated with them. The only inquiries that seemed legitimate for us to make were in regard to "medicines" considered specific for lactation and babies. As reported in Chapter 6, most of the mothers seemed ignorant of any traditional "medicines" pertinent to lactation or neonatal sucking difficulties, although a fair number (as reported in Chapter 7) used traditional herb baths for their babies, at least on occasion. Those few who admitted to some knowledge of traditional remedies professed little faith in their efficacy. Only twice did I directly observe evidence that resort had been made to ancient "medicine." One day Muhamidi's sister, who was chronically ill and miserable, was encrusted with a grey coating of ashes; her mother was desperate

DOI: 10.4324/9781003629337-13

with anxiety for her and was simultaneously arranging to take her to hospital. Another day we found Alima in a similar state. We made no comment in either case—nor did the mothers.

Infant mortality is undoubtedly higher in Buganda than in Western countries, although reliable statistics are lacking. It was my impression, however, and this impression is supported by Welbourn's findings,[1] that Ganda babies tend to thrive well during the first half-year of life. It is in the second half-year of life that difficulties begin to arise—difficulties that become more numerous and serious in the second year of life, after the child has been finally weaned from the breast. Welbourn found that the growth curves for height and weight approximated American norms during the first half-year but began to lag behind at about six months—at the onset of what she calls the "weaning period" when, even though the child is still suckled, the mother's milk supply is no longer adequate as the sole source of nutrition. Although—as noted in Chapter 6—it has been the custom in Buganda since ancient times to supplement breast feeding with solid foods, the foods considered appropriate for young children are protein deficient—and, indeed, the adult diet tends to be seriously protein deficient. It is also after the first six months of life that the Ganda child begins to be vulnerable to infection, particularly to malaria and respiratory disorders.

It had been hoped to observe details of the physical examination of the babies when they visited the clinic, and to note the interchange between doctor and mother. This was possible at first, but later it became impossible. For the research team, clinic days became increasingly occupied with shuttling mothers and babies to the clinic from several different villages and back home again, with three or four round trips required to deal with everyone—even with two vehicles. It was subsequently possible to copy clinic records, and so we were able to obtain records of height and weight, together with prescribed treatment, and scattered notes of the doctor's findings. These records are summarized at the end of each case report in Chapters 12 to 18, except for the babies who did not attend the clinic. But we were not able to get the doctor's opinion of the baby's general health; therefore, the classification of health reported in Table 11 is impressionistic.

Eleven babies seemed to be in a good state of health and nutrition, ten in a fairly good state. Eight babies, however, were in poor health throughout all or most of the research.

The eight babies in poor health had had serious difficulties before the research began. Three were severely malnourished. Kulistina, who had been bottle-fed from the beginning, was in a precarious state. She improved considerably as

1 Hebe F. Welbourn, "The Danger Period During Weaning: A Study of Baganda Children," *J. trap. Pediat.*, 1955, *1*: 34–46.

TABLE 11 Health and medical care

Name	*Health*	*Attendance at Clinic*	*Other Medical Care*
SECURE – ATTACHED			
1. Paulo	good	occasional	private physician
2. Sembajwe	good	none	none
3. Juko	good	regular	none
4. Petero	poor	occasional	private physician hospital
5. Senvuma	good	occasional	
6. Mutebe	good	occasional	none
7. Nakiku	fairly good	regular	none
8. Alima	fairly good	occasional	none
9. Aida	good	occasional	hospital [a]
10. William	poor	regular [b]	hospital
11. Senkumba	fairly good	regular [c]	none
12. Kyimba	good	occasional	none
13. Samwendi	good	regular	none
14. Maryamu	fairly good	regular	none
15. Lusiya	fairly good	occasional	none
16. Nabatanzi	good	occasional	private physician
INSECURE – ATTACHED			
17. Muhamidi	poor	occasional	none
18. Magalita	poor	regular [b]	private physician
19. Kasozi	fairly good	occasional	private physician
20. Sulaimani	fairly good	regular	none
21. Nakalema	poor	none	hospital
22. Waswa (1)	poor	regular	hospital
23. Nakato (1)	poor	regular	none
NON – ATTACHED			
24. Nora	fairly good	regular	none
25. Kulistina	poor	regular	private physician
26. Waswa (2)	fairly good	regular	none
27. Nakato (2)	fairly good	regular	none
28. Namitala	good	occasional	none

[a] For examination only.
[b] Even before the research started.
[c] Regular before parents separated, then not at all.

a result of the nutritional program instituted by the clinic but was retarded in her development throughout the period of our observations. The older twins were said to have thrived for the first four months of life, but by the time we encountered them at fourteen months of age they were in a pathetic state and were severely retarded in development. They were helped by the nutritional advice of the clinic and by the dried skim milk we gave them, but their health could be described only as poor throughout our observations.

The five other children in chronic poor health all suffered from severe, recurrent diarrhea, with fever, weight loss, and weakness. Petero was said to have been "born weak." When he was four months old he had an attack of diarrhea, and after this he failed to gain normally; when he was nearly seven months old he had a very severe recurrence, which was nearly fatal. William was said to have been "very tired" when born, but seemed to be in good health for the first three months or so of his life, after which he began to have repeated colds and fever. Between thirty-one and thirty-seven weeks of age he had a constant slight fever and then became very ill with diarrhea, vomiting, and loss of weight; this state continued for another two months until finally he had to be hospitalized. Muhamidi was said to have been "very sick" for a while after birth but then seemed in good health until about five months of age. From that time on, throughout the remaining period of research contact, he had a succession of complaints—malaria, colds, conjunctivitis, diarrhea—and did not gain weight well. Magalita was severely ill with diarrhea from two to four months of age, and subsequently this recurred with fever, weakness, and weight loss. By the time she joined our sample (at forty-nine weeks of age) she had had another bout with diarrhea from which she did not recover throughout the entire time we observed her. Her mother also believed that she had been underfed at the breast, claiming that there had been insufficient breast milk from the beginning. Nakalema was said to be ill often and she had had a prolonged bout with diarrhea which required hospital treatment. She also coughed and vomited frequently.

Even among the relatively healthy babies minor illnesses were frequent—more frequent, of course, among those whose health was classified as fairly good than among those whose health was classified as good. Nearly all of these babies had colds from time to time, often accompanied by coughing and some fever, but none of these respiratory disorders seemed to incapacitate the child or set him back in his development. Almost as many had diarrhea at one time or another during the period of research, or before it, and even these relatively healthy babies tended to be set back by isolated attacks of intestinal infection associated with diarrhea—although not nearly as severely as were those babies in the poor-health group who suffered from chronic or recurrent diarrhea. Malaria is endemic to Buganda. Nineteen babies of our sample were known to have had at least one bout with malaria. The fact that none of them suffered severe or prolonged attacks of "fever" is probably attributable to the availability of antimalarial drugs distributed at the clinic. Daraprim was given to any child currently suffering from malaria and to any others whose enlarged spleens indicated that they had had repeated attacks; prophylactic doses were continued regularly for these babies, and I was responsible for dispensing the drug during the week between clinic visits. Daraprim was not used as a prophylaxis for all clinic babies because once it is stopped the child is as susceptible to malaria as any unexposed person; Dr. Welbourn preferred to let healthy children go through the inevitable exposure while still under supervision of the clinic in the hope that a natural immunity might be built up.

In addition to colds, diarrhea, and malaria, there were a few other common complaints, including skin rashes and infections, conjunctivitis, middle-ear infections, and, more distressing and serious, stomatitis, which discouraged the child from eating. Except for Nabatanzi, who suffered a painful burn which took a long time to heal, no child experienced physical trauma of any significance during the span of the research.

One complaint that has been observed with some frequency in my current sample of American babies is "spitting up"—i.e., regurgitating milk with no apparent sign of distress or illness. Although vomiting occurred occasionally in this Ganda sample, and invariably in conjunction with illness, there was only one instance of "spitting up" observed—Kulistina, who was bottle-fed. Three major differences between the Ganda sample and the American sample occur to me as being possibly relevant; the Ganda babies were breast-fed (except for Kulistina); they were not overfed; and most of them were given considerably more physical contact than were babies of comparable age in the American sample.

Nearly all the families who participated in the research used the transportation services we provided to the child welfare clinic. Fourteen babies were taken regularly, perhaps not every fortnight but at least once a month, and two of these had been regular patients even before they joined the research sample. Twelve babies were taken to the clinic occasionally, usually because of an illness, but they did not attend regularly. Only two mothers—Nakalema's and Sembajwe's—did not take advantage of the opportunity we provided (see Table 11).

Our offer to transport to hospital any baby who needed urgent treatment was helpful to only one of our sample; Aida, whose mother was desperately anxious about her, was taken to Kampala for examination; she was judged not to be seriously ill and returned home. Other emergencies cropped up in the periods intervening between clinic days and at times when I was not available to help. William, Petero, and the older Waswa all had illnesses severe enough that they were admitted to hospital when taken by their mothers for examination and treatment. Magalita, Kulistina, Nabatanzi—for her burn—and again Petero were taken to private Indian physicians in or near Kampala when attention seemed urgently necessary.

Safety

Our information about safety practices was gained by asking the mothers what dangers they feared on behalf of their babies. Although illness and malnutrition were clearly the chief sources of concern, these were not considered "dangers." A danger was an environmental hazard against which precautions could be taken.

Before the baby could crawl there was little that could harm him, but after he was able to get about on his own initiative fire and hot liquids were the chief hazards that he might encounter. These were real dangers, as demonstrated by the fact that burns and scalds were the most frequent injuries treated at the clinic.

The cooking was usually done on a fire at ground level in a separate kitchen or kitchen hut. The mother attempted to keep the baby away from the kitchen. If a baby was left in a room unattended, it was usually while his mother was in the kitchen. Since few of these babies were content to be left alone, their mothers found it difficult to get their cooking done unless there was someone else around to care for the baby. In some households a Primus stove was brought into the living room and placed on the earthen floor when it was time to boil water for tea; then there was the problem of keeping the baby away from it. In any event, there was a danger from tea and other hot liquids at the time they were being served, even though they might have been prepared elsewhere, for almost everyone sat on the floor to eat or drink. Simple vigilance and holding the baby so he would not crawl toward the danger were the only safety practices used, except in one household where the babies were kept in their cribs most of the time.[2] Despite this danger, only one baby in the sample—Nabatanzi —suffered from a burn.

Few other dangerous things were mentioned. One baby was intrigued by his mother's knife and played with it whenever she laid it down. Since tables and shelves were rare in these households, it was indeed a problem to find a safe place for a forbidden object. More mothers were concerned, however, with safeguarding precious breakable objects from the baby's assault than with safeguarding him from dangerous objects—except, of course, for fire and hot liquids.

Although the baby was in most instances permitted to crawl about freely inside the house, except when cooking was going on, he was rarely, if ever, permitted to go outside the house out of sight. Most mothers did not verbalize what dangers they feared the baby might encounter outside. Two, however, mentioned mango worms as a danger—the larvae of an insect which burrowed

2 Although sixteen of our sample lived in households acculturated enough to provide cribs for the baby, none of them had playpens, jump seats, or other items of equipment in which a baby can be confined to keep him safely out of the way.

in under the skin to form a swelling resembling a boil. Three mothers feared their babies might fall, but in each instance there were unusual circumstances. In one case, post holes had been made for the posts of a new house into which the baby might tumble. In another case, the danger was that trees had been felled, over which the toddler might fall. Finally, Nora's mother was afraid that she might fall down the front steps—theirs was the only house with this hazard.

PART III

Case Summaries of the Infants and Their Families

Introduction

In the next seven chapters, summaries will be presented of each of the babies in the sample, giving an account of the family background and the child's development, and noting any special variations of infant-care practices which seem pertinent.

Each chapter will deal with a cluster of families, each representing a group of neighbors, friends, or relatives, who are together frequently, and who influence one another in regard to infant-care practices. It was hoped to reduce redundancy by grouping the cases in this way. The first group consists of three relatively unacculturated Muslim families chosen to be presented first because the babies were very young when first visited, and because they represent as well as any cluster the traditional methods of infant care. The second group is a large group of Protestant families, some of whom are relatively acculturated and who have influenced each other considerably in regard to infant care—and all of whom wanted help. The third group, although living in the same village as the second, are Muslims little influenced by their Protestant neighbors. The fourth is another Protestant group—all of whom are related—led by William's mother, and more influenced by clinic recommendations than any other group. The fifth group, although living in the same village as the families of the fourth, are not close friends with them and follow more traditional practices; this is also a Christian group. The sixth group consists of three Catholic families who are characterized by being relatively well-to-do, and all of whom know each other. Finally, the seventh chapter deals with one child, who is to be distinguished from the rest both because he was the oldest in the sample, and because his mother avoided

DOI: 10.4324/9781003629337-14

contact with the other three groups in the village and was highly idiosyncratic in her methods of infant care.

At the end of each summary is a very brief list of the findings of the child welfare clinic, including only weight, and presenting symptoms, if any. After some of the summaries are condensations of the reports of the Gesell Developmental Schedules provided by Dr. Marcelle Géber.

12

THREE CHILDREN FROM UNACCULTURATED MUSLIM FAMILIES

Aida, Juko, and Muhamidi

In response to my request for introductions to less highly acculturated families than those to which we had first been introduced, the chief took us to visit Aida's and Muhamidi's mothers. Later Aida's mother asked us to include Juko in the sample.

Aida

Aida was the youngest of three living children, all daughters, and the only child living at home when we first began to visit the family. Her parents are Muslims. Their wattle-and-daub house was shabbier and more sparsely furnished than most of those we visited. Her father, whose occupation we did not ascertain, was at home only occasionally. For a while the father's sister lived in the household and could look after the baby if the mother had to be absent; later, neighbors sometimes looked after her.

Aida's mother was very serious and tense at the time of our first visit. She told us that she had had four babies who died before they were two years old and implied that she would cooperate in the research in the hope that this might help keep this baby alive. She did not know the cause of death of the other children, saying only that it was "fever." Two of them had died in hospital; one had died two months after being discharged from hospital as improved; a fourth died a week after being refused admission to hospital. We knew that traditionally the

DOI: 10.4324/9781003629337-15

mother is blamed for the illness of the baby, since it is assumed that she had broken some taboo during pregnancy. We suspected that an irrational fear of having unknowingly done something wrong contributed to the grief this mother expressed over the loss of her babies and to the anxiety she felt about Aida's welfare.

The mother told us that she had sent her eldest daughter—now adolescent—away to live with relatives when she was two years old, and when the other babies died she had thought it best for her firstborn to remain away from home. The other daughter—now nearly six—was living with her grandparents nearby. This information contributed to our conviction that this mother was afraid that she somehow was the cause of the children's deaths. Further confirmation came when I checked the records of a survey that had been conducted the previous year to investigate the fertility of a sample of Ganda women; this woman had reported that she had never been pregnant!

On our second visit we found Aida's mother in a panic. Aida had been ill for a week with frequent vomiting, diarrhea, and a fever. Although the baby looked strong, plump, and well-nourished, we offered to take her to hospital for examination. Her mother agreed and immediately made arrangements to leave. At the hospital we took her to one of the doctors we knew, who gave her prompt attention. He found her very strong and well-developed for her age and attributed her illness to her mother's anxiety. He gave the mother a bottle of medicine for the baby—bicarbonate of soda and water colored pink—to make her feel that something was being done, and advised her to hold the baby upright after feeding, to help her get rid of wind. His main advice was to us—to visit the mother frequently, to give her much reassurance, and to urge her to take the baby regularly to the child welfare clinic.

From that time on—except for occasional diarrhea and one bad cold—Aida was healthy; she gained well and developed rapidly. Her mother was much less tense and was very cooperative in gratitude for the help she felt we had been to her. Perhaps as one sign of her renewed confidence in herself as a mother she brought her other daughters home to live with her.

Aida was born at home. She was given the breast "whenever she is hungry"—but not every time she cried and not merely for comfort. She slept in her mother's bed so that when she awoke at night they could both lie comfortably during the feeding. Although the mother's milk flowed freely at first, before long she thought it to be insufficient, despite the fact that the baby was gaining well. By the time she was fifteen weeks old, Aida was receiving supplementary bottle feedings of an imported formula, and by the time she was twenty weeks old her mother was so sure there was not enough milk that she offered the breast but rarely and gave three full bottle feedings a day, using dried skim milk from the clinic. Two weeks later Aida's mother said that she really had no breast milk left but that she put Aida to the breast anyway, "to make her feel she is having something." At night, however, Aida still woke to suckle, usually three times. By this time she was getting a variety of solid foods—porridge, vegetables, fruit, and eggs—all °f which seemed to agree with her. By the time Aida was thirty-one weeks old, her mother at last seemed satisfied that she was well-nourished. Cup feedings were started at thirty-three weeks, but the breast was still suckled occasionally.

Our first glimpse of Aida was when she was nine weeks old, when we came to ask her mother's cooperation in the research. She seemed strong, and her skin was satiny smooth and of good color. She was lying on the floor of the house on a heap of ragged cloths, quite naked except for a string of blue beads around her waist. She was crying when we arrived. There were several other people in the room, but the mother was not there. Presently one woman picked Aida up and tried to comfort her, but she continued to cry. Soon her mother came in and promptly put her to the breast. She stopped crying immediately and sucked readily.

A week later when she was ten weeks old, as previously reported, she seemed ill and we took her to hospital. During the physical examination it was ascertained that she weighed thirteen pounds and was nearly ready to sit unsupported. When she was held in a standing position she seemed very strong, and the tonus in her muscles was good. She seemed passive and unresponsive, however, and surprised the doctor by not protesting when he manipulated her muscles. Eventually he elicited a quiet whimper.

She slept through our brief visit when she was twelve weeks old. She was on a mattress in the living room, with two adults also present, while her mother worked in the garden. She did not awaken when her mother returned.

On another visit at sixteen weeks, Mrs. Kibuka found the mother out of the house and Aida lying naked on a mat near a woman visitor. When her mother came in Aida made no special response; her mother picked her up and held her sitting on her lap for a while. When she was placed on a mat on the floor she tried very energetically to crawl and managed to push herself off the mat. Her mother said that she could not keep her on a mat any more. She could not yet sit alone, was disinclined to try, and the mother had not tried to "train" her.

Her mother said that she held Aida in her arms for a while after each feeding. When she was put down she sometimes cried; knowing nothing to be wrong, her mother did not pick her up but let her cry. She usually then dropped off to sleep.

When we visited at twenty weeks we found the usual cluster of unexplained children outside and two women—also unexplained— in the house. Aida was sitting on the floor near one of them, naked except for a string of little cloth bags worn like a bandolier (containing "medicine") and a string of blue beads around her waist. As we visited, three children were in and out of the house, as were several chickens with a brood of cheeping chicks. Aida's mother fussed with a Primus stove and began to boil water. Aida stared very intently at us and then, after a while, began to creep about actively on her hands and knees. She spied her bottle on the floor with some milk left in it, crept to it quickly, picked it up in both hands, and drained it to the last drop. She was then brought over and placed on the mat in front of my chair. I put my hands out, and she leaned forward to grasp them and pulled herself to a standing position. She was fairly steady on her feet but obviously needed some support. I took her on my lap and she immediately reached for my glasses, the comb in my hair, and my pencil, grasping these things strongly and persistently. Wishing to take notes, I finally put her down on the floor, and she cried. I tried to encourage her to crawl, but she seemed frustrated and whimpered a little. Mrs. Kibuka then picked her up, and Aida transferred her interest, remaining on Mrs. Kibuka's lap until she wet; her mother then rushed her out of the house to hold her down.

When her mother brought her back she placed her on the floor where she lay on her side sucking her thumb. Noticing her long inactivity and apparent drowsiness, the mother asked the other women, "Has she had her bath?" Receiving an affirmative answer, she then said, "Then she will go to sleep." She put Aida down on a "bed" apparently consisting of a pile of burlap bags covered with old cloths. Aida went to sleep quickly, with her thumb still in her mouth and the other hand loosely clenched.

The mother gave us the following information. When Aida is left with someone else, as she was that day while her mother was at the mosque, she accepts the attention of others and can be given her bottle feeding. She can sit unsupported, and, said her mother, she has been able to do so since three months of age. (This was inaccurate, for when she was visited at sixteen weeks of age she still was unable to sit.) She makes cooing noises, especially in response to her mother when she speaks to her, and also when she first wakes in the morning. She squeals when excited, laughs aloud, and makes "much noise." She takes naps both in the morning and afternoon and now sleeps well during the day and at night. She receives baths two to four times a day; she is always given a bath before being put to bed, for otherwise it was believed she would not sleep.

Suddenly, and to our surprise, dinner was served, although it was midafternoon. (It was *matooke* served with a tasty sauce, followed by thin, very sweet coffee. We found out that the mother had not expected our visit, not having received the message we sent to say we were coming. She showed no sign of having been ruffled by unexpected dinner guests.) Aida slept soundly throughout dinner and through subsequent conversation, apparently being not at all disturbed by the noise in the room. Toward the end of the visit I suggested taking photographs. Aida was wakened and immediately was taken outside where she passed urine as her mother held her down. Her mother brought out a little navy blue dress and, while she dressed her, Aida smiled up at her and vocalized—the first vocalization we noted in the visit. She sat alone while I took some snaps, not protesting at being separated from her mother outside of the house.

I noted in my field notes after this visit: " Aida's mother is very cooperative. She seems to have been extremely appreciative of our help and continued interest. She answered questions readily and expanded her answers in an informative way."

Two weeks later we gained additional information. Aida was sucking her thumb more. She still wet the bed, but her mother kept a close enough eye on bowel movements that she usually caught her and avoided smearing.

The six-year-old sister, now living at home again, helped "mind" Aida while the mother worked in the garden but was too young to do anything else for her. Sometimes Aida was left with neighbors, but at times she was taken with her mother. She seemed content with any of these arrangements; "she is happy with everyone." Nevertheless, her mother said, she was likely to cry when her mother left the room and to try to follow her, especially if she was hungry. When Aida was taken along to the garden, her mother carried her there on her back but then put her down on a mat on the ground. Whenever Aida was left with someone else she gave her mother a good greeting when she returned, smiling and lifting her arms toward her mother. Her mother's face lit up as she described this response. She said that the sister gave Aida affection, and so did she, holding her after her day's work was finished. When Aida cried her mother said she soothed her by bouncing her about over her back.

While we were talking I could watch Aida myself. I took her on my lap when I first arrived and she was very responsive to my attention. Soon I gave her a piece of hard candy. She accepted it readily, put it to her mouth, and then transferred it from hand to hand, sucking it occasionally, getting very sticky, and vocalizing happily. I set her down on the floor and she sat happily, squealing from time to time as though she liked the sound of her own voice. Her mother then took her on her lap and soon gave her the breast without any noticeable signal from Aida. She suckled quietly for a while and then seemed sleepy. Her mother took her outside and gave her a quick bath in a tub of water (see page 69 for a description of the bath.) She brought her inside while still dripping and gave her the breast again. She suckled a bit and then was put to bed where she remained quietly throughout the rest of our visit.

When we visited at twenty-four weeks, Aida had a bowel movement on the mat near the door soon after we arrived. She had had diarrhea for several days, and perhaps because of the excitement of our arrival her mother did not notice any signals. The mother did not fuss, but cleaned up the floor with leaves. Then she went outside to fetch water to give Aida a bath. The baby cried when her mother left but stopped as soon as she returned. Then she was bathed outside in a tub, just as before.

Once back inside after the bath, Aida cried again when her mother left for a moment. Mrs. Kibuka took her on her lap and tried to comfort her, but she continued to cry until her mother returned. Back on her mother's lap, she quieted, then became drowsy, and finally fell asleep. Her mother said that whenever she was left with someone else, even a familiar person, she cried for a while and then stopped, but when the mother was present Aida was friendly with other people, both men and women—and, indeed, she was friendly with us. She did not yet recognize her father for he was so rarely at home.

The mother got up to put Aida to bed, but she awakened immediately and was given the breast instead. She suckled a while, then fell asleep again and was put to bed.

Our next long visit was at thirty-one weeks. Aida was away visiting her maternal grandmother for the day, and her eldest sister, who had also returned home by this time, was sent to get her. While we waited the mother told us that Aida could now stand alone. She sometimes said *mama* and *taata* (presumably to her paternal uncle who was often there), and could imitate sounds. She responded to her name but did not yet heed *neno* ("no, no!"). When she was happy to see someone, she greeted them by clapping her hands. She had not soiled the bed for a long time and only occasionally wet it. She was still friendly with strangers and was said to treat all people the same way.

When Aida returned home with her sister, she seemed subdued and had tears in her eyes. The sister said that she had been awakened from a nap to be brought home. I offered to take photographs, and the mother put Aida into a new dress. This time when Aida was set on a mat alone and left by her mother, she cried. She could not be consoled until her mother returned to her side.

At thirty-four weeks Aida had a heavy cold with a cough, but she seemed cheerful and active. I invited her to come to me, but she would not come, even when I offered her candy. The mother rose with her in her arms and put her down on the floor halfway across the room from me and returned to her mat. Aida scuttled back to her mother and buried her head on her lap. I then crossed the room to her, held out the candy, and she took it hesitantly. This was the first time that she had seemed shy of me. The mother thought it was because I was European, for she was still usually friendly with strangers. The mother also said that Aida followed her about more consistently than before. Nevertheless, she spent much of her time with her six-year-old sister and did not seem to mind her mother's absence. She did not appear to get hungry while her mother was gone, but when her mother was near she often tried to get at the breast, even though breast feeding was now infrequent during the day.

Aida began to eat the candy messily, dribbling sticky saliva all over her body. After finishing the candy she became quite active, crawling about on the floor, mostly in the corner near her mother, and playing with a cloth. She vocalized for an extended time, making a "brrrrr!" sound, trilling her lips. She then played near another baby —Juko—who was there, and when he went to his mother Aida did also. She crawled about some more, seemingly fascinated by the process of emitting "brrrrr!" For a while she scrambled over her mother, who was sitting

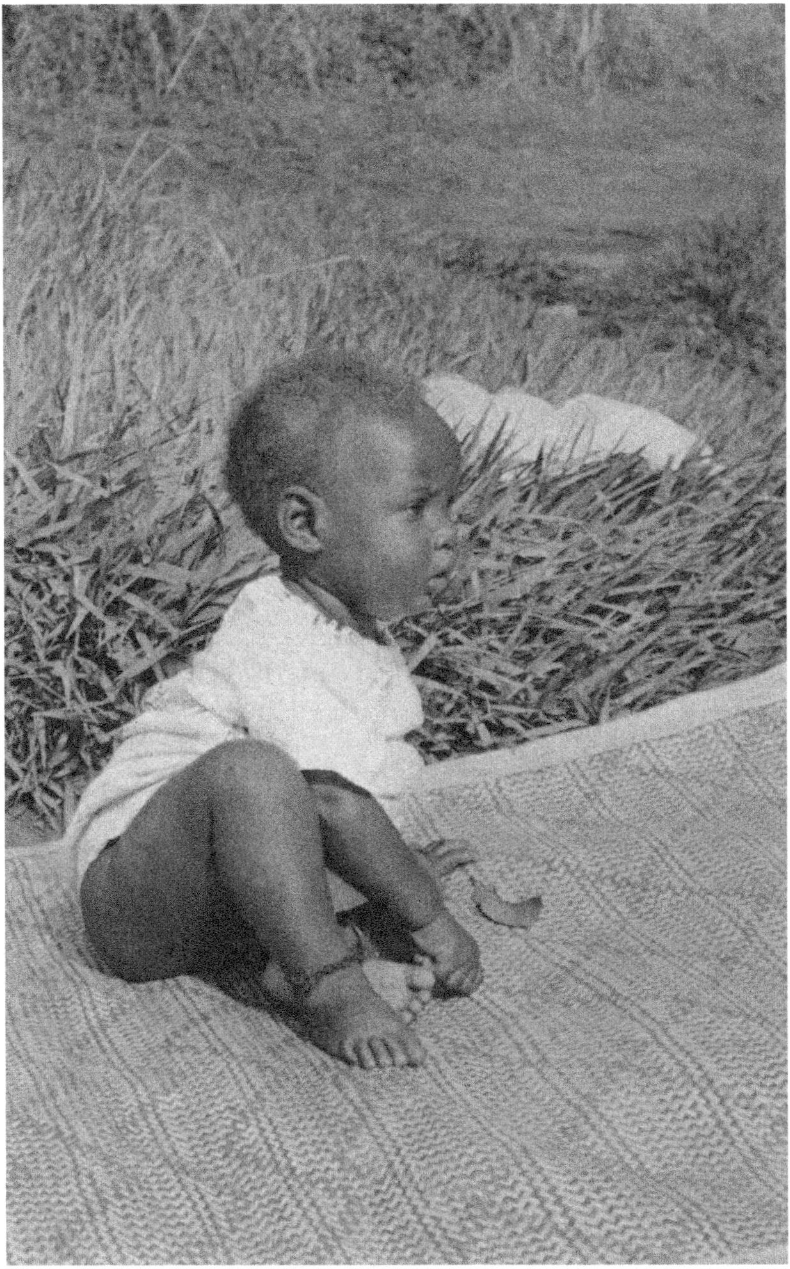

FIGURE 2 At thirty-one weeks Aida cried when left alone to be photographed and could not be consoled until her mother returned to her side.

on a mat on the floor, but then she left her for other explorations. The little boy was playing with a corncob, banging it on the floor, but when Aida came near he banged her on the head with it several times, and she accepted this without protest. Both children went together to the door, which had been propped open with an empty bottle. The boy kept removing the bottle so that the door swung shut, and his mother kept replacing it. Whenever the door swung shut, Aida swung it back and forth repeatedly. After a while she returned to her mother and sat sucking her thumb on her mother's lap. The mother finally gave her the breast, but she did not suckle long. When we got up to go, I picked Aida up, and she did not protest this time but began to play with my glasses. When I put her down she did not protest. She was carried on her mother's hip to the car to see us off.

Visits to the Clinic

Age *wks.*	*Weight* *lbs.*
10*	13.0
13	13.7
17	14.5
21	15.5
27	16.5
31	17.7
33	18.2

* Visit to hospital.

Juko

Juko's father was Aida's mother's brother. The father was a handsome young man, whose manner combined dignity and an easy friendliness. He worked in the Department of Health on mosquito control and was able to commute to work, returning each evening. The mother was pleasant, rather shy, and seemed very young. She had reached the fourth grade in school before she stopped. Juko was their first baby; they seemed proud, pleased, and happy—with him and with each other.

It was Aida's mother who brought this family into the sample. She said they were eager to participate, and certainly they wanted the transportation to the well-baby clinic which we provided. We saw their house once—a typical wattle-and-daub hut with a thatched roof. The road that led to it, however, was quite impassable after the rainy season started, so it was arranged that we would visit with Juko and his mother at the same time that we visited Aida. Although his mother took him to the clinic four times, we had only two good visits with them. Fortunately, she was a good informant, so our interview schedule is fairly complete, although I observed his behavior much less frequently than I would have wished.

Juko was born in hospital a week later than Aida and Muhamidi. Suckling was well-established within two days, but from the beginning Juko's mother feared that she did not have a good supply of milk. Despite these misgivings, she enjoyed breast feeding, the child gained well, and she did not begin supplementary feedings until he was about six months old. He was given the breast whenever he cried—to comfort him if he was unhappy and not just when he was hungry. From the beginning he slept in a crib so that his mother had to get up to feed him at night; but by thirty weeks he woke only once during the night. After feeding him, even during the day, his mother put him down—although she said that she held him and played with him a great deal at other times. His first supplementary feeding consisted of milk and tea given by cup. Then came papaws and sweet bananas, which he liked from the beginning. He had three baths a day at first but later only two. He was said to have stopped soiling his bed by four months of age. He was held down after feeding and when he awoke from sleep, but he still wet the bed and passed stools in the house.

Juko had his first visit to the clinic when twenty weeks old. He weighed 17.5 pounds. His spleen was found to be enlarged from malaria, so Daraprim was prescribed. Otherwise, he was judged to be strong and well-developed.

At thirty weeks I had my first long visit with Juko. He was asleep in a corner of the room when we arrived and slept through half the visit. Our conversation did not disturb him at all. Mrs. Kibuka noticed his eyes open finally and she picked him up. His mother took him immediately, to "hold him down" outside. When they returned I noticed that he was a plump, well-nourished baby. He was naked except for a string of white beads around his waist and black strings tied as though to hold the little cloth bags that Aida and Muhamidi sometimes wore, but the bags were not attached. His mother held him on her lap as she sat on her mat, and he scrambled over her, seeming quite cheerful. Mrs. Kibuka took him onto her lap presently, and he seemed cheerful there too. When he was put down he moved toward his mother, creeping vigorously and efficiently. He vocalized often—loudly and happily. Whenever one of the adults present made an overture he was friendly and responsive. In due course his mother gave him a drink of water from an enamel cup. He took the cup and managed the drinking himself, dribbling only a little water down his bare tummy. He crawled about for a while, very actively, exploring the room and the people in it. Aida's mother brought in a Primus stove placed it on the floor, and began to prepare tea. Juko took great interest in the preparations. Time and again he crawled toward the Primus stove and the hot kettle and had to be lifted away. Finally the repeated frustration made him fussy. One of the women present playfully offered him her breast, although it was covered by her dress. She then picked him up and bounced him about quite roughly and he seemed to enjoy this. Down on the floor again, he found a little glass bottle, with which he played for a while, mouthing it and manipulating it. His mother left the room for a moment, and Juko immediately crept after her, without crying. Before he reached the door, however, she returned. After tea we took some photographs of the babies outside. Juko was cheerful throughout, both when with his mother and when on a mat by himself, although he tried to crawl toward his mother when left on the mat. As we left at the end of the visit, he was playing just outside the door of the house, standing, holding on to a large four-gallon tin, beating it with one hand, and saying "da-da-da-da." There was something very enchanting about this sturdy, vigorous, responsive baby.

While Juko was exploring his world, we sought information from his mother, some of which was reported in an earlier section. His mother said that she did everything for the baby herself. She had no one with whom to leave him, so she took him with her wherever she went. She carried him usually straddling her hip but put him in a sling on her back if she was going a long distance. She said that he cried whenever she left the room, and that he had been doing this ever since he could crawl. He had also tried to follow her as soon as he could crawl. Whenever his father was at home, however, Juko was said to "want to be with him." He was friendly with strangers, at least when his mother was present, and so indeed it was with us.

He was said to have begun to sit unsupported at four months of age and to crawl at five months. He was helped to learn to sit by being put into a basin with cloths wrapped around him for support. He could stand by thirty weeks, supporting himself with his hands against the wall—indeed, we saw him standing holding onto the big tin, and he must have pulled himself up.

His mother had recently begun to give him *matooke*, corn meal porridge, sweet potatoes, and squash to eat; he received this food at adult mealtimes and was not given the breast for quite some time after eating. He fed himself with his fingers, but it was his mother who always gave it to him. His mother said that he could hold his own cup when drinking, and this, too, we witnessed.

He was said to do most of his sleeping during the night and to nap little during the day. He was impervious to noise if very sleepy, but otherwise he was kept awake by noise. His mother said he cried very little, usually only when hungry, and never from anger. He sucked his thumb rarely.

When he was thirty-two weeks of age he was ill with diarrhea, vomiting, and a fever. Despite his illness, he was quiet and contented at the clinic, sitting on his mother's lap or close to her. She gave him the breast only once. Later in the week he was said not to have recovered completely, but he seemed cheerful and active. He was crawling about the floor when we arrived, vocalizing, with a loud and emphatic "da-da-da-da." Soon he crept over to his mother's lap and she gave him the breast. After he seemed satisfied she put him down, but soon he was back on his mother's lap, making his demand for the breast clear by grasping her clothing

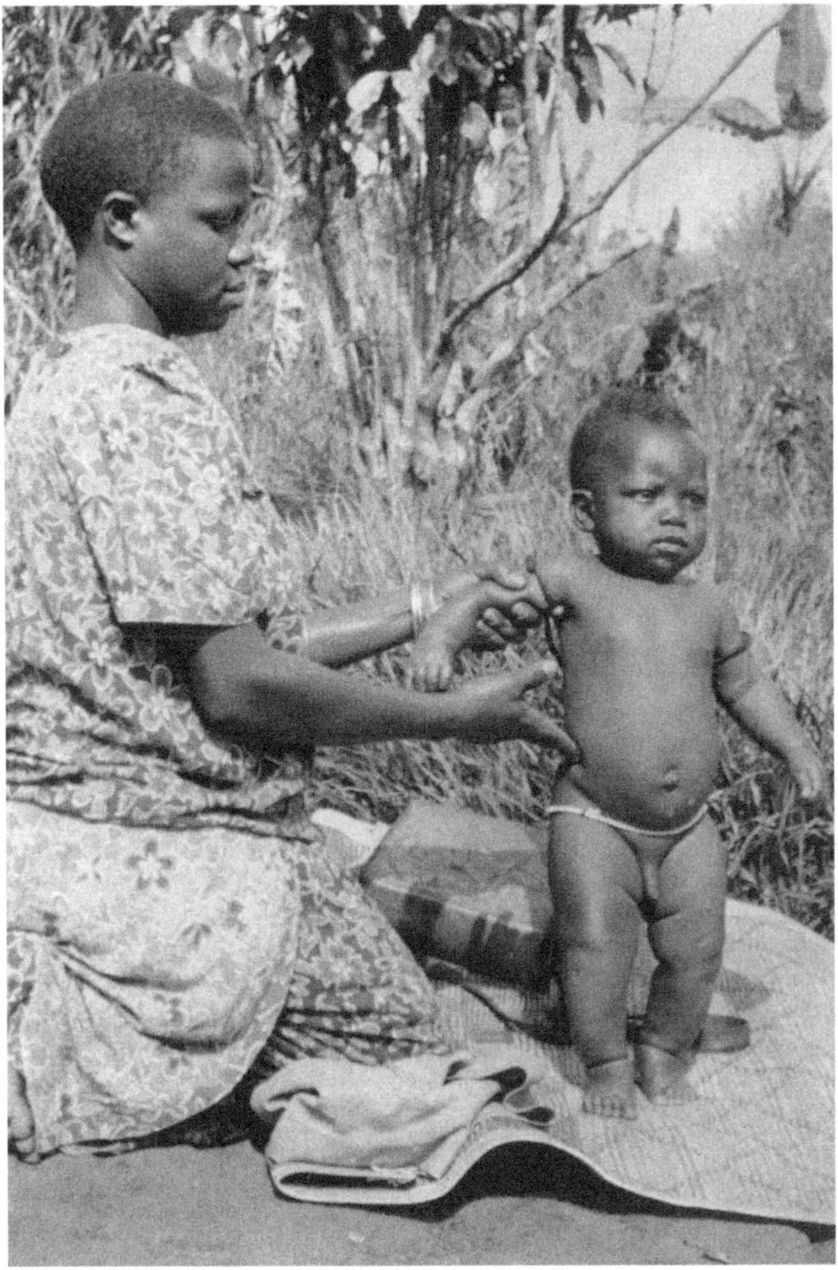

FIGURE 3 Juko is a sturdy boy at thirty weeks. He is content here, but when his mother moves off he creeps after her.

over the breast and trying to get it for himself; she gave it to him again. After he was finished suckling this time, I offered him a piece of hard candy, holding it out and inviting him to come to me. He would not come. I crossed the room and offered the candy again, but he buried his head in his mother's breast and would not look at me. (His mother said later that she thought that his shyness was because I was a European; he was usually easy with strangers.) I left the candy with his mother, and he accepted it, enjoying it messily. After getting sticky all over with the candy, he began to crawl about his mother's lap, scrambling over her person, exploring her. He remained near her for quite a while. At one point his mother held him by the hands in a standing position, smiling at and talking to him. He smiled back most responsively. And then, in response to no signal that I could perceive, she gave him the breast a third time.

Aida, who was also present, was crawling about on the floor. She approached Juko and his mother, and soon Juko was down on the floor also and the two babies began playing together. As described earlier, he found a corncob on the floor and hit Aida over the head with it several times, in the same spirit that he banged on other things. Next he found an enamel basin on the floor and began to roll it about, making much noise and enjoying himself thoroughly. Then he and Aida began to play with the door. He kept pulling the bottle away from the door and his mother kept replacing it. After several repetitions he tired of this game and found the basin again; he began to beat it rhythmically as though it were a drum.

Finally he returned to his mother, reached for the breast, and received it again—for the fourth time. He suckled briefly, left her for a few minutes, returned, and took the breast again, managing it himself. Before we went, I picked Juko up to see what he would do. He did not protest and seemed mildly interested as well as slightly tense and apprehensive. He sat on my lap for a while, and then I got up, took both of his hands, and led him over to his mother. Mrs. Kibuka then took him, and he sat on her lap without complaint.

While all of this was going on I interviewed Juko's mother. She answered my questions shyly, with covert glances at Aida's mother, as if acknowledging her seniority. Since this was to be my last long visit, I pressed the questions, and she responded with no apparent impatience. Whenever Juko came close to her, she was responsive, gentle, and affectionate—and she managed to respond thus to him without any obvious diminution of her attentive responsiveness to Mrs. Kibuka or to me.

The mother told us that she was giving the breast to Juko as often as ever; she explained that since he was the only child and was with her all the time, he had much more opportunity to demand the breast than a baby who is sometimes left with other people. She admitted that he had begun to handle his genitals at about five months of age, especially after urinating, and that she had "tried to stop him"; but she never smacked or "beat" him for this or for anything else. He had stopped soiling his bed, and he never had smeared.

He rarely cried, and never merely to be picked up. Nevertheless, when he did cry his mother always picked him up to comfort him. He vocalized a lot and could imitate sounds. He could say *taata* (daddy) and *jjajja* (grandparent) but, strangely enough, not *mama.* He responded to his own name and understood phrases like *jjangu* (come here!), *vaawo* (get out! get away!), and *lekerawo* (stop what you are doing!). He played with anything he could get hold of.

Visits to the Clinic

Age wks.	*Weight lbs.*	*Comments*
20	17.6	malaria, enlarged spleen
24	18.4	conjunctivitis
28	18.5	scalp infection
32		fever, diarrhea, vomiting

Muhamidi

Muhamidi's father was a farmer. To reach the house we had to leave the road and walk along a narrow path for about fifteen minutes, winding through long grass and finally through fields of cotton. The house was made of wattle and daub, the roof of tin. The front room was large but was crowded with sacks of coffee beans. It contained only two folding chairs and a few dusty mats on the earthen floor.

The household was Muslim and polygynous. Although the place usually swarmed with people, we could rarely identify the adults present. When we first visited this mother, Muhamidi was the only one of her children at home. There were, however, four other living children, who had been sent away to live with the maternal grandmother in another county. A sixth child, a three-year-old daughter, had recently died, and the mother wept when she told us about her.

This was a very disrupted, unstable household, and the mother was extremely anxious and troubled. It seemed to me that one of her reasons for wishing to participate in the research was that she longed for a sympathetic ear. She had had more than her share of misfortunes, but, as we got to know her better, it seemed that she was a masochistic person who always did things the hard way and who compounded the difficulties that a malign fate had visited upon her.

One of this mother's chief concerns was the illness of her four-year-old daughter, Asa. Much of our visiting time throughout the research was spent talking about Asa and trying to make plans for hospital treatment. The clinic diagnosed sickle-cell anemia—a genetically determined disorder—with osteomyelitis, which was particularly resistant to treatment because of the underlying sickle-cell condition. The child was crippled, helpless, and usually very ill and miserable. Our contact with the family was interrupted during the first three months because the mother took Asa to hospital and stayed with her for a while, then took her and Muhamidi to visit the maternal grandfather. When contact was renewed, Asa was taken to the clinic and Dr. Welbourn urged hospitalization. We made repeated arrangements to take the child to hospital, but something always intervened. The father refused permission for a while. One of his reasons for refusing was that they already owed a large sum of money to an Indian physician in private practice who had been treating the child, and he seemed to feel it was unethical to take her to hospital when they still owed the doctor money. Another time she seemed better, and her parents decided she would recover without further treatment. After hospitalization was finally arranged, there was a dismaying series of disappointments and misunderstandings, which discouraged the mother so much that she took Asa away—still without treatment. This mother clearly was not capable of being sent with a chit from the examining doctor to the X-ray department and of arriving at the proper time. But since she had to carry the crippled four-year-old, as well as the baby, from one building to another in a setting that was quite incomprehensible to her, she won my sympathy.

A hint of marital discord was given at our first visit. The mother said that she was glad that the other children were being cared for by the grandmother because her husband did not help with the children. On the contrary, he expected her to help with the coffee harvest, and this, together with a new baby and her usual duties, was too much for her without having the other children there also. One day, five months later, she stopped us on the road and asked for a ride to her father's house. She had quarreled with her husband, the occasion of the quarrel being the return of another wife who had been away for some time. She was determined to leave him. She could take Muhamidi with her, but the father claimed the other children. They had a bitter quarrel over Asa, and the mother finally got his permission to take her with her also, since she so clearly needed her mother's care. After this separation the father refused to give the mother any support. Any money she received was from her father, who already was providing school fees for two of her children.

The maternal grandfather seemed to be a man of some substance and importance, with enough money to undertake a pilgrimage to Mecca (for which plans were then being made). He had separated from the maternal grandmother and had taken several young wives—younger than his daughter. The mother was close to her father and felt she was his favorite. Perhaps she incurred the jealousy of the young wives, but in any event she felt neither happy nor comfortable in her father's household. The place teemed with children; the other women were busy with their own families; and she still had no one to help her with her two helpless children—Muhamidi and Asa. To pile misery on misery, she herself became ill.

As implied in the foregoing account, all the children but Muhamidi, who was still unweaned, had had repeated separation experiences. Each time a new baby was born the older children were sent away to live with relatives; the mother visited them from time to time but did not bring them home quickly. All were away when we first visited the family. Then Asa and another daughter returned home, but the latter stayed with her father when the mother left home. A third daughter was staying with the maternal grandmother; she was temporarily reunited with her mother when the maternal grandmother came to visit the maternal grandfather. A son, whom we never met, lived elsewhere with other relatives.

All of this misfortune and instability, feeding the mother's anxiety as it did, seems significant as a background for the relationship Muhamidi and his mother built up between them.

Muhamidi was born at home. It was said to have been a quick, easy birth, which was fortunate because the mother was alone. He was "very ill" when he was newborn, but the mother had forgotten what "they" said was wrong. Because of this illness he did not suckle well at the beginning. As far as I could ascertain he received no European medical attention until his mother first availed herself of our transportation to the clinic—when he was twenty-three weeks old.

He was breast-fed on demand—and indeed, it seemed to us, on the slightest signal. He slept with his mother and woke about five times each night to be fed; this continued throughout the period of our contact with the family. When he was thirty-four weeks old I asked his mother whether she enjoyed breast feeding or felt it to be a duty; she did not reply directly but later admitted that she had enjoyed it when he was younger.

When Muhamidi was five months old supplementary foods were started. By the time he was thirty-two weeks old he was receiving milk with tea in the middle of the morning; his mother fed him this liquid mixture with a spoon! At midday and evening mealtimes he received what the adults ate—*matooke* or potatoes well-mashed. He also ate corn meal porridge, papaw, sweet bananas, and squash, feeding himself with his fingers.

Until he was five months old he received two or three baths a day—at midday, in the evening, and sometimes also in the morning—but after the fifth month the morning bath was omitted. His mother said, when he was ten weeks old, that she had begun to hold him down when he was one month old.

At our first brief visit Muhamidi at nine weeks seemed healthy and well-developed for his age. His hair was very thick and black. He had a handsome, responsive, and somewhat comic face; his heavy eyebrows were shaped like a circumflex accent, which gave him a look of chronic surprise. He was given to Mrs. Kibuka to hold. He smiled at her, and then made little grunting vocalizations and worked his mouth. When he was given back to his mother she gave him the breast straightaway, although he had not cried, and he nursed vigorously.

When we arrived again a week later Muhamidi's mother was working in the yard, spreading coffee beans out on the ground to dry in the sun. She had Muhamidi in a sling on her back as she worked. She told us later that she took him wherever she went, usually carrying him on her back. She came into the house with us, took Muhamidi from her back, and held him in her arms. He seemed to be asleep, with his head lolling and his eyes closed. He was naked except for little cloth strings about his ankles and waist and another string with little bags tied to it, worn like a bandolier, like Aida's.

After we had chatted for a few moments, his mother took him into her room. She had scarcely settled herself on her mat back in the living room when he started to whimper, and soon he cried in earnest. She picked him up, and as soon as she had settled herself again on her mat she gave him the breast. He sucked slowly with his eyes closed, and his mother held her breast in position for him while he lay passively in her arms. Finally he went to sleep. After a while his mother roused him and "held him down," not bothering to take him outside. She held him under one arm, and firmly pressed him into a squatting position, where he remained as long as she held him, his back straight, his head erect, and seeming remarkably strong. He looked up at his mother and smiled at her, but he did not oblige her by urinating. Then the mother sat down again on her mat, holding him beside her in a standing position, supporting him with one hand. He tipped his head back and smiled up at his mother, and then he smiled across the room at me. After this visit, the mother took Muhamidi away with Asa, first to hospital and then to visit her father. We did not see them again until the baby was twenty-two weeks old. We met them on the road, Muhamidi in a sling on his mother's back. She looked anxious and explained that he had a fever. Indeed, his forehead was very hot and he was listless and unresponsive, even when his mother took him from her back and held him in her arms. I gave her Daraprim and aspirin for him.

About an hour later we came to their house, after visiting another family. We found Muhamidi sitting outside the house crying bitterly. His sister was lying on a pile of cloths near him, appearing very ill and paying no attention to the baby. The mother appeared from behind the house where she had been working. She ushered us into the house, giving first attention to the polite greetings. She then went out to get him and put him to the breast immediately, without stopping to wipe his nose, which was streaming, or to wipe his face, which was muddy. He suckled for a while, and then the mother removed him briefly from the breast and wiped his nose and face with a rather rumpled, dingy cloth. He suckled a bit more and then was ready to look around. He became very active and seemed quite a different child. His fever seemed to have vanished, and certainly he was no longer listless. He bounced about actively on his mother's lap, scrambling over her, frequently smiling at her, and sometimes hiding his face in her lap. He vocalized a great deal. His face expressed so much animation that it invited an exchange of smiling and vocalization. He responded readily to Mrs. Kibuka and to me, although in the course of the visit he smiled more frequently at his mother than at us.

He did not leave his mother's side, but when at a later visit we inquired when he had begun to crawl his mother replied: "When he was four and a half months old, and he began to sit at the same time." He was certainly able to sit unsupported and for an indefinite period when he was twenty-two weeks old, so I give credence to the mother's statement, which sets the milestone for both sitting and crawling at twenty weeks, approximately. The mother said that she had not trained him to sit, nor did she entice him to crawl by offering attractive objects out of reach. She felt, however, that he had been stimulated to crawl by himself, seeing objects out of his reach that he wanted.

We did not inquire about elimination control until a later visit; the mother then told us that he stopped soiling the bed when he was five months old, at about the same time that he had begun to sit alone and to crawl.

During the next nine weeks we saw Muhamidi and his mother ten times but we were unable to arrange a real visit. He was judged to be well when he visited the clinic at twenty-three weeks of age, but two weeks later he had conjunctivitis, a cold, and fever. He had, however, gained eight ounces in two weeks and weighed 16.5 pounds. Two weeks later, when twenty-seven weeks old, he still had conjunctivitis and had gained only two ounces. He was very fussy throughout the whole time at the clinic and was still fussy a week later when we saw him briefly. His mother was concerned that he was not getting enough milk and attributed the dimunition of her milk supply to the Ramadan fast.

Another visit to the clinic occurred when he was thirty-one weeks old. As soon as they arrived, Muhamidi was suckled. After this he stood on the ground holding onto his mother's knees, looking quite cheerful. Despite his good appearance, he had gained only seven ounces during the month and was found to have malaria. The results of a blood test were available; some sickle cells were present, but there were few enough to suggest that he had inherited the disorder through only one recessive gene rather than through two genes as his sister presumably had. When Asa was examined she screamed and struggled, so her mother gave Muhamidi to me to hold while she tried to comfort and control Asa. Muhamidi sat on my lap without protest, but he was tense, with his whole body oriented toward his mother, whom he watched intently.

As mentioned earlier, Muhamidi, Asa, and their mother had gone to live with the maternal grandfather. A few days later, we came to give them transportation to hospital so that Asa could be treated there. We came earlier than expected and had to wait a half hour while the mother made her preparations for the trip. She gave Muhamidi to one of her father's young wives to hold. He fussed continuously while his mother was away getting ready. The woman tried to comfort him, first bouncing him up and down on her lap, then holding him on her back while she bounced him about vigorously. Muhamidi cried for about twenty minutes and then settled down. The woman kept wiping his runny nose, first on the skirt of her dress and then on her head scarf, which she removed for that purpose. Finally he fell asleep in her arms. He was content during the trip to hospital, sitting on his mother's lap. We stopped at a shop briefly, and his mother took him in with her rather than leave him with us in the car.

Finally, when Muhamidi was thirty-two weeks old we made a long visit again. I suggested sitting outside on the grass, instead of going into the house, hoping thus to avoid the interminable greetings that would be necessary with all the members of the grandfather's large household. Gradually, however, everyone came out to sit with us—two of the young wives, the maternal grandmother, and a large number of children.

Muhamidi sat on the grass near his mother for a while, and then, when the other children came out, he crept over to join them. One little girl gave him a lot of attention. I noticed her kissing him with her lips much protruded and her mouth open, and Muhamidi kissed her right back, full on the mouth, in the same way. Then he moved closer to his mother, then right to her, and began to play with her hair while she talked to us. As he did so, another little girl kept tickling him. He laughed, but kept his attention oriented toward his mother. Presently he began to chew her hair, standing behind her as she sat on the grass. He remained mostly near his mother throughout our visit but from time to time made a little excursion to see someone else. Another child kissed him. Finally one of the children pulled him onto her lap, and he let out a howl. He was comforted only when his mother picked him up, and he stayed close to her for the rest of the visit.

His mother said that he had been crying a great deal. He wanted to be with her all the time. Whenever he was parted from her, for even a moment, he cried and tried to follow her. He had been following ever since he could crawl (at twenty weeks), but he was crying more now. Even when he was with her he was often fussy and frequently tried to get at her breast. Whenever he fussed his mother held him in her arms until he was quiet, and she gave him the breast if that seemed to be what he wanted. In this big household it was the mother who did everything for him, and she took him with her nearly everywhere she went. He was responsive to other people as long as his mother was present; otherwise he cried persistently and could not be comforted. He was occasionally held by other people, but chiefly by his mother, who held him a lot. Before they left home he had been friendly with his father, but he no longer saw him and had not become that friendly with anyone else.

A few days later we encountered Muhamidi and his mother as we passed in the car. He was very fussy throughout our chat with the mother, even though she held him in her arms.

When he was thirty-three weeks old we visited the grandfather's home again. I hoped that we could have our visit in the car, and for a while Muhamidi and his mother sat beside me. He seemed content and played with my handbag. It emerged that the mother had prepared us dinner—*matooke* with peanut sauce—so we went into the house. When she left the room to get the food she took Muhamidi with her and left him behind the scences when she returned. A little later one of the young girls in the household brought him in with her and put him down on the floor. He immediately scrambled across to his mother, smiling and crowing with pleasure. The mother picked him up and gave him the breast. After suckling for a while, he was put down on the floor where he sat close to his mother for quite some time. He obviously had a cold, and his nose was running. His mother wiped his nose on the cloth in which she usually carried him on her back. Another little boy came in for a while. He too had a cold, and Muhamidi's mother attempted to wipe his nose on the skirt of his grubby little dress; the dress was too short to reach his nose, so she took it off him and had him blow his nose on it. Presently Muhamidi crept out the door, presumably toward the other children who were playing outside. He returned in a moment with a kettle lid and spent most of the rest of our visit playing with it, banging it aganst the cement floor, seeming to enjoy the noise it made.

The mother told us that Muhamidi had had diarrhea for several days. The cold had begun the previous day when he had been quite sick. He was said to have a poor appetite. Just recently, she said, he had begun to stand alone, but the diarrhea and fever seemed to have weakened him so that he had not done so during the last few days.

He was not sleeping well. It took him a long time to get to sleep at night, and once asleep he woke easily. He still slept with his mother, who still gave him the breast whenever he woke. By this time he took only one nap a day but was very sensitive to noise and would not sleep if anything was going on.

Although he had not soiled the bed since he was five months old, he still wet the bed, especially when his mother was asleep and did not wake up to hold him down. He had not yet learned not to soil and wet in the house and occasionally smeared feces if he had a bowel movement while unattended.

His mother said that he had been enjoying the company of the other young children in the household and spent quite a lot of time "playing" with them, She said he could imitate sounds now. I heard crowing and quite a variety of vocalizations, but his mother said that he could say appropriately *mama, taata* (daddy), and *jjajja* (grandmother or grandfather). He also could understand *jjangu* (come!), *vaawo* (get out! get away!), and *lekerawo* (stop doing that!) and acted accordingly.

The following week—when he was thirty-four weeks old—I came prepared to take photographs, and all the household hurried to get into their best clothes for the occasion. Muhamidi's mother wanted one picture of him by himself, but every time she attempted to move away from him he cried and tried to get to her. After the photographing we went into the house to talk. The rest all disappeared to have a meal, but the mother said she did not feel well and did not want to eat, so we had a peaceful visit alone with her and Muhamidi. Muhamidi sat on her lap and fussed until she gave him the breast. He sucked briefly and fell asleep in her arms. She held him while he slept for a long time and then gently laid him down on some cushions which were on the floor. He woke immediately and whimpered and struggled to get back to her. She persisted in her efforts to make him lie down and bent over him in a reclining position so that he would feel her close to him, but he still struggled and fussed, so she picked him up again. Toward the very end of our visit she laid him down again. This time he did not protest. She reclined near him, leaning over him as he rested.

Our conversation ranged over a wide variety of topics pertaining to Muhamidi—and to the other children as babies, which will not be reported here. The mother said that he was very attached to her, and was not friendly to anyone else in her absence. Recently, while she was ill, he would not play with the other children—although he enjoyed playing with them when she was nearby. He insisted on being in bed with his mother. The maternal grandmother, who was still visiting, helped take care of him, and he accepted her attentions as long as his mother was present also. He was generally friendly with other people as long as his mother was there, but he did not "know" other people, such as his grandfather—by which the mother seemed to imply that he did not make differentiated responses to other people.

The mother felt that her milk supply had been further diminished by her illness since she herself had not been able to eat much. She offered Muhamidi milk as a supplement, but, although he had previously accepted it, he now refused. He used also to eat *matooke* and sweet potatoes but he now ate just a little of them.

Despite these difficulties, she said she did not intend to wean him until he was fifteen months old. This plan was contingent upon receiving money from her husband so that she could buy milk for Muhamidi. She felt that since Asa needed her help so much, it would be a relief to wean him earlier than eighteen months, the age at which she had weaned the other children. She planned to wean him abruptly, dropping both daytime and nighttime feedings at once. She had done so with the other children, and they had all been very disturbed for some weeks, crying a lot and demanding the breast, but she felt they would have been even more frustrated if they had been weaned gradually.

I inquired about what made Muhamidi angry and how he acted. His mother said he occasionally got angry when he was with the other children and they took away something that he was playing with. He would begin to scream and hit out at them, although he did not succeed in actually hitting them. I inquired whether he ever got angry with her, and she said that he did when he wanted the breast. She responded to his angry demand by giving him the breast.

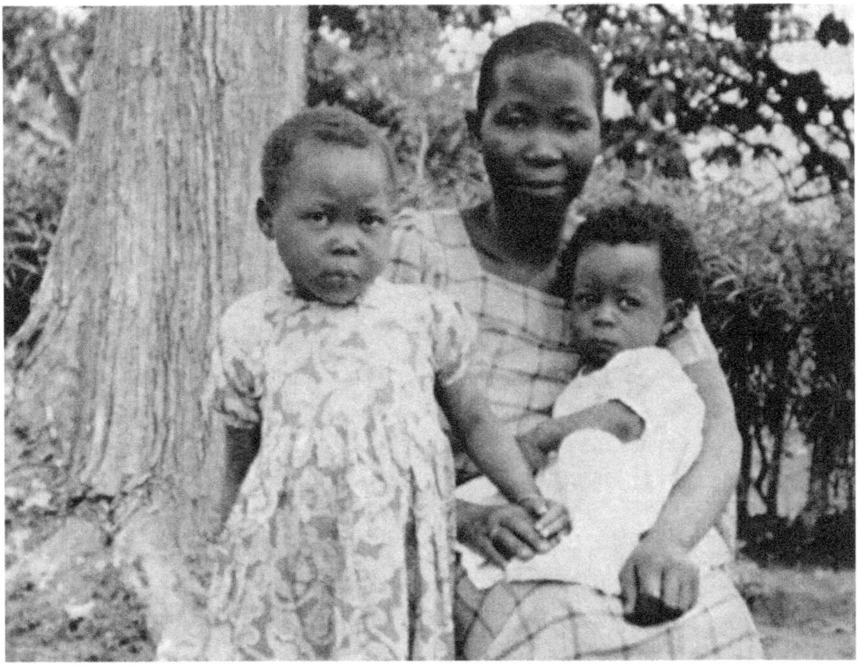

FIGURE 4 Muhamidi at thirty-four weeks clung to his mother and looked at us mistrustfully. His sister, Asa,is to the left.

He, by this time, was occasionally trying to suck his thumb, although he had stopped trying to put other things in his mouth. I inquired what the mother did when Muhamidi smeared feces, and she said she "beat" his hand to make him know that what he did was wrong. I inquired under what other circumstances she would "beat" him, and she said she did so when he was reaching toward hot water or breakable things. She gave him a light tap on the hand "to teach him." She had just started to do this recently when he began to move about more and get into things that were dangerous or which he could spoil. I inquired about masturbation. She said that she had occasionally noticed him fingering his penis, usually after urinating. This had not happened often, and she had "stopped him."

He played with empty tins and things that make a noise. His favorite activity was banging these playthings.

Our farewell visit occurred when Muhamidi was thirty-six weeks old. He was fussy and kept scrambling over his mother. He showed no real interest in anyone else, although all of us tried to evoke a friendly response from him. Every time his mother went out of the room she took him with her.

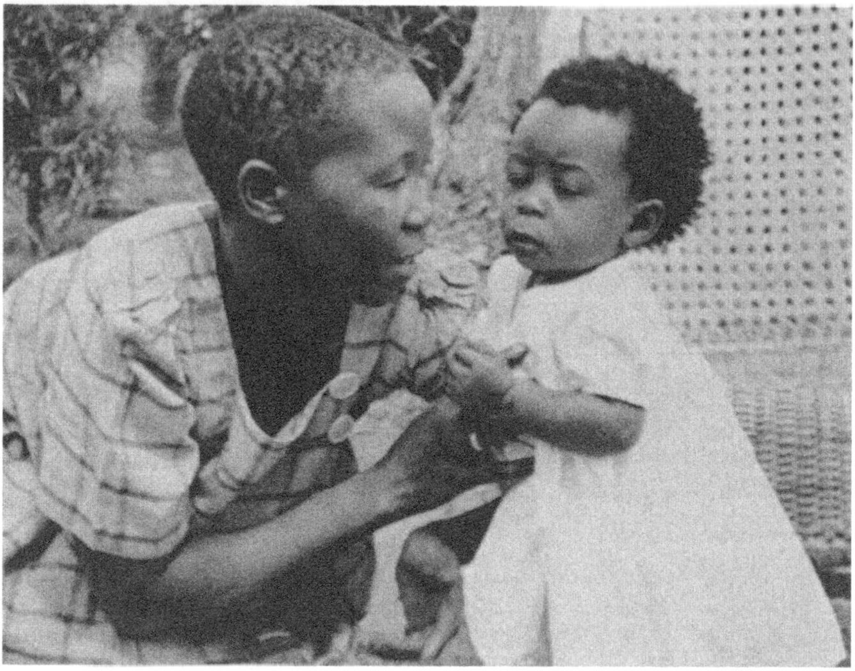

FIGURE 5 When his mother put him down, Muhamidi would not let her go.

At this last visit we introduced Dr. Marcell Géber, who arranged to administer the Gesell Developmental Schedules to him a few days later. She found him to have a global DQ of 130 and reported that he was active and *dynamique* during the testing. When he was twenty-two months old he was retested; he was interested in the test but was much less *dynamique,* and his DQ had dropped to 109. At thirty-four months of age he was retested again; he seemed sad and dull, and his DQ had dropped to 96. At the same time Dr. Géber tested Muhamidi's new baby brother, who was then seven months old, joyous, and *dynamique,* with a DQ of 142. Two years later when Muhamidi was nearly five, he was living with his grandmother and was not available for testing; his little brother was tested and was found to be sad and apathetic; he received a DQ of 76.

Visits to the Clinic

Age *wks.*	*Weight* *lbs.*	*Comments*
23	16.1	none
25	16.6	conjunctivitis, cold, fever
27	16.7	conjunctivitis
31	17.1	fever

13

EIGHT BABIES FROM RELATIVELY ACCULTURATED PROTESTANT FAMILIES

Waswa, Nakato, Nora, Kulistina, Senkumba, Nabatanzi, Nakiku, and Kasozi

The *muluka* chief was very helpful to us in finding the nucleus of our sample; he was motivated not merely to help us but also to help some of the families in his *muluka* who lived close to him and whose needs he knew. He first directed us to Nnalongo, the mother of twins who were already fourteen months old. Although these babies were outside of the age range in which I was most interested, they were still unweaned and thus met the major criterion I had mentioned to the chief. Nnalongo, mother of five children, had been deserted by her husband. She had no money for extra protein foods, and the twins were suffering from malnutrition. Next the chief directed us to the mothers of Nora and Kulistina, who were as affluent as Nnalongo was poverty stricken and who were wives of the same man, living in the same house with a large brood of children. Kulistina's mother was the senior wife, and particularly wanted to participate in the project because Kulistina was severely undernourished, breast feeding having failed. I had intended to limit the sample to breast-fed babies, but again I could not refuse to include Kulistina, both because she obviously needed the help the clinic could give her and because I wanted to observe Nora, who met all criteria and who lived in the same house.

At the same time the chief directed me to the mother of two-month-old Senkumba. The mother was a young girl and this was her first baby. She sought guidance both from Nnalongo who lived nearby and from the clinic. Another of the nuclear group was Nabatanzi, whose mother was unmarried and without support other than what she herself could provide. Finally there was Nakiku, who met all criteria and whose parents seemed to have a stable marriage and adequate though modest resources. But Nakiku had frequent colds and was delicate; her parents much wanted whatever help they could obtain from us and the clinic.

DOI: 10.4324/9781003629337-16

Nakiku's mother was a good friend of Kasozi's mother and worked quietly to bring us together. Kasozi's mother had been deserted by her husband and was struggling to survive. She too was concerned about infant nutrition and had looked to Nakiku's mother for guidance.

Waswa and Nakato: the older twins

Especially favored by God are the parents of twins; such is the Ganda belief. If one child is a treasured gift from God, twins represent great bounty. From the time of the birth of twins, the parents are no longer addressed by their own names but as *Ssalongo* and *Nnalongo*— father of twins and mother of twins. The twins themselves are given special names, according to sex and order of birth. If the first-born is a boy, he is Waswa; if the second-born is a girl, she is Nakato. Furthermore, the name of the next older sibling is changed to a special one, and the name of any later sibling designates whether he is first after twins, second after twins, and so on. The parents of twins seem to feel more bound to observe traditional customs than do the parents of single babies. For example, the mother of these twins felt that they should have been weaned when younger, but it seemed particularly important in the case of twins that the father be involved—and the father was unavailable to give the permission for weaning that seemed to be all important.

Nnalongo had five children, two boys aged ten and six years, a girl aged three and a half, and the twins. Her husband, with whom she had lived for many years, had been married before, and the first wife was considered the "legal" wife. When the twins were about two months old, he was appointed as chief in a distant *ggombolola.* He presumably believed that he could not take an *omukwano*—a "friend," or common-law wife—with him to his new post. So he abandonned Nnalongo and took his legal wife with him. His appointment was to a distant place, and, although he had promised to provide some support he had not done so, and, indeed, Nnalongo seemed to have lost touch with him entirely.

Living nearby, practically in the same household, was Mukulu (an old woman) whose relationship to Nnalongo was never clarified, and her daughter, a pleasant woman of about Nnalongo's age. The three women cooperated, worked the same garden, and to some extent shared the care of the children. The garden was their only resource. They were able to raise a small cash crop of millet from time to time, but the money from this was soon exhausted, and there was not enough to buy clothes for the oldest boy to wear to school, or for school fees, or for the extra milk that the twins needed so badly.

The twins themselves were thin, with heads too big for their bodies. Their skin was too pale, and their hair was too scanty, soft, and straight. They were sitting quietly, with their little legs tucked properly to the side, quite naked, beside a woman who was caring for them in their mother's absence. Soon the mother returned from the garden. The twins both cried immediately, crawled to their mother, who had seated herself on the floor, and clung. Throughout the rest of this brief initial visit they cried almost continuously, competing for her attention, clutching at her, trying to reach her breasts. Nakato, the girl, seemed especially frustrated and kept throwing herself backward as she cried. Nnalongo did not feed them, since, as it gradually emerged, she was reluctant to do so in my presence.

The twins had been born in hospital. They were breast-fed on a schedule set by the clock. Nnalongo implied that they had been fed four times a day at regular intervals—but it was not clear that this schedule had been used from the beginning. Supplementary feedings of milk were begun when they were four months old since then there was some money from the sale of millet with which to buy milk. Solid foods were begun at six months.

At first the twins developed normally, but they became increasingly undernourished and their rate of development slowed down. By the time our visits began the mother's milk was obviously inadequate for their needs, even with the supplementary solids, and there was no longer any money with which to buy dried milk to give them the protein that was so obviously lacking in their diet. In order to try to meet their needs, their mother now was feeding them every two hours, but they were chronically hungry and crying and clutching for the breast. In between feedings, the mother tried to comfort them by holding them, holding one on her lap, the other slung over her back, and jiggling them about as they fussed.

The twins slept in the same bed, one at one end and one at the other. They were restless at night, and when one woke up he wakened the other. They cried for long periods during the night, and were each given the breast two or three times. Nnalongo began " holding them down" at about two months of age. By fourteen months they had accomplished bowel control and rarely wet their bed, but they still wet in the house. During one of our early visits Nakato started to wet while on her mother's lap. Her mother held her out by one arm so that the trickle went on the dirt floor. Later, Waswa also wet the floor; the puddle threatened a mat on which the women were sitting; they held the mat up until the puddle had been absorbed by the dirt floor.

Both twins were said to have sat unsupported at four months. Nakato crawled first at about five months, Waswa a month later. Nakato could stand alone at thirteen months, but Waswa did not until nearly fifteen months.

A week after our first brief visit we paid a long visit. The twins sat close to their mother, scrambling over her restlessly, especially Nakato, who kept trying to open her mother's dress. For a while she sat on her mother's lap playing with two strings of beads, smiling, and swinging the beads around. Waswa, meanwhile, sat nearby quietly playing with a smaller string of beads, absorbed in them and not looking at anyone. Throughout, Nakato's play seemed oriented more toward people while Waswa's seemed withdrawn. Once the mother picked Waswa up and bounced him around. Nakato set up an outcry. Nnalongo put Waswa down and picked Nakato up, first taking her on her lap, where the little girl buried her face; then Nnalongo put her over her back and bounced her about as she held Waswa in her arms. Although there were lulls during the visit, the twins were demanding attention from their mother for at least half the time. Occasionally someone else would pick up one of them. The child would sit quietly when held, but as soon as he was put down he would creep to his mother.

Nnalongo said that while she worked in the garden she left the twins in care of one or the other of the two women because she could not work and look after them. They were said to be content while she was gone and "very happy" to see her come back.

At the clinic it was confirmed that they were undernourished. Nakato weighed 14.5 pounds and Waswa 12.5. The mother was given instructions about supplementary feedings, and we had already promised to give them a regular supply of dried skim milk. Both had chronic colds, running eyes and nose, for which they were treated, and Nakato also had an ear infection. Within a week they looked remarkably improved—more cheerful, more active, and more responsive.

At this visit the boys were home; each of them held a baby throughout at least half of our visit, affectionate, interested, and playful. I noticed the older of the boys kissing the baby he was holding. Nakato, in particular, seemed responsive to people. As one brother held her and bounced her about she smiled. Later, the other rocked her back and forth while holding her facing him on his knees, and she laughed gleefully. While Waswa was trying to cling to his mother, Nakato walked a few steps—nearly her first—and smiled and responded to the encouragement everyone gave her. She was active throughout the whole visit. Several times she walked, and several times she fell, but she did not cry. She permitted me to hold her for a while; she sat quietly, looking solemn. When I handed her back to her brother she smiled at me. For a while she played with a large tin funnel, for a while with an empty shoe polish tin. Then Waswa got hold of the funnel; Nakato dropped her tin and tussled with Waswa for the funnel; she won it. As she played with these objects she kept looking up at the people in the room.

Waswa was less responsive when held by his brother and finally he cried. He crept to his mother, and clutched at her, fussing for about ten minutes. Finally she soothed him by jouncing him on her back. When he was on the floor playing with an empty tin, he was completely absorbed in it and did not look up. Nevertheless, he paid some attention to others. For a while he sat looking around, saying "da-da-da-da," and for quite a long period he accepted being held by his brother. But he sat quietly, and once when rough play was begun he cried.

I inquired how the twins responded when the mother left the room. She said that they did not protest unless they were hungry. At one point, however, she did leave the room, and Waswa cried and began to follow her, despite having been left with familiar people.

On several subsequent visits the behavior of the twins was much the same. Nakato was active, exploring, creeping about, and demanding relatively little attention, while Waswa clung to his mother and seemed passive, even listless. Nnalongo attributed the difference to the fact that boys tended to cling to their mothers more than girls. Consequently, when they went to the clinic or elsewhere, it was Nakato who would be carried by someone else while Waswa clung to his mother.

At seventeen months of age Waswa began to walk; by this time Nakato was running about actively, her ankle bells tinkling. Waswa would not show off his new accomplishment for us, however. When his mother put him down he let his legs go limp and would not even stand. Nakato had begun to say *mama* appropriately. Each now held his own cup and was beginning to feed himself. Nakato weighed 17.5 pounds and Waswa 16.

Despite this general improvement in development, both babies still cried more than most of the other babies in our sample, and, according to the mother, more than their siblings had done at a comparable age. The crying was especially noticeable at feeding time. When one was suckling the breast, the other clamored for attention. At other times, also, the crying was largely for the mother's attention, there being much competition between them.

At eighteen months both babies had a setback—stomatitis. They cried a great deal and were disinclined to eat or drink. They had scarcely recovered from this when both had severe and persistent diarrhea, with vomiting and a fever. Nakato recovered fairly quickly and continued to gain; Waswa continued to be ill for about two weeks and lost weight. One unfortunate consequence of this illness was that the twins began to refuse to drink their supplementary milk. They refused it even when mixed with porridge. At a brief visit that we made when they were nineteen months old they had returned to the same kind of behavior they had shown five months before—both clutching at their mother's dress, trying to open it to get the breast, fussing and crying, and pushing each other away. Once the mother left the room for a moment. Waswa followed her but was stopped by a high doorsill and stood there screaming. At the next clinic visit it was found that the twins had each gained, despite their illnesses.

Nakato got diarrhea again and lost weight; Waswa escaped the illness and caught up with her at last. By twenty months both children were well again. Both

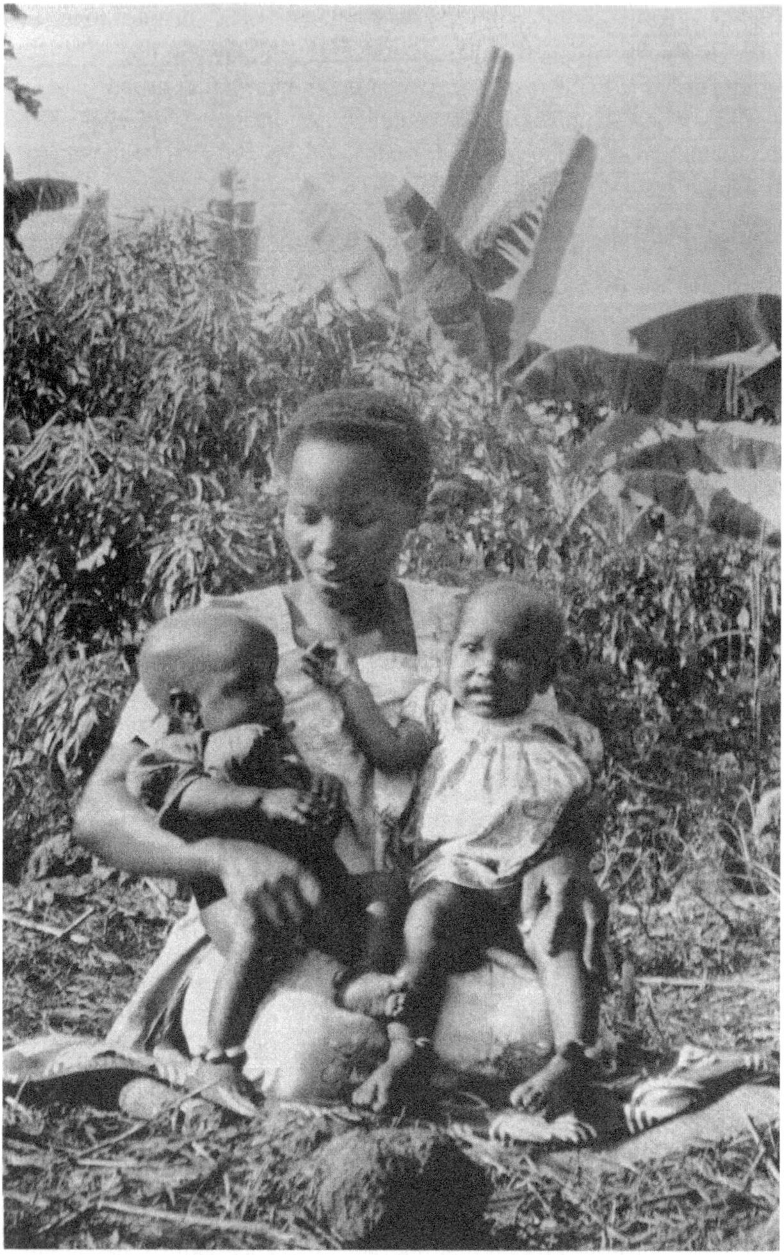

FIGURE 6 The older twins, Waswa and Nakato, with Nnalongo at sixteen and a half months. They are still undernourished and retarded in development.

knew three words, and could understand simple commands. Nakato was trying to say *aba* (bye-bye) but it did not always come out well. Nakato had been going out of the house on her own initiative to have bowel movements; Waswa still had his in the house. Bedwetting had long since ceased, although both still wet in the house. They were sleeping well.

Waswa was more responsive than I had seen him before. I coaxed him to come to me by holding out a candy. His mother urged him to go and gave him a little push from behind. To my surprise, he came, offered me an empty powder tin that he was holding, took the candy, and then took it straight to his mother and offered it to her. He came back for another, and when I said it was for his four-year-old sister, he took it to her, and so on until all members of the family had been given a piece of candy. Nakato was quieter than usual and played with some empty spools on the floor. She had two temper tantrums, one because something was taken away from her that she wanted to keep. Later she fussed a little and her mother jounced her on her back. She soon went to sleep and was put to bed. She woke in a while, and by the end of the visit both twins were clambering over the mother, fussing, and trying to get at her breasts.

Their mother said that they still followed her whenever she left the room, Waswa crying, although recently Nakato had stopped crying when following. Although their strongest attachment was to the mother, Nakato was strongly attached to the older of the two brothers, and Waswa to the younger. They both—but especially Nakato—showed attachment to the woman who lived in the hut next door, who had always helped care for them. Neither liked their four-year-old sister.

We had two further visits with this family, the last when the twins were twenty-one months old. At one clinic visit, both babies fussed almost continuously. Whenever Nnalongo picked one up the other would cry. Nakato had one tantrum so violent that it took her a long time to quiet down, even in her mother's arms; meanwhile, Waswa cried because he was not being held. Neither could be comforted by anyone else. Finally the mother strapped Nakato onto her back and held Waswa. At our final visit Nakato had three tantrums, all caused by her mother's interference with her taking something away from Waswa that he wanted to keep. She was soothed either by her mother or by her brother. When not fighting with Waswa or throwing herself about in a tantrum, she was active, responsive, smiling. Waswa, meanwhile, was reponsive to us only when candy was distributed. For the most part, he sat near his mother quietly. When Nakato tussled with him or hit him he did not fight back but cried helplessly until his mother comforted him.

Visits to the Clinic

	Waswa		Nakato	
Age mos.	*Weight lbs.*	*Comments*	*Weight lbs.*	*Comments*
Birth	5		6	
14	12.6	malnutrition, chronic cold	14.8	malnutrition, chronic cold
14.5	13.6		15.8	
15	14.0		16.0	diarrhea
16	15.7		17.0	
16.5	15.6	diarrhea	17.4	
17	16.0		17.6	fever
18	16.7		18.2	
18.5	18.3	stomatitis	18.3	stomatitis
19	14.7	fever, diarrhea	18.4	
20	17.1		18.6	cough
20.5	17.9		18.0	diarrhea
21	17.5		18.1	

Nora and Kulistina

Nora and Kulistina are half-sisters. Their father, a university graduate, had two wives. Indeed, he had three wives, if one counts an earlier one from whom he subsequently separated. There were several children of the first marriage, who visited the household during school holidays. Kulistina's mother was the second wife and she bore six children—a girl (seven and a half), a girl(five and a half), a boy (four), a girl (three), a girl (one and a half), and Kulistina, who was sixteen weeks of age when we began to visit. The eldest girl had started school, but the other five children were at home. Nora's mother was the third wife, and she had two children, a boy (two and a half) and Nora, who was twenty weeks old when began we to visit. In the household also was the child of a relative, a boy, who appeared to be mentally defective. He was said to be deaf and dumb. He was not deaf, but he was unable to talk. In total, therefore, there were eight children regularly present during our visits, plus a school girl and an assortment of half-siblings who were there during holidays.

This household was the most affluent that we visited. The house was made of brick and stucco and it had a tile roof. Inside, the floors were made of the same smooth cement that was used in the houses occupied by Europeans in Kampala. The house was built on the side of a small hill and therefore there was a flight of rather steep cement steps leading to the small veranda outside the front door. There was a garden, but it was not visible from the house. Despite its relative grandeur, this house lacked the grace of the wattle-and-daub house in which William lived. It looked rather like a new house in an American suburban development before there had been any shrubs or trees planted and before the lawn had become properly established.

The ladies did not have to spend their time gardening in order to raise food. They had enough money to employ men to work for them. Occasionally they complained that while labor cost more than it used to cost, the workmen did less and were so much less dependable than they used to be.

The father was a surveyor, and, although his work made it impossible for him to live at home, he managed to get home on weekends and usually once in the middle of the week. He owned a car, which made it possible for him to get home more frequently than other fathers who worked elsewhere. His university studies were evident from a bookcase full of textbooks which graced the living room.

There was a cooperative and pleasant relationship apparent between the two women—the mothers of Kulistina and Nora. Kulistina's mother was clearly the senior; she took the lead, both in determining how the household would be run and in our visits. Nora's mother accepted her leadership without apparent resentment, although on the few occasions when we saw her alone we found her much more communicative than when Kulistina's mother was also present. They shared the responsibility for the household and for the children. Both enjoyed sociability, and they found it convenient to spell each other off. One afternoon one would go visiting and the other would take care of all the children. Another afternoon the roles would be reversed. Whatever resentment they may have felt for each other was submerged beneath their keen appreciation of the advantages of the freedom implied in having a built-in baby-sitter.

With Kulistina's mother taking the lead, these ladies very much enjoyed our visits—as an opportunity to air their European refinements and to talk of matters which enlarged their horizons beyond the mundane affairs of the household. They liked to serve us tea, with all the proper English appurtenances. They gave us information about their babies and their child-care practices but were really more interested in talking about other things.

With Kulistina's mother again taking the lead, they were eager to be as Europeanized as they could. They had cribs for the babies, each being placed in the mother's room, and the babies—like proper European babies—spent much of their time in their cribs. They had learned that Europeans used scheduled feedings, so they followed suit. There was a complicated spiral here. On the one hand, they obviously valued being progressive and acculturated, but, on the other hand, they unerringly selected from among the infant-care practices that they observed to be European those which would give them freedom from being tied to a baby in the same way that traditional Ganda practices tied a mother to her baby. Even with all that they had done and could do for each other to make for flexibility and freedom, they —with Kulistina's mother as spokesman—said that life was difficult with the father away so much, and with the need to spend so much time at home with the children.

The house was indeed full of children. The children were active and spontaneous. They did not sit quietly during visits with their toes tucked in politely. They could manage the traditional Ganda child role for a while, but then their controls relaxed and they became rambunctious. Kulistina's mother asked our advice repeatedly; she wanted to know how to get the children to be obedient and disciplined. In our sample she was almost unique in feeling discipline to be a problem. I could not take her concern too seriously because, by conventional Western standards, the children did not seem to be unduly uncontrolled. Indeed, the older children seemed more polite and controlled than children of comparable age in the West.

Cleanliness was emphasized in this family. The women were fastidious in their own dress, and the children always were clean and well-dressed when we visited. The house was clean and well-kept.

Kulistina was the only baby in the sample who had been bottlefed throughout. Her mother tried breast feeding for the first three days but said that she gave it up "because the milk did not come." She said the same thing had happened with two of the other children. Kulistina weighed 6.5 pounds at birth; when our visits began she weighed 8.5 pounds. She had been fed through an imported, commercial baby formula; probably the mother made it too dilute, for Kulistina had not gained well. She was fed five times during the day and once at night and also received orange juice. At first she cried a great deal but by sixteen weeks she cried less, although still more than her siblings had at a comparable age. Her mother said that she slept most of the time; in any event, she spent most of the time in her crib in her mother's room, alone except at night.

Throughout our first visit she lay quietly in her mother's arms, sometimes sucking her fingers. She was extremely thin, with arms and legs like pipestems. She was not apathetic, however. She seemed to take an active interest in her environment. Several times she smiled widely at me from across the room, although I had done nothing to elicit a smile.

Her mother was concerned about her, and at the next clinic visit the doctor confirmed that she was undernourished, although nothing else appeared to be wrong. She recommended that the mother discontinue the imported formula, and, until the baby had pulled out of her undernourished state, a formula of fresh cow's milk was to be used. Kulistina responded to the new formula and started to gain at a steady rate of about a half-pound a week. Other foods were gradually added to her diet. At the last clinic visit, when she was forty-six weeks old, she weighed 17 pounds.

Kulistina had become so accustomed to being left alone in her crib that she did not cry when put down and left, nor did she cry to be picked up—and this continued to the end of the project. Her mother felt too busy to hold her after feedings except in the afternoon after she had finished her work. When the baby cried her mother did not pick her up unless the crying continued persistently. Since someone was always at home to "mind" the children, Kulistina was rarely taken anywhere, and, indeed, she was rarely carried. Nora's mother shared in her care, and the other children gave her some attention, even the three-year-old sister.

Although the mother had used a potty in training the other children, she did not with Kulistina, but, rather, "held her down." She did not do this consistently, however. Since she often woke up alone, her mother, being elsewhere, did not know she had awakened and did not "catch her" before she soiled. Since bowel movements often went unnoticed, Kulistina sometimes smeared her feces. Her mother took this as a natural outcome of not being cleaned up immediately. When finally she was taken up and dressed, she usually was diapered with *amerikani* cloth and sometimes had an additional diaper of waterproof material on top.

The visits came to have a characteristic pattern. We were usually met by the children first, who rushed out turbulently and then dropped to their knees for the traditional greetings. Then the ladies appeared, cordial and gracious. Each woman had her own special place in the room to sit. After unrolling her mat she would settle down, and the children would sort themselves out so that Nora's brother sat by their mother, and the other children sat with theirs. After a while, tea was usually served, and the children began to play, sometimes outside but sometimes in the living room. We tried to steer the conversation to the babies, but Kulistina's mother, especially, preferred to talk of other things. In due course, first one, then the other, would disappear to get her baby, and after a delay while the baby was being dressed in her best clothes, they would reappear and sit down, each holding her own baby.

When we visited at twenty-one weeks, Kulistina was brought in by her half-sister, who was visiting during school holidays. The half-sister held her throughout the visit; for a while Kulistina sat supported and for a while she stood supported. She seemed more active than before. She smiled across the room at me, at her mother, who was closer, and at her sister, who kept making affectionate little faces at her.

She continued to smile frequently and indiscriminately. At a brief visit when she was twenty-seven weeks old, I held her for most of the time, and she responded to me as readily as she responded to her mother or to anyone else.

When she was twenty-nine weeks old she could sit with the soles of her feet together, propped up by her hands. She sat in this position for quite a while, looking about, seemingly interested in everything. She did not vocalize at all, however. Indeed, I had not yet heard her make a sound, except when crying. But by thirty-one weeks vocalization had begun. She sat on her mother's lap, making baby sounds, smiling at her mother, and—and this was new—playing with her mother's face and dress. About this time she began to crawl and within a week she was able to pull herself to a standing position in her crib.

When we visited at thirty-three weeks, Kulistina sat on her mother's lap for a while and then on Mrs. Kibuka's. Wherever she sat, she smiled cheerfully at the person holding her and at others in the room; she did not appear to smile more fully, more readily, or more frequently at her mother than at anyone else. She was also held by her two sisters, who seemed very fond of her. She responded readily to them also. She was most active with her mother, however. When her mother held her standing, she waved her arms and seemed very pleased with herself. And for a while she played with her mother's face. Once during the visit she spat up quite a bit—the only baby in the sample who was observed to spit up. We inquired whether she had begun to follow her mother when she learned to crawl and were told that she very rarely had.

When we visited at forty weeks we inquired whether Nora's mother ever fed or bathed Kulistina, and vice versa. The women were shocked that we might think a woman would look after her own baby only. Whoever prepared the food

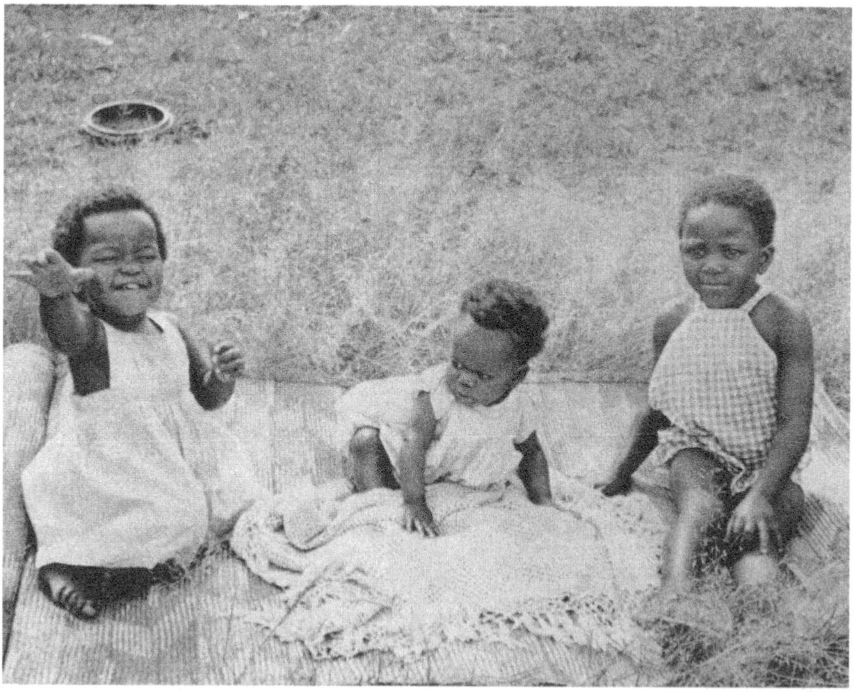

FIGURE 7 Kulistina in the center is thirty-three weeks old. Her sisters are one year and three years old.

for one would feed both, and so it was with baths. Sometimes one of the older children helped feed the babies. Kulistina was said "to know her own mother" and also to know her father when he came home. She accepted being cared for by other people and was not at all afraid of strangers. She was still said to sleep most of the time but by this time she cried very little.

During the visit she sat on Mrs. Kibuka's lap, and, although she smiled frequently as usual she was very quiet. Finally she wet and was handed to her mother. Kulistina continued to wet while her mother held her in a standing position on the floor. The children were sent to get her dry clothes. As her mother took off her "waterproof" panties, Kulistina sucked her thumb. Her mother told us that she could stand supporting herself with her hands on the wall, and that if one held her hands, she could support her weight and bounce up and down, enjoying herself very much. Although she told us about this while she held Kulistina, she did not demonstrate this accomplishment. Her mother said that she was given toys to play with, but she did not play with them much—not nearly as much as Nora.

At our last visit at forty-seven weeks, Kulistina was said to have been quite ill. She was taken to a doctor in Kampala, received an injection, and was much better the next day when we visited. When her mother went to her room to get her up we heard crying, which was unusual. During the visit she sat for a long time on the lap of a visitor and was very friendly. She became increasingly active, and when placed on the floor she kept pulling herself up into a standing position. She could stand unsupported and had been able to for two weeks. She fell twice but did not cry. She vocalized a lot but spoke no real words yet. She could respond to her name and to several simple commands. Her mother said that she had not established bowel control and still soiled the bed.

We inquired about "beating." Her mother said that she had spanked her once, when she was crying continuously and "would not stop." Her mother got so angry at the crying that she spanked her hard, and, of course, Kulistina cried harder than ever.

Despite her initial malnutrition, Kulistina was judged by the doctor to be in good health and to be developing normally. She was notable in this sample, however, for her lack of differential response to her mother. She was friendly with everyone. She did not cry when her mother left the room nor did she follow.

Nora was reared in the same way as Kulistina, except that she was breast-fed rather than bottle-fed and suffered no malnutrition. The breast feeding was scheduled in the same way as Kulistina's bottle feedings, about every four hours, and once during the night. She weighed 6.5 pounds at birth and by twenty-eight weeks of age weighed 16 pounds. She had received no supplementary feedings by that time. She could sit unsupported by three months of age. During our visit at twenty-one weeks, she gurgled and cooed in her mother's arms, living up to her mother's description of her as a "very happy child." For a while she stood supported on her mother's lap while her mother nuzzled her affectionately. For a while she chewed her own hands and her mother's as well. When I held her in my arms she did not babble as much as when held by her mother. Her mother said that she was "good" with all people and as happy with Kulistina's mother as with her own.

When she was six months of age solid foods were begun—*matooke*, porridge, papaw and sweet bananas—not every day, but several times a week. Nora seemed to like these but rejected milk that her mother tried to give her as a supplement to breast feeding. She continued to refuse milk, although her mother managed to get her to take a little—from a cup.

On our visit at thirty-three weeks, there was a long delay before Nora was brought out by her mother. She looked fat, well-developed, but had rather a sober expression. She sat quietly on her mother's lap for a while and then, when put on the floor, began to crawl quite actively, although still very flat on her tummy. Her mother tried to keep her on the clean mat, but she kept getting onto

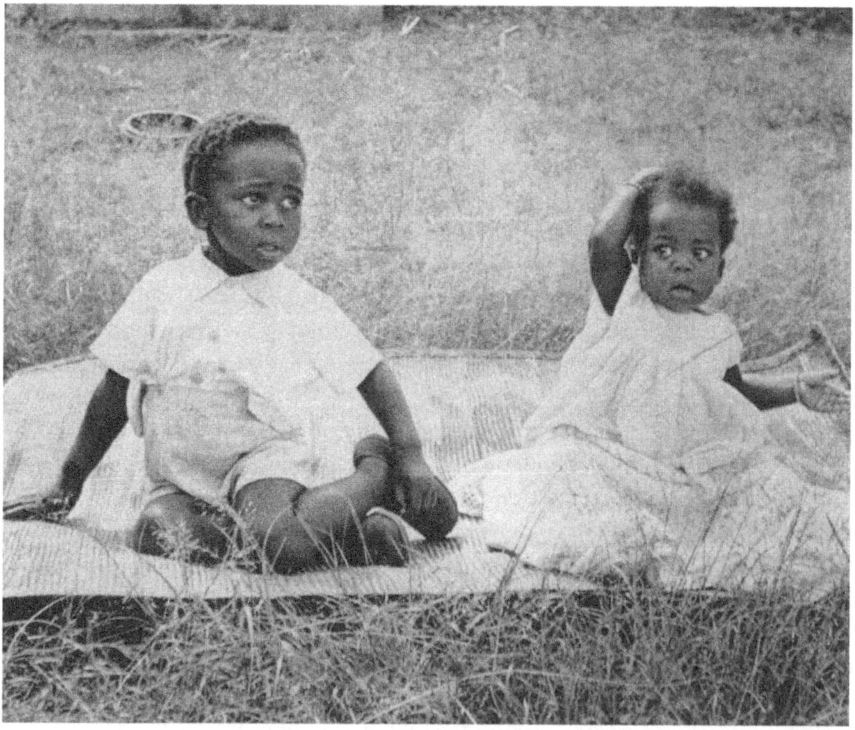

FIGURE 8 Nora at thirty-nine weeks with her two-and-a-half-year-old brother. This makes five children under four years of age in this household.

the floor and had to be pulled back. Her mother said that she had been crawling for a week.

At thirty-nine weeks she was held by Mrs. Kibuka. She seemed quite content and interested in Mrs. Kibuka and in the pencil with which I was writing. She kept grabbing for it. She was handed to her mother when she started to wet. Her mother removed her panties, and then lugged her outside, holding her by her arms. When they returned she was placed on the mat beside her mother, but she was anxious to creep about—sometimes on hands and knees and sometimes on all fours. She was wearing a pretty little smocked dress, but she kept stepping on her skirt. Perhaps because of her dress, but also because of the danger that she might go out to the veranda and fall down the steep steps, her mother kept pulling her back to the mat. Nora protested each time she was pulled back and several times hit out at her mother. As soon as she was released, she escaped again; if she was held on her mother's lap, she cried. Her mother said she could pull herself to a standing position and could cruise while holding onto the railing of her crib.

Like Kulistina, Nora was "held down"—after feeding and when she woke, but, like Kulistina, she spent so much of her time alone in her crib that she often was not "caught" and smearing was a problem.

Like Kulistina, Nora did not cry when her mother left the room. Although she could creep, she did not follow her mother unless she was very hungry. Similarly, she did not cry to be picked up except when hungry. Her mother usually held her for a while after feeding and after her bath—perhaps somewhat more than Kulistina was held. Moreover, Nora was picked up by her mother when she cried but Kulistina was not.

At this visit the mother said that she planned to wean Nora in about a month; she promised to give us advance warning. Meanwhile, some new foods had been added to her diet, and she had begun to feed herself solids after a fashion, although her mother preferred to feed her by spoon. The daytime feedings were dropped when she was forty-three weeks old—but we received no advance warning. When we visited a week later, her mother was absent, and it was from Kulistina's mother that we received the news. We heard Nora crying in her room throughout the visit, but no one went to her.

When we visited again at forty-five weeks her mother said that Nora had not cried much when her daytime breast feedings were stopped and that her behavior was much the same as before. She did, however, try to reach her mother's breasts, and her mother had to hold her in a position so that she could not reach them. This effort had continued. The only other change was that she wet the bed more frequently than before. Her mother said that it was a relief to wean the baby.

Nora smiled at me several times during the visit—for the first time. She sat on her mother's lap for a while, and then began crawling about. As before, her mother kept pulling her back. Nora seemed frustrated and protested. Her mother said that she was crying because she was hungry. Finally her mother tucked her pretty little dress into the string of beads she wore around her waist and she crept around without interference. For a while she sat on Mrs. Kibuka's lap and seemed content. She was said to have stood alone a month before. I noticed her taking a couple of steps unsupported, but her mother insisted that she could not yet walk.

Final weaning took place at forty-eight weeks. On the first night when Nora had wakened to be fed, her mother had held and cuddled her without feeding her. Since then she had slept through the night without waking. Her mother said that she had not been crying during the daytime and then corrected this to say that she had been fussy but that this was because she had a cold. Moreover, she had cried a lot the first night, but that was because she had a fever. I wondered why the mother had selected a time when Nora was ill to begin her final weaning.

When we visited at fifty weeks this information was confirmed. Since final weaning, however, she had not tried to get at her mother's breast. Indeed, when ever she caught sight of it she gave her mother the impression that "she did not care for it." There had been no change in her behavior otherwise. She put playthings in her mouth but no more than before. She did not follow her mother and, indeed, had rarely done so. She was eating well. She wet, but not more than usual. She regularly got angry when anyone interfered with her activities, but this also was characteristic of her previous behavior.

Nora was in her bed when we arrived. When her mother went to fetch her we could hear intermittent crying behind the scences. After she was brought in she was quiet for a moment on her mother's lap and then squirmed to the floor and began to creep about on all fours. Her skirt was long enough that she kept stepping on it, but it was not long enough to cover her. It hitched up over her bare bottom, and fell away in front so that her long and pendulous umbilical hernia was quite visible. For a while she seemed to want to get out into a back room, from which issued the voices of the other children who had not been permitted to come in because they had not yet had their baths and hence, presumably, were not fit to be seen by visitors. Nora stood at the door and said "da-da-da-da" quite fiercely to her mother when she was dragged away from the door, but she did not cry. She smiled at her mother from time to time. Her mother presently went out of the room, but Nora seemed to pay no attention to this. When her mother came back she crept towards her eagerly, laughing. I thought she was welcoming her mother, but she continued past her mother through the open door, to the back room where she had wanted to go all along. Her mother pulled her back. Nora protested. Nora was very active, and her mother kept interfering; once Nora bit her hand. Finally, she got hold of a child's exercise book and played with it roughly, trying to tear it through. Her mother took the book away. Nora was determined to have it back and tussled with her mother for it. Her mother gave in and permitted her to have it. Nora then came over to offer it to me and did not take it away until I offered it back to her. There were no playthings in the room to give her instead of the book.

She did a little walking during the visit, having begun to walk two weeks before. She could say *mama*, *taata* and *laba* (look!). She understood *jjangu* (come here!) but often would not come. She seemed to know *mpa* (give it to me), but when asked to surrender something she was holding, she would hold out the other, empty hand.

Her mother said that she still soiled the bed and she felt that it was taking an unusually long time to train her. She said that she did not soil anywhere else in the house, but shortly after that Nora had a bowel movement in the corner of the room.

Nora was said to treat Kulistina's mother much as she did her own. She followed neither, and did not cry when either left the room. She smiled at her mother from time to time but smiled at us equally often. She behaved quite independently of her mother during our visit, and this was said to be characteristic of her. Her biting of her mother when frustrated was also said to be characteristic—either biting or hitting. She was said sometimes to bite or hit her brother, who is two years older, and to reduce him to tears. She was said to play with Kulistina, often cheerfully and laughing, but sometimes they would fight, and Kulistina, although smaller, could fight back. She was said to get on with the other children in the household, but she was especially fond of one older half-sister who visited the house only on school holidays. This half-sister and her father were her favorite people. When her father was at home Nora awoke at night calling *taata.* And during the day she was exceptionally active, going to him, going away, and coming back, laughing. She was said not to be afraid of strangers and, indeed, she sometimes responded to our advances, sometimes smiled spontaneously; for the most part, however, she paid little attention to us. She paid little attention to her mother, for that matter, except when her mother interfered with her activity.

Her mother had begun to "beat" her, giving her little slaps on her arm to correct her, but a cupped hand was used so as not to hurt or sting. Nora understood the words "I will beat you," and whenever her mother threatened to do so, she would hit her first.

Visits to the Clinic

	Nora		Kulistina	
Age wks.	*Weight lbs.*	*Comments*	*Weight lbs.*	*Comments*
Birth	6.5		6.5	
18			8.6	cold, malnutrition
20			9.6	
24	16.3	fever	10.8	cold
26			11.2	
28	17.3		12.5	
30	18.3		12.9	cough
32	18.5		13.2	
34	18.5	cold	14.0	
36			14.3	
38			14.9	
40	19.4			
42	19.7		16.1	
44				fever, diarrhea
46	20.5		17.0	cold
50	21.5			

Senkumba

Senkumba's mother was a girl of sixteen, the second wife of a driver who commuted in the evenings from his work in town. She had been married for only a year when Senkumba was born and seemed inexperienced and insecure in the role of mother. She was, however, eager to learn and thus was a willing participant in the project. She lived close to Nnalongo, the mother of the older twins, and often sought help and advice from her.

When we first visited the family, the first wife was also present, but before we had an opportunity to sense what kind of relationship there was between the two women, the first wife went away for a long visit. She returned after a month's absence, and not long after that Senkumba and his mother went away. We saw the first wife on several occasions; she was the least friendly of all the women we had been seeing, and it seemed that she was jealous of our interest in Senkumba and his mother. It emerged in time that Senkumba's mother had taken him to live with her own parents. Mrs. Kibuka got the impression that there had been a quarrel with the husband and with the first wife. It was two months before we found out how to contact her, but then we visited her at her parents' home. A month later she had returned to her husband.

Senkumba was eight weeks old when we first visited him. He was ill with a fever, which was diagnosed the next day at the clinic as malaria. He weighed 12.5 pounds.

We were told that he had been born at home but that three days after his birth his mother had become ill and had spent three weeks in hospital. Senkumba accompanied her, and although for a time her milk gave out, the flow resumed and he was totally breast-fed. His mother was concerned about him, feeling that he was a small baby because of her own illness at the beginning.

She tried to feed him according to a schedule. She believed that if a baby was fed on demand, that is, when he cried, he cried more, ate less, and gained more slowly than if fed on schedule. But Senkumba's schedule was flexible. He was fed upon waking, again in the morning before his mother went to work in the garden, and again when she returned. During the afternoon he was fed at intervals and he was fed whenever he woke during the night, which was usually only twice. He slept with his mother in her bed.

When we arrived for this visit we found Senkumba alone in the living room crying, lying on the floor on a damp cloth which looked like an old dress. He stopped crying when I picked him up and held him in my arms. He did not cry again during the visit, and his mother said that he cried very little. His mother returned and bustled around to make us comfortable. Mrs. Kibuka suggested that the cloth upon which he had been lying was too wet and cold (it was raining hard that day), and that she should find a dry one. His mother took this suggestion willingly and found another cloth. Then we settled down. For most of the visit the mother held Senkumba in her arms, patting him, slowly, regularly, and rather hard, on his legs. Shortly after we arrived, she gave him the breast, and he fed eagerly and steadily. After his feeding he was cheerful and smiling.

His mother told us that she usually worked in the garden while Senkumba was having his morning nap; she sometimes left him with her neighbor, Nnalongo. He usually cried when left with other people, however.

Two weeks later Senkumba was ill again. His mother had misunderstood the doctor's instructions and had not given him his weekly antimalarial drug when it was due. Three days later when we visited, she said that his fever had subsided as soon as she had given him his medicine. During the visit he was very active, scrambling over his mother while she held him on her lap, babbling a great deal. He seemed hungry, but his mother did not feed him.

Again, when he was twelve weeks old, he was active and cheerful. He was active on Mrs. Kibuka's lap, kicking vigorously and blowing bubbles. When returned to his mother's lap, he became very fussy, seemingly hungry, but she did not feed him. His mother told us that after he had been fed she put him down in his crib (a new acquisition) and left him to cry until he went to sleep.

He had just begun to sit. His mother demonstrated this for us, arranging his feet with the soles together in front of him and propping him forward on his hands so that he could not fall over. It was not, of course, setting erect and unsupported. He was said to know his father, who liked to hold him and play with him. The father helped to give Senkumba his bath if he had not already had it when he came home in the evening.

A period followed during which our visits were either very brief or confined to the clinic. At the clinic Senkumba's mother usually did something to bring disapproval upon herself. Once, when Senkumba was only eight weeks old, she was scolded for picking him up by one arm, as Ganda women often pick their babies up, even the tiny ones. And once she allowed him to play with and finally eat the clinic chit. Moreover, he had two more illnesses. Through this period, he struck us as being sober and subdued.

At twenty-one weeks, however, he seemed very well, active, responsive, and he was babbling a lot. His body was plump, well-shaped, and his color was good. He was dressed in a little gold-colored sun dress—his usual garb for special occasions—and he had blue beads around his waist and ankles. He had lost the very sober, almost sulky look that he had seemed to have for some weeks. By this time he could sit erect indefinitely. His mother held him on her lap for a while, holding him in a standing position. He hummed and made happy noises. Later he began to fuss and finally to cry. His mother patted him, rocked him, talked to him, and finally succeeded in soothing him. He sat on her lap, babbling, rolling about actively, trying to put his foot in his mouth, and occasionally smiling at me. I held him for a while when his mother was out of the room, and he was cheerful and responsive.

There were two problems. He had a profuse discharge from his eyes, which had not responded to the drops that his mother had been given at the clinic. His mother kept wiping the discharge away with her fingers. She listened attentively while Mrs. Kibuka explained the importance of using a clean, white cloth for this purpose. Also, he had begun to cry, for no apparent reason, in the middle of a breast feeding. She wondered whether he was not getting enough milk and was angry.

Supplementary foods had been started recently—bean soup from a small glass, papaw by spoon, and *matooke* with sauce given from his mother's fingers. His mother said that he sucked two fingers frequently, especially when crying from hunger. "Holding down" had begun at three months of age, after each feeding.

Senkumba was just beginning to crawl—flat on his tummy but making headway.

Despite the crying in the midst of feeding and his spell of crying during the visit, his mother said that he cried little. His mother said: "He is a good child who lets me do my work." He was said to accept being left with the other wife, but when his mother returned he lifted his arms and shouted.

Our next real visit with Senkumba did not occur until he was thirty-seven weeks old; he was then living with his maternal grandparents. This visit was very difficult at first. The grandfather first inquired whether I had permission from the chiefs to visit African families. Then he said he did not welcome me in his home because I was English, because the English had taken his *Kabaka* away. He then strode from the room. Assuming he could still hear me (and could understand English), I asked Mrs. Kibuka to explain that I was not English. He came back with a manner that was pleasant and courteous—as, indeed, it had been all along, despite the content of our exchange—and said that I was European and it amounted to the same thing. He explained that he would have welcomed Europeans to his home before the *Kabaka* was exiled, and he would again welcome them after the *Kabaka* returned, but he could not welcome them while the *Kabaka* was away. I said that I did not wish to offend him and made a move to go, whcreupon he said that I could stay if I liked and added that his daughter had agreed to answer my questions. He had just wanted to make it clear how he felt. Meanwhile, Senkumba's mother and grandmother sat nearby, undisturbed by the whole exchange.

Senkumba was said to be developing well. He crept about very actively and could now pull himself into a standing position, holding onto someone or something. He had stopped soiling his bed when six months of age but was still wetting the bed occasionally. He could imitate noises and vocalized a lot—"ja-ja-ja-ja" and "brrrrrr." He responded to his name and understood simple commands. He had become a very active child who liked to make noise and he was particularly fond of beating an empty oil tin as though he were beating a drum.

When we arrived Senkumba was out in the yard, crawling about actively. He was taken away to be dressed, and returned in a sundress with a very full, long skirt. At first he sat on Mrs. Kibuka's lap where he remained quiet for a long time. Finally he whimpered and was returned to his mother. He stopped crying and soon was smiling and crawling about near his mother. He got up on all fours and began to shake his head from side to side, almost as though he were imitating an animal. He made happy sounds and became increasingly vocal. At one point he knelt before the door and patted it happily. He was active in his creeping about but then he returned to his mother, lay back against her knees, and smiled up at her. We went outside to take photographs. When he was settled on a mat for a solo, he explored a handbag that had been given him and did not fuss when his mother moved away. Before we left he sat on my lap for a while and was moderately responsive to my attention, but without the spontaneity he showed his mother.

His mother told us that he was still breast-fed but that he was getting, in addition to solid foods, tea with cow's milk in it, by cup. He was said to cry very little, and not unless hungry, tired or unhappy. He ordinarily did not protest when his mother left the room. He would follow her if she was leaving him alone, but often he did not if he was left with someone else. His mother

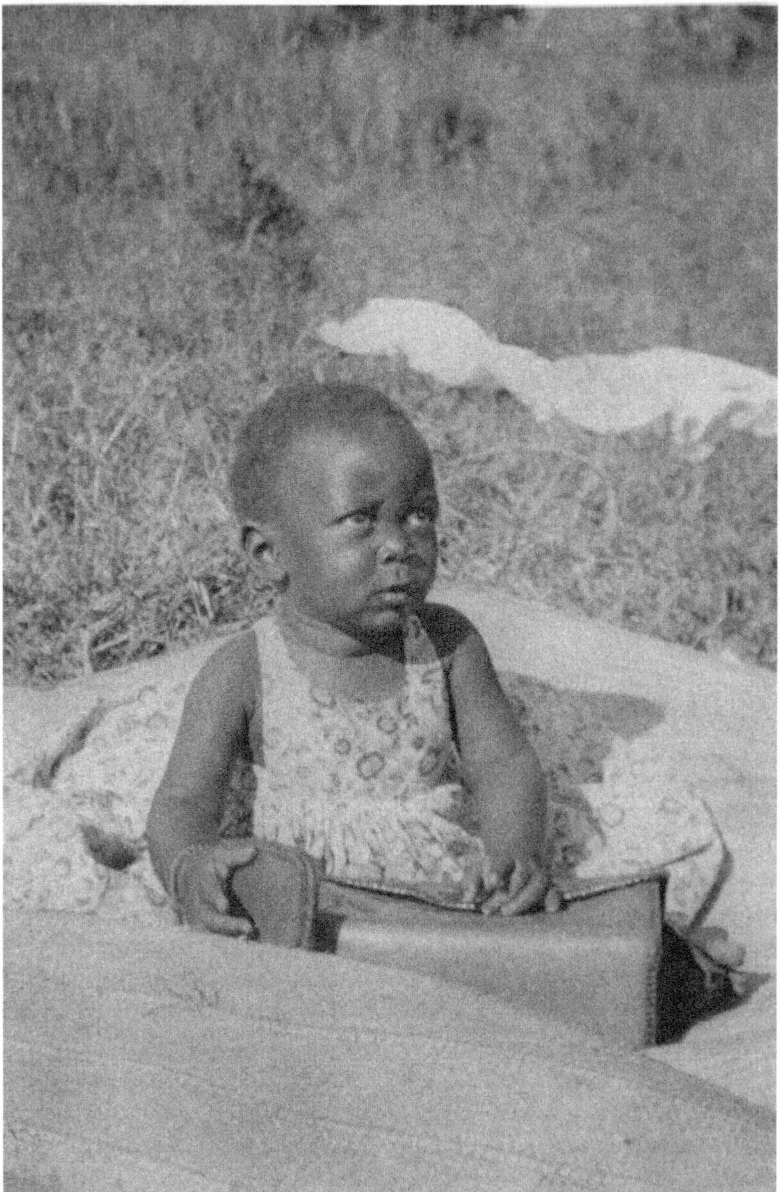

FIGURE 9 Senkumba at thirty-seven weeks did not fuss when his mother moved off—but he watched her as he fingered a handbag. Notice his full skirt.

rarely left him for any period of time, but one day she left him for the entire morning, and he did not cry at all. He was said to like people; he was quite willing to leave his mother to cross the room when someone else invited him to play.

He had become capable of real anger. He became angry when prevented from having something he wanted. When angry, he cried hard and was not easily soothed. Sometimes he became so upset that he would refuse the breast. His mother had begun to "beat" him. Sometimes she spanked him when he became very angry. She smacked his fingers to stop his masturbating.

This was the last long visit we had with Senkumba. Shortly after they returned home, the project ended.

Visits to the Clinic

Age wks.	*Weight lbs.*	*Comments*
8	12.4	malaria, enlarged spleen, conjunctivitis
10	13.5	improved
12	14.6	
16	14.6	
18	15.5	
20	16.0	
22	16.0	
24	17.2	

Nabatanzi

Nabatanzi's mother was a big, robust, cheerful teenager; she was unmarried. She and Nabatanzi lived in a tiny two-roomed hut across the compound from a larger house occupied by the maternal grandmother, maternal great-aunt, and two children. One child, a six-year-old boy, was the son of the maternal great-aunt, and the other, a three-year-old girl, was her granddaughter. The maternal grandmother was frail and could do no heavy work. Most of the cultivation of the food crops was undertaken by Nabatanzi's mother. The older women took charge of the children throughout much of the day, although most of the routine care of the baby was still her mother's responsibility. They were very poor, for there was no regular cash income. The maternal grandfather worked as a houseboy in a town thirty miles away, but presumably made little contribution to the household. Nabatanzi's father, a driver in a distant town, visited occasionally, and after Nabatanzi was weaned he contributed some money to buy milk for her.

Whatever the disgrace attached to unmarried motherhood, it rode lightly on this mother's broad young shoulders. She was delighted with her baby and played with her joyously. She welcomed our visits for the opportunity they gave her to talk about Nabatanzi and to soak up the pleasure given by our admiration of her attractive, plump, responsive baby. The older women also enjoyed the baby and were bound in ties of mutual affection and interdependence with each other and with the young mother. Despite their poverty and worry about the future, this seemed to be a solid, happy family.

Nabatanzi was born at home, with the assistance of the maternal grandmother. She was breast-fed "whenever she was hungry," and her mother enjoyed the feedings. Supplementary feedings of solid foods were begun when she was five months old. She slept in her own bed, which was placed so close to her mother's that when she awoke at night her mother could take her up for feeding without getting out of bed. "Holding down" began at four months of age. Nabatanzi was said to have sat alone at three months and to have begun to crawl at five and a half months.

She was thirty weeks old when we began to visit. She looked healthy and well-nourished. She coughed slightly from time to time, but her mother was not concerned and said that the baby was rarely ill. She wore a single garment, a faded little dress, and a double string of blue beads around her waist.

We crowded into the front room of the tiny hut for the visit—mother, baby, Mrs. Kibuka, and I, and the two older children, who sat quietly and properly in a corner. There was no room for the great-aunt, who sat on a mat outside the door. For a while she held Nabatanzi, who seemed happy, squirming about and grunting. The baby appeared to be equally comfortable with her mother and her great- aunt and showed her preference chiefly by the fact that when put down on the floor, she spent most of the time close to her mother, although she crept about vigorously and made several excursions away from her mother. She was said to be content when left either with the great- aunt or with the grandmother, both of whom played with her affectionately and sang to her. She was said to have no use for the other children, however. During our visit she smiled frequently and responded cheerfully to our advances, showing no shyness of strangers.

When we visited at thirty-one weeks the mother went to fetch Nabatanzi from the other house, where she was being looked after by the great-aunt. As they returned across the compound, the mother paused, held the baby high in the air, and smiled at her, making affectionate faces. Once in the hut, she held Nabatanzi on her lap. The baby was very active in scrambling over her mother, babbling happily, and occasionally looking curiously at me. After a while she began to slap at her mother's dress, trying to reach the breast. Finally her mother gave it to her. Nabatanzi sucked greedily, snorting with pleasure, squeezing the breast with her hands. She was given only one breast, although her mother had said that she usually gave both in a feeding. I could only assume that the mother was too modest to let her dress down to give the other breast. Nabatanzi was said to be very active. When tea is being served she creeps about and picks up the cups and would break them if not watched constantly. When she is given solid food she is so eager that she grabs the food before it can be fed to her and feeds herself with her fingers.

I asked the mother what infant-care customs her own mother had taught her. She first replied that her mother had told her about supplementing breast milk with solid foods, but then she went on to tell of other things her mother had taught her: how to greet visitors, how to sit properly when having food, how to do all that she can to help others, how to wash dishes and clean the house, and to give to other people and not to hold everything back for herself. This list was given quickly and readily and seems to sum up many of the feminine standards esteemed by the Ganda.

By thirty-seven weeks Nabatanzi had begun to stand alone. Her mother had encouraged this development by standing the baby up and singing a little song, accompanied by clapping her hands: "She can stand by herself without falling down." This was demonstrated for Mrs. Kibuka, who visited by herself that day. Nabatanzi was with her grandmother when Mrs. Kibuka arrived. The grandmother went off to fetch the mother, leaving the baby behind with the stranger. Nabatanzi sat quietly and did not cry. When her mother arrived, however, Nabatanzi crept to her quickly, crowing with delight. Later in the visit the two women went out to the garden to find some fruit to send to me, and Nabatanzi was again left behind. Again she sat quietly until her mother returned. On the occasion of another unannounced visit, Mrs. Kibuka found Nabatanzi in the care of the six-year-old boy; all the women were absent. She was asleep on a mat, covered with a cloth.

At forty weeks, when the women accompanied the visitors into the house, leaving the baby behind outside, she followed them, creeping quickly. She sat on her mother's lap for a while, then crept over to the little boy to play with him for a moment, then back to her mother. Her mother sang the little song to prompt her to stand up, but Nabatanzi was too busy eating a piece of candy to respond.

At forty-two weeks Nabatanzi began to walk—quite on her own initiative and without "training." When we visited two weeks later, however, she did not demonstrate her new accomplishment. She was quiet throughout the visit. Her mother believed she was quiet because she had just wakened from a nap, but I sensed that she was subdued because of the presence of a white stranger, for I had not been able to visit for two months. Admiring her plump legs, I touched her foot gently, and Nabatanzi responded with a whimper. She sat quietly on her mother's lap and fixed me with an intent stare. After a while she clutched at her mother's dress, trying to reach the breast, but did not persist in this when her mother did not respond. She then lay back against her mother, still watching me intently. I offered her a piece of candy, which she accepted readily. Her little fingers busied themselves in an attempt to remove the paper wrapper. Her mother took the candy away to remove the wrapper; Nabatanzi cried in sharp protest but stopped as soon as the candy was returned to her. She spent the rest of our visit happily with the candy.

All the women agreed that Nabatanzi was not usually shy of strangers, but as she continued to be subdued during the visit, they agreed that she was, in fact, shy of me, presumably beccuse I was a European. The brief cry of protest when the candy was taken away from her was the first cry I had heard from Nabatanzi. Her mother confirmed that she cried very rarely. When I inquired whether she understood any words, her mother's face lit up and she explained that Nabatanzi responded to *vaawo*—"stop!"—but usually only if it was repeated.

Nabatanzi's excellent health continued. She did not often go to the clinic, but when she did the doctor always commented on how plump and healthy she was. By forty-six weeks of age she weighed 21 pounds.

By this time she could walk well. She could get to her feet by herself without pulling herself up on anything. Sometimes she fell, but this did not disturb her. She could not yet run, but she seemed to be trying to do so and could walk very quickly. At the front door there was a high doorstep, like the doorsteps on board ship, and similarly intended to keep water out. When Nabatanzi negotiated it she stepped over it, holding on to the door jamb, rather than crawling over it. She did so with some difficulty because the step was a very high one for her—but she did not regress to a more baby-like mode of locomotion. When her mother demonstrated for me the little song that she had sung to encourage Nabatanzi to stand, Nabatanzi not only stood but clapped her hands rhythmically, keeping time with her mother's clapping. Her mother said that Nabatanzi always clapped her hands when anyone else clapped.

This young mother was more overt in her demonstrations of affection to the baby than any of the other mothers in the sample, and she also seemed to play with the baby more than the others did, despite the fact that she had so much garden work to do that she had less time with the baby than moist of the other mothers did. She told us that she often sang to the baby, singing the songs that she had learned in school. Most of the playing was said to occur right after feeding. Nabatanzi also played by herself. She liked to hold two objects, one in each hand, and to bang them together; she also occupied herself for long periods putting little objects in and out of a container.

By this time she had two words that she could say appropriately—*jjajja* for her grandmother or great-aunt, and *tyo* as a greeting. She could not understand simple commands like "come!" and "go away," and simple statements like "I'll come back." She now could give up an object in to response to a verbal request. She had begun to imitate sounds. After riding in the car to the clinic the day before, she made a prolonged "vvvvuuuu" sound and bent over to imitate the progress of the car. She could not only feed herself solid food with her fingers but could also held her own cup to drink.

During the visit Nabatanzi was again somewhat shy of me. She cried briefly several times, apparently in response to my presence and to the unfamiliar situation of having her photograph taken. She was dressed in a new pink rayon dress for her picture. Her mother tried to get her to sit by herself on a mat, and she seemed very distrustful. We gave her a piece of candy to distract her; she was very interested in this and picked away at the paper wrapping, trying to remove it. Several times her mother tried to move away, and Nabatanzi protested. She also protested when her mother tried to push her into the desired position. When we returned to the house she sat close to her mother, although for a while she was content to sit with her grandmother and great-aunt just outside the door. She smiled and talked with them. Once, while she was standing outside, trickles of urine ran down her legs, but no one paid any attention. Once back inside she sat on her mother's lap and began in a determined way to get at her breast. The mother's dress was held fastened by snaps below the buttons. When Nabatanzi pulled sharply at the dress the snaps popped open; her mother pushed her hand away and fastened the snaps and Nabatanzi protested. This was repeated several times. Perhaps to distract her, the mother began to play a game with a ten-cent coin (one-tenth of a shilling), handing the coin to her, saying, "Here is ten cents to get some bread." Nabatanzi would take the coin, only to drop it—and this was repeated over and over. Then she returned to her efforts to get the breast, and mother finally relented and fed her.

Since Nabatanzi showed much more clearly than before a reluctance to be parted from her mother, we inquired about this aspect of attachment. Her mother said that for many months Nabatanzi had cried when she left the room. As soon as she could crawl she began to follow her mother, crying. She still cried when her mother left and sometimes followed or attempted to do so. I could not believe that her crying when her mother departed was consistent, for we had not observed it on previous visits, and she was regularly left with one or the other of the older women while her mother gardened. Nabatanzi had always been described as content with these other caretakers. Moreover, at the end of the visit, the whole group started to accompany us to the car; halfway up the path the grandmother, carrying Nabatanzi, turned back, and the mother continued on with us; Nabatanzi did not cry at this parting. The older women occasionally gave Nabatanzi solid foods when she was left in their care, but most of the feedings and always the baths were given by the mother.

When Nabatanzi was forty-eight weeks old she got too close to the cooking fire and burned her foot. The burn was a severe one, which caused her much pain, both at the time and for a few weeks afterward. It hurt her to walk, and since she was characteristically an active child, the burn caused her much discomfort. She cried almost continuously for a few days, and even a week later, when we visited, she fussed intermittently throughout our visit. She sat on her mother's lap, squirming about and crying until she was given the breast. After a brief time of suckling she fussed again. She quieted for a while after being given a piece of candy but then resumed fussing and clutching at her mother. Her mother cuddled her and tried to distract her. Just before we left, her mother went to get us a pineapple as a gift. She took Nabatanzi with her, straddled on her hip. When she returned she put Nabatanzi down outside the door, where the grandmother and the two children were sitting. Nabatanzi started to cry loudly and continued until her mother again picked her up.

The burn put an end to Nabatanzi's regular weight gain. At the clinic she was given some medicine to put on the sore, but the bottle was broken and an infection developed, then fever. Nabatanzi was taken twice to another doctor in the interval between clinics, but it was not clear what treatment was given.

At our visit at forty-nine weeks we were given the following information. Feeding had changed little, except that occasionally Nabatanzi received an egg to eat and daily she got a pint of milk to supplement breast milk. Bread had also been added to her diet, which she liked very much—better than the other solid foods of which she was said to eat relatively little. She was said not to suck her thumb—and, indeed, we have never observed her to do so. She was said to have stopped soiling the bed as soon as she began to walk—at forty-two weeks. She had one bowel movement a day, in the early morning, and always waited until she was "held down." By this time she had nearly stopped wetting the bed. During the day, Nabatanzi tried to go outside by herself to urinate, although she did not always quite make it. At night her mother held her down twice, first when going to bed herself, and later at midnight. If Nabatanzi wakened, wanting to urinate, she cried until her mother took her up to "hold her down." By this time, also, it was clear that Nabatanzi did not like strangers; her previous friendliness had given way to distrust of strangers, whether men or women, Africans or Europeans.

The next week at the clinic Nabatanzi was quite ill—a cold, sore throat, fever, and stomatitis. She had been refusing food and had lost weight. She continued to be ill, despite the medicine dispensed at the clinic. Fortunately her father turned up and was able to drive her to Kampala where she was given penicillin. She began to improve, but her appetite was still poor.

On a brief visit when she was fifty-one weeks old Mrs. Kibuka found her sitting quietly in the care of the boy, who was by this time seven years old. Mrs. Kibuka tried to pick her up, but Nabatanzi protested, crying. The boy picked her up, and Nabatanzi quieted. Soon the grandmother came in from the garden, and Nabatanzi crept to her with a warm greeting.

At our second visit, when Nabatanzi was thirty-one weeks old, we had asked the mother when she intended to wean her. She answered, "When she is a year old." At a later visit, when Nabatanzi was ten months old, we explained that we were especially interested in weaning and wished to visit more frequently during the weaning period so that we could observe the baby's reactions to it.

The mother seemed to understand and agreed to give us advance notice. A month later I was making plans to be away for two weeks. The mother readily agreed to postpone weaning until after my return.

Despite all this discussion, when I visited Nabatanzi after my return I found that weaning had already begun. The mother told us that she had dropped the daytime feedings three weeks earlier when Nabatanzi was about forty-nine weeks old. This landmark had not been mentioned to Mrs. Kibuka, who had visited twice during my absence. A further puzzling circumstance was that weaning had been started when Nabatanzi was ill—which seemed an inappropriate time, especially since the mother still had plenty of breast milk.

By this time Nabatanzi was used to a varied diet—oranges, sweet potatoes, squash, porridge, *matooke*, bananas, papaws, white potatoes, eggs, bread, and a daily pint of milk—but, on the other hand, her mouth and throat were too sore for her to want to eat. Her mother said that she had tried to behave as usual toward Nabatanzi, giving her no more and no less attention than she was accustomed to giving. The baby's response to the partial weaning was undoubtedly complicated by her illness, but she wanted to be close to her mother all the time; she sat beside her mother a lot, although she got no special cuddling. The mother said that Nabatanzi did not seek the breast, but it was not clear whether this had been the case from the beginning or only after the lapse of three weeks.

During our visit at fifty-two weeks, Nabatanzi had a temper tantrum—the first that we had witnessed. The tantrum began when she lost a piece of candy that she had been sucking. She began to kick at the young boy and then threw herself back against her mother, repeatedly, screaming at the top of her voice, too angry to notice that her mother had found the candy and was offering it to her. She finally saw the candy and quieted down, sitting on her mother's lap. When her mother got up at the end of the visit and put Nabatanzi down, she howled. A week later, a visit to the clinic confirmed the mother's impression that Nabatanzi was gaining. She had gained over a pound in two weeks. At the clinic the mother left Nabatanzi with me while she went to assist with an injection to be given to the little girl who lived with them. Nabatanzi cried when her mother left but calmed when I took her on my lap—she was turned away from me. She sat quiet for some time, then whimpered to be put down. When her mother returned she made a cry face but did not actually cry.

For seven weeks Nabatanzi was given the breast when she woke at night but not during the daytime. Finally, when she was thirteen months old, weaning was completed. The first night she awoke crying; her mother heated some cow's milk and gave it to her. Nabatanzi accepted it and went back to sleep. Later she wakened again and cried. This time her mother did not give her milk but cuddled her. Warm milk was ready for her when she woke in the morning and she accepted it. The second night she slept through without waking.

When we visited on the second day after final weaning the mother said she could notice no change in her behavior. I asked whether she tried to get at her mother's breast during the day. The mother laughed and said that she did, although a month previously she had said she did not. She always asked Nabatanzi, " What are you doing?" and Nabatanzi always laughed in reply.

During this visit Nabatanzi, although solemn at first, became active and very gay. She sat on Mrs. Kibuka's lap at first, but when put down she walked across the room to her mother with arms outstretched and climbed up on her lap. Her grandmother, sitting on the doorway, called to her, and Nabatanzi went to her, offering a piece of candy that we had given her. She smiled at me charmingly and several times during the visit laughed out loud. She enjoyed hearing her mother tell me how Nabatanzi sometimes threatened "Stop it! I will hit you!" When her mother told how she could greet visitors, she gave me a greeting, putting her hand in mine, and laughed. Then she rushed over to her grandmother, still laughing. She offered her mother her candy, saying, " 'Say thank you!" Then she quieted and sat by her mother. When her mother went out of the house for a moment, Nabatanzi followed her without apparent anxiety but stopped at the door. She stood in the doorway smiling at her grandmother.

Nabatanzi was a plump, healthy little girl, with very dark skin and large clear eyes. On the occasion of this visit she wore a blue sun dress with a full skirt, which looked nice on her. She wore silver bangles on her wrists and quite an assortment of things on her ankles —a string of large bells, an anklet like a large curtain ring, and a couple of thin bangles. We took some photographs. It was somewhat difficult to get her into the right pose, for she was either very active, or very absorbed in a flower that she was holding, her head down and her face hidden. But she did not protest our efforts to pose her and she did not protest when her mother moved away.

When we left, the grandmother carried her part way up the hill, accompanying us. When the grandmother turned back with Nabatanzi and the mother continued to accompany us, she did not protest. It seemed to us that she had behaved throughout the visit much as she had done before she had burned her foot and before weaning had started, although perhaps she was a little less inclined to be close to her mother than previously. Her mother said, however, that she still cried and followed whenever she left her alone in a room, although she did not do so if left with one of the familiar figures of the household.

The mother said that Nabatanzi still wet the bed, but no more frequently than before weaning. (Yet two months previously bed-wetting had been described as very infrequent.)

All the talk of beating and hitting prompted me to ask whether the mother did, in fact, discipline Nabatanzi by smacking her. She said that she did spank her if she was crying "for nothing" and smacked her fingers lightly if she was holding something her mother did not want her to have. Nabatanzi always replied to a verbal threat of a smacking by threatening to hit back. She was said to get angry

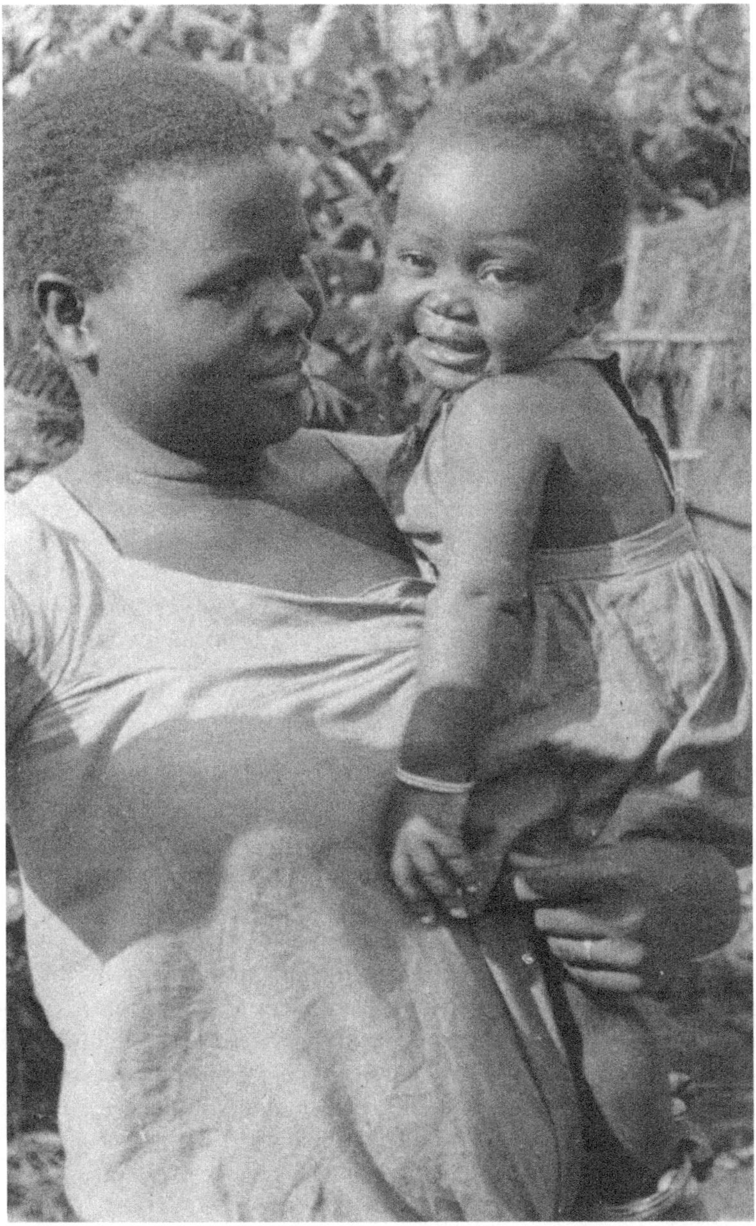

FIGURE 10 Nabatanzi's mother played with her more than did the mothers of the other children. Here she is at thirteen months just after weaning. Her weaning disturbance is not noticeable here.

when frustrated by having something taken away from her or by having her activity interfered with. Sometimes she accepted the frustration, but sometimes she became angry and cried. Usually her mother tried to comfort her, and only rarely did the crying continue long enough to warrant a spank. Occasionally she cried when she was hungry, and her mother responded by feeding her as soon as she could get the food ready. But on the whole she was still said to cry very little.

We inquired about language development, and her mother beamed with pride, telling us about her new acquisitions. In addition to the words we had heard her say, she could ask *kik?* (what is it?), respond to a call with *wange!* in the conventional way, and say an approximation of *weeraba* (good-bye) and *weebale* (thank you).

Two weeks later Nabatanzi's mother reported more disturbance than had been evident immediately after weaning. She wanted to be with her mother all the time and cried and followed whenever her mother left the room for a moment. She was eating less well than before. Previously, the only food she had been reluctant to eat was *matooke*, but now she rejected everything but fruit and milk, and porridge, provided it had plenty of milk on it. She was said no longer to try to get at the breast. "She does not care for it." But she flew into tempers when she was hungry and her mother could not prepare the food quickly enough to suit her. She was sleeping well. If she became restless during the night, this was a signal to her mother that she needed to be held down. Bedwetting was thus usually averted.

During our visit Nabatanzi at first sat across the room from her mother. I gave her candy, and she immediately crossed the room to offer it to her mother, then sat on her lap. She ate the candy with concentration, and when it was gone she began to search, as though not believing it was gone. She searched in the open neck of the boy's shirt. Her mother told her to stop and then tried to pull her hand away, saying, "I will beat you." Nabatanzi retorted, aggressively, "I will beat you." After she had calmed down from this exchange I took her on my lap where she sat quietly but as though she were simply tolerating it. When I put her down she was sunny for a while, then became tempery for no apparent reason. When her anger showed no sign of abating, her mother told her to quiet down and smacked her lightly with her cupped hand. Nabatanzi became furious at the smack and hit her mother back with all her strength. The mother repeated the gentle smack, and Nabatanzi continued her tantrum with renewed vigor, throwing herself about and hitting out wildly, Finally she buried her head in her mother's breast and then began fumbling at the fastening of the dress in an attempt to get to the breast, continuing to cry loudly.

I asked what had made her so angry, and her mother said: "She is angry when she remembers the breast." Then she said that she thought Nabatanzi might be hungry. Meanwhile, Nabatanzi had quieted. She spied a package of tea that I had brought as a gift and grabbed it. Tea was too precious for her to be allowed to play with it, so her mother tried to take it away from her. There was a tussle, with more loud crying. She crept to her mother and calmed when held on her lap, her crying subsiding to the occasional whimper. Her mother said, for no apparent reason, and in a quiet voice: "I will beat you." At this, Nabatanzi began to cry loudly again.

Her mother said that Nabatanzi did not like strangers, although she seemed to be accepting us better than she had for some weeks. Her mother also said that she did not like men, and, of course, there were no men in the household.

When we left, the mother, carrying Nabatanzi straddled on her hip, accompanied us for a while. When she said she would go no further, Mrs. Kibuka took Nabatanzi in her arms, and began to carry her up the path away from her mother. Nabatanzi looked back at her mother but did not protest at being taken away. I caught up with them and walked along; Mrs. Kibuka turned Nabatanzi so that she could not see her mother, but there was no distress. Finally we took her back to her mother, who stood waiting and expressed surprise at Nabatanzi's lack of distress. The mother astonished us by saying "She will go with anyone who is well-dressed."

Two days later at the clinic the mother complained that Nabatanzi had lost her appetite and refused all food but orange juice. On our last visit, when she was fourteen months old, she seemed much as usual, except that she seemed to want to be close to her mother even more constantly than before. She had regained her appetite. Her mother said that she still had tempers but insisted that these were no more frequent than they had been before weaning.

It is difficult to sort out the discrepancies between Nabatanzi's postweaning behavior as we observed it and her behavior as her mother reported it. It seemed to us that her relationship with her mother was much more ambivalent and that her temper tantrums were more frequent than they had been before weaning, although her mother denied this. Her mother also denied that she sought the breast, although it was obvious that nine weeks after weaning she still sought it occasionally. Her mother reported that she wished to be closer to her than before and that she more consistently cried and followed when left. This appeared to be the case during our visits; yet there were two occasions when she did not protest our pretending to take her away with us. Perhaps she did not believe our pretense!

Visits to the Clinic

Age wks.	*Weight lbs.*	*Comments*
31	18.6	
45	21.3	
47	21.5	burn
49	21.2	stomatitis, fever
51	21.3	
53	22.4	
59		

Nakiku

Nakiku was a quiet, gentle little girl, who, although she was developing normally, was slight and fragile in appearance and prone to colds. Her parents were concerned about her development to the point of being overanxious. It was undoubtedly this concern which led them to be among the first families to volunteer their cooperation in the research. Nakiku's mother had acquired two pamphlets on child care and nutrition written in Luganda by Dr. Welbourn. She had pored over these and had tried to put the recommendations into practice, but she sought further advice from us, especially about feeding; she was concerned that Nakiku was not plump and robust. Of special concern was the baby's susceptibility to respiratory infections, which recurred despite the apparently excellent care she received. On one of our visits Nakiku's father was also present. He asked thoughtful questions about the research, about the possibility of the continuance of our services after the research project was over, and about infant-care practices. His questions covered much of the same ground as had the mother's but extended to the issues of the right age for weaning and the advisability of separating the child from his mother after weaning. He himself answered the last question by saying that he thought separation to be a bad practice because no one could take as good care of a child as the mother, but he added that he wanted to do the best thing for the child.

The father was a shoemaker who worked in Kampala and returned home every evening. Nakiku was his only child, and his pride in her and his affection and concern for her were intense. In the evenings and over the weekends he enjoyed helping to care for her. He played with her and sometimes gave her her bath, but only her mother fed her.

Nakiku's mother was quiet and pleasant, soft of voice and gentle in manner. She talked freely to us but was not as outgoing and vivacious as some of the mothers in the sample. On the other hand, she never strayed from the point during our interviews and was conscientious and dependable in being available at the appointed times for visits. Nakiku was her second child. The first child, a daughter, had been born out of wedlock and was left to be reared by the maternal grandmother when the mother married seven years later. The mother often spoke longingly of this elder daughter. Her husband was quite willing to have the child with them, but the maternal grandmother did not want to give her up.

Nakiku was not the only child in the household, however. There was a twelve-year-old boy, Pantaleo, the child of a relative, who lived there in order to attend primary school. He was a pleasant boy and was helpful to his foster mother. He helped by looking after Nakiku and especially in carrying her if any expedition had to be made.

Despite the relatively high degree of acculturation of this family in regard to child-care practices, they had few European possessions. Their wattle-and-daub house was small and was thatched with straw. There were no chairs and tables, no china cups and saucers, and no cross-stitched table covers. On the other hand, there was no apparent lack of money for things considered essential for Nakiku's welfare.

Nakiku was twenty-eight weeks old when we began to visit her. We were told that she had been born in hospital. She was a healthy newborn who sucked well from the beginning. Her health continued to be good except for the frequent colds. She was breast-fed according to a four-hour schedule during the day and twice during the night when she wakened. Supplementary feedings of orange juice and *ensujju* (summer squash) had been begun at about six months of age, and in addition Nakiku received supplementary milk from a cup. She was never given the breast—or foods— for comfort; they were offered only at scheduled feeding times. Upon the advice of the clinic, supplemented by advice sought from Mrs. Kibuka, further solid foods were added to Nakiku's diet, and soon she was receiving quite a variety. She was said to enjoy them all.

Nakiku slept in a crib in her parents' room and was said to sleep well. She also had naps both in the morning and in the afternoon. The morning nap was on a mat in the shade in the garden where her mother worked. She had two baths a day, which she was said to enjoy so much that she protested at being taken from the water. "Holding down" began at about six months of age and was a resounding success. Nakiku very soon learned not to soil or wet her bed, and even the "housebreaking" aspect of the training was precociously successful. Further, her mother said that she sat alone at four and a half months of age without any special training and that she began to crawl at six months.

Nakiku was said to be a happy child, crying only if she was about to become ill. Whenever she cried, for whatever reason, she was picked up and comforted. Wherever her mother went Nakiku was taken along. She was never left alone, although sometimes she would be left in the house with either her father or Pantaleo while her mother worked elsewhere. She was said not to cry when her mother left the room, but as soon as she could crawl she went to her mother if she were sitting apart from her and tried to crawl up onto her mother's lap. She would attempt to follow if her mother left the room. She was said to be fond of her father and to greet him enthusiastically when he returned from work. She readily accepted being held by visitors. All of this information matched closely what we observed on our first and subsequent visits.

During our first visit at twenty-eight weeks Nakiku sat for most of the time near her mother on the mat on the floor. She bounced about, gurgling and smiling at the visitors. Once she crawled onto her mother's lap and buried her face in it. For a while she sat on the lap of a woman visitor who was present and smiled across at her mother from this vantage point. Once she crawled toward me, seemingly attracted by my sandaled feet. Her mother thought that the fact that my feet were white made them attractive playthings. For a while her mother held her in a standing position. Her legs were straight and close together while her mother supported her around the arms and shoulders. For a while she played with a small tin that rattled. Her mother said that all her playthings were like this and she sounded apologetic as she said it.

Throughout the visit the mother directed her attention toward us rather than toward Nakiku. Nevertheless, for a while when she was holding Nakiku standing, she kissed her repeatedly and tenderly on the cheek or the back of the neck, seemingly absent-mindedly. This did not strike me as unusual at the time, but later I came to realize that this kind of display of affection was unusual in the mothers in this sample.

At thirty-three weeks of age Nakiku was creeping efficiently and quickly and was very active during the visit. Every now and then she returned to her mother, but she did not go to Pantaleo, who was sitting nearby, nor to the visitors. When questioned, her mother said that she gave Nakiku much cuddling and patting, although this was chiefly after feeding and before being put down to sleep. Nevertheless, during the visit, whenever Nakiku went to her mother there was contact—holding, cuddling, caressing. Her mother also reported that she had begun to feed herself with her fingers; she had started this on her own initiative, picking up any food within reach and popping it into her mouth.

At this visit, and off and on for the next two months, Nakiku had colds and at one visit to the clinic she had conjunctivitis and stomatitis. Her weights gains were irregular, slowed down by each cold. Nevertheless, at forty-three weeks of age Nakiku began to walk alone.

At forty-four weeks Nakiku seemed better. She looked very clean in a faded red dress. Underneath, she had a string of beads around her waist, and she also had beads around her wrists and ankles— to keep these parts slim. She seemed well, although she was not plump. She was no longer a baby but a pretty little girl, slender and dainty. She sat for a long time on her mother's lap at the beginning of the visit, quiet and watchful. She then stood up holding onto the pedal of a bicycle that was standing in the room. I tried to persuade her to walk by holding out a piece of candy. She looked interested and reached; finally she took a few steps. Her mother took it away to remove the paper wrapping and Nakiku protested. When the candy was returned she ate it, dribbling syrup on her dress; she often took it out of her mouth and fingered it, getting herself thoroughly sticky. I thought that perhaps her mother might have wished I had not given it to her, but she was watching the whole scene with an affectionate expression and said that Nakiku was very fond of candy; her father sometimes brought her treats of candy. The mother reached behind her for a basket in which she had oranges and a papaw as gifts for us. Nakiku picked up the oranges and let them drop to the floor, continuing the game as fast as her mother could retrieve them and put them back in the basket.

We inquired about crying. Her mother said that whenever she had fever she cried more and that this happened with each cold. Otherwise, she cried very little during the day, but she had begun inexplicably to awake crying during the night. She still did not cry when her mother left the room. If left with her father or Pantaleo, she was content to stay, but when her mother returned she gave her an excited greeting. If left alone in a room, she would follow her mother. She also had begun to cry occasionally when first put down to sleep; this appeared to be a signal that she wished to urinate, for after being "held down" she was content to go to sleep.

One cold followed another, then a fever, and still another cold. Again, at forty-seven weeks of age she had a cold with fever. Despite this, she looked well and seemed her normal self. There were other visitors; for a while Nakiku sat on the lap of one while her mother held another baby. Nakiku accepted this, showing no jealousy. When the visitors left she was put on the floor. She walked over to me first, then to her mother, and then to her father, who was present during this visit. She walked back and forth a lot during the rest of the visit but was quiet in her movements and did not seem overactive. She did not vocalize much during the visit, but her parents said that she called them *mama* and *taata* appropriately and had names for other familiar people too. She also responded to the command "come back."

The crying at night had stopped. She still woke twice at night to be fed, however—once while her parents were still up and again later. Each time she was held down as well as fed. During the day she was no longer held down; she was able to go outside by herself and on her own initiative. She was said not to have had a bowel movement in the house since she was eight months old; wetting was very infrequent, occurring perhaps only once every two weeks. Perhaps the chief change in her behavior was that she now became angry at times, and when she did she expressed it by throwing things about. The cause for anger was being refused something she wanted. Her mother said that she dealt with the episodes by holding her close and comforting her until she was calm again.

When Nakiku was fifty-one weeks old her mother began to wean her, stopping the daytime feedings. We had talked of weaning plans earlier. At eight months Nakiku was eating so well that her mother said she was considering weaning her at ten months of age. Then, when Nakiku was ten months old, her mother had changed her mind and planned to wait until she was a year old. She agreed to inform us before she began the weaning, but, as it turned out, she did not.

Nakiku did not cry when the daytime feedings were discontinued, but she did try to get to the breast. Her mother discouraged this by holding her on the side opposite that on which her dress opened. After three days she no longer sought the breast. By this time she was accustomed to a wide variety of solid foods and she continued to eat well. She did not wet her bed. She did not seem to want to be with her mother more than usual or closer to her than usual.

A week later, and the day before her first birthday, we began our visit by taking pictures. Nakiku seemed a little subdued by the strange situation but she accepted being put down by her mother and did not protest when her mother moved away so that she could be photographed by herself. When we went into the house she sat for a while on Mrs. Kibuka's lap and played with her ankle bells, making them jingle. When she was put down she went to her mother and played beside her on the mat. For a while she chewed at a yellow tomato that she had been given to amuse her while her picture was being taken. Then she sprawled on the floor near her mother, rolling about and vocalizing happily. Occasionally she smiled up at her mother or across the room at us. Soon she got up, walked to the doorway, and then looked back, smiling. Her mother called her back and she came. Then she played with a green pepper, with the tomato again, and with a forked stick. I took her onto my lap; she looked at me intently, did not relax, and soon indicated that she wanted to be put down.

During the visit her mother told us of new accomplishments. She could now say good-bye and could call to a person. She had her own idiosyncratic words for different foods, but her mother found them difficult to understand. Her understanding of simple commands had increased. When told to put down something she was holding she obeyed; when told "don't go there" she obeyed. Her mother said that she could not yet say "no" or give greetings. Soon after this she surprised her mother by suddenly saying *otyanno*, the simplest form of greeting. Everyone exclaimed approvingly, so she repeated it several times. She had been feeding herself for some time with her fingers but she could not yet hold a cup by herself.

The reported change in her crying was that she now sometimes cried when her mother left the room. This occurred only when she tried to follow and was prevented from doing so by a closed door; sometimes she accepted the frustration without crying. Her mother did not remember her ever crying to be picked up; instead she indicated her wish by holding up her arms. When her mother would return after an absence from the room, Nakiku characteristically laughed joyously and trotted toward her. Despite this obvious attachment to her mother, Nakiku was said to prefer her father whenever he was at home. This was said to have been the case ever since she started to crawl—from about six months of age. The preference held even if Nakiku was tired or ill. She was said also to like Pantaleo very much. She knew no men except her father. She was friendly with women that she knew well, but was said not to be good with strangers. Nevertheless, she did not seem shy with us during the visit, except for her tension while I held her. She did not cling to her mother during the visit; she played close to her for quite a while but showed no hesitation in moving about the room and toward the door. Mrs. Kibuka and I both received smiles from her, but only when there was some distance between us. Nakiku was said to "play with" other children who came with their mothers to visit.

The rosy picture of elimination control given a month earlier was somewhat modified at this visit. She was now said never to soil the bed, usually (not always) to go outside the house for bowel movements, never to wet the bed unless ill, and still to urinate in the house. Even so, this is a remarkable degree of control for a year-old baby by contemporary Western standards.

We visited again four days later, the day after final weaning. The night before when Nakiku woke as usual, her mother, instead of feeding her, took her out to hold her down and then put her back to bed. Nakiku went back to sleep and slept through the rest of the night. (At this point we learned that lately she had been fed only once a night, instead of twice.) The next day when we visited, we were told that she had been crying a lot. Also she had developed another cold. She sounded quite miserable and her breathing was labored. She had a fever and had vomited twice, which she usually did not do with a cold. It was difficult, therefore, to judge how much of her disturbance was attributable to weaning and how much to illness. She was said to be eating well. Apart from the crying, her behavior appeared to be unchanged.

Mrs. Kibuka took Nakiku onto her lap soon after we arrived, and she did not ask to get down. When put down she played on the floor with some berries. She seemed cheerful and vocalized a little. She then sat on her mother's lap for a while, and just before we left I held her for a while. She did not cry while we were there.

We inquired about her diet. Her mother said that she had breakfast at ten in the morning—mashed papaw, porridge, and milk. Sometimes she also received an egg, sometimes bananas. Lunch consisted of *matooke* with nut sauce and orange juice. Dinner came at four o'clock in the afternoon—porridge and milk. At bedtime she received another cup of milk.

Two days later—the third day after final weaning—we took Nakiku and her mother to the clinic. Nakiku still had a slight cold and had not regained the weight that she had lost two weeks before, but the doctor thought she was very well. Her mother said that on the previous night she had wakened twice, crying and wanting to be fed, although the night before she had slept through without waking. Her father gave her some milk and she quieted. During the day she had not been crying since the first day after weaning.

A week later when Nakiku was fifty-three weeks old, we visited again. We were told that she had had one more disturbed night, the fourth night, and that since then she had settled down. During the day she cried only occasionally, if her mother was taking an especially long time to prepare food. The chief change that had taken place was that Nakiku no longer wanted to be with her mother all the time as she had before weaning. Now she was content to remain in a corner of the room, lying on an old *busuuti* of her mother's, while her mother was out of the room. Although she still followed her mother about sometimes, she did so less consistently than before. Two weeks later at the clinic Nakiku had lost

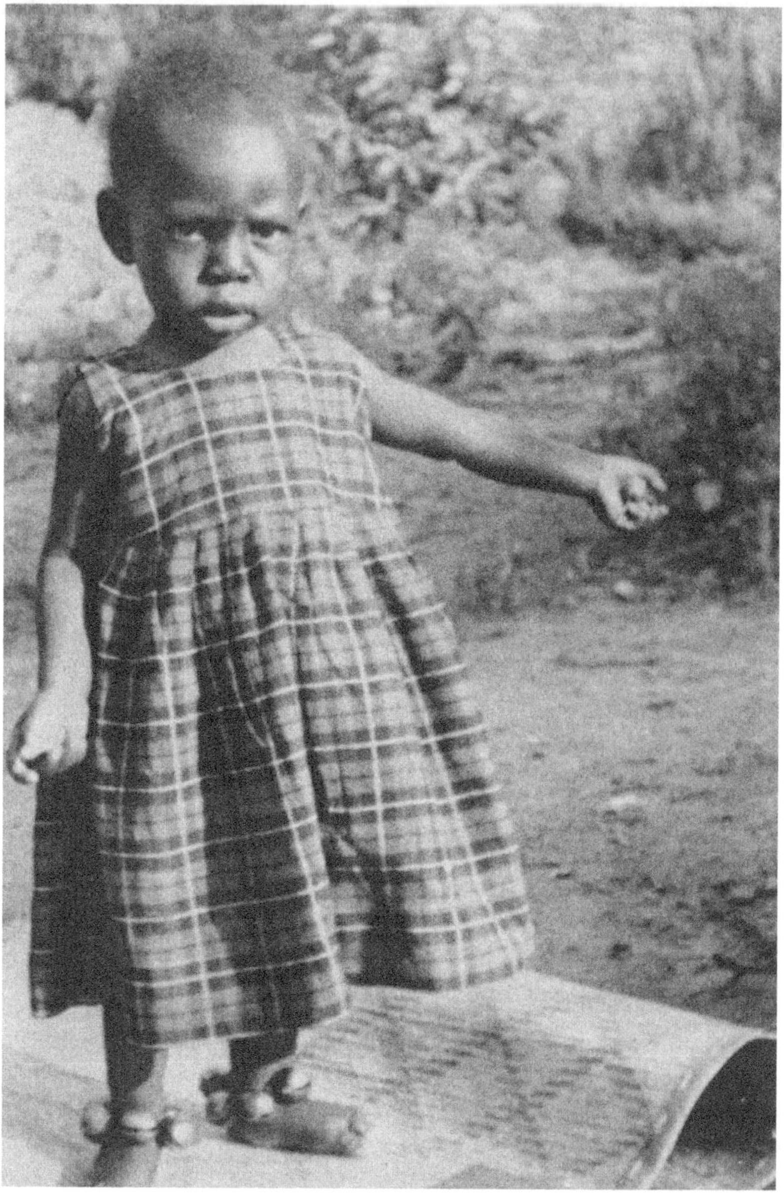

FIGURE 11 Nakiku at fifty-three weeks is reaching toward her mother, whom she does not follow so much now that she has been weaned.

another ounce of weight. This was a blow to her mother, who had been trying so hard to feed her well.

When Nakiku was fifty-six weeks old she developed another cold accompanied by vomiting. She lay on the floor near her mother and occasionally smiled up at Mrs. Kibuka. Presently she began to play with some berries she found on the floor and put them in her mouth. Then she climbed onto her mother's lap and lay back against her. She got hold of a large white handkerchief, put it over her head, and initiated a peek-a-boo game with Mrs. Kibuka. After a while I invited her to come to me, holding out a piece of candy. Nakiku was shy and held back. I deliberately looked away while still offering the candy; she came quietly, took it from my hand, and returned to her mother. There was a sick child in the house, left by a neighbor to be looked after. Nakiku wanted to go into the room where he was; her mother prevented her from going, and Nakiku cried angrily for a few moments. On the whole she seemed more subdued than usual—but she was not well.

We asked about any changes in behavior since the last visit. The mother reported that Nakiku was no longer following her about as she used to. When Pantaleo was present, Nakiku appeared quite content to see her mother go. But she still gave a characteristically warm greeting when her mother returned and seemed to enjoy her company. Her behavior with her father had not changed; she still ran toward him when he returned home and still preferred his company. Her mother further reported that Nakiku had begun to suck her fingers much more than she had before weaning. She also was more frequently angry than before, crying when frustrated in having or doing something that she wanted.

We saw Nakiku briefly five more times before the end of the research. For a while she did not gain and then she gained a pound—her first since weaning, and despite another cold. Her behavior was amiable and she seemed secure. She smiled readily at us and on one occasion accepted the attentions of a white visitor who was a complete stranger. She did not cling to her mother, but, on the other hand, she did not stray away from her.

Gesell Testing

Dr. Géber first administered the Gesell Developmental Schedules to Nakiku when she was sixty-two weeks old. She was delighted with the testing. She was very interested in the toys and manipulated them skillfully with quick, economical movements. She was in easy communication with her mother, the examiner, and everyone else present. She showed her mother the various test objects, and she was particularly interested in one of the male visitors, glancing at him frequently and smiling. She took great pleasure in exploring the adaptive possibilities of the bottle with its pellets, pencil and paper, and the blocks. She was entranced with the ball, throwing it and trying to catch it when it was thrown to her. She looked at the picture book with great interest. Her mother was warm and responsive to her, and Dr. Géber judged their relationship to be excellent. When the steps were presented to her she hesitated for a moment, but when encouraged to climb, she did, and climbed up and down with excitement and delight in her new accomplishment.

Her Developmental Quotient (DQ) was 120. She was particularly advanced in locomotion (136) and social reactions (136) and least advanced in language (110) and manual ability (114).

When retested at twenty-seven months her active delight and sociability had given way to a grumbly reaction, and her DQ had dropped to 99. At three years of age she was again cooperative in the testing and received a DQ of 105. The following summer she was not available for testing; her two-year-old sister had died and the mother had gone away. When she was five years old she seemed sad and subdued; her DQ was 80.

Visits to the Clinic

Age wks.	*Weight lbs.*	*Comments*
29	13.7	cough
33	14.8	cold
37	15.0	
39	15.5	
43	15.6	conjunctivitis, stomatitis, diarrhea, recurrent cold
45	16.3	
47	16.7	mucus in stools
49	17.8	cold
51	17.3	cold
53	17.3	cold, cough
55	17.2	
57	17.1	
59	18.0	cold, vomiting

Kasozi

Kasozi's mother asked to join the research sample by seeking an introduction to us through Nakiku's mother. On the occasion of our first long visit she told us about the difficult time she was having. When she was pregnant with Kasozi, her husband informed her that he wanted a new wife and asked her to leave him. She did so, taking Kristina, their pretty little three-year-old daughter, with her. When Kasozi was about seven months old she set up a new household with her twenty-year-old brother who works near Kampala. He built the house and she made the garden. She had been laboring hard on this new garden for four months and it was just beginning to produce food. The house itself was bare and unattractive; it was a wattle-and-daub shell with a metal roof. The floor was rough; the doorsteps between the rooms were rough; the only floor covering was an old piece of burlap. There had been no time to make mats, and when we visited, chairs for our use were borrowed from a neighbor.

We met the brother twice, but he was too shy to talk with us. He preferred to remain in a little shed near the house, playing an accordion.

Kristina looked very well cared for in a red jumper dress that her mother had made for her. She always sat quietly, in proper Ganda fashion. Whenever her mother wanted something from another room or from a neighbor, she sent Kristina for it. Kristina, out of sight, would call to her mother and carry on what sounded like quite an adult conversation. They seemed to have a close, companionable relationship, which must have been a great comfort to this unfortunate woman. Kristina was responsive to us, even at our first visit, and managed several friendly smiles. She seemed quite feminine and very much mother's little helper.

Kasozi was eleven months old when his mother first approached us. He was a very well-developed, healthy-looking baby. He was born at home with the help of a woman who had been a midwife. He was described as a very small newborn baby and "tired." He was breast-fed on demand and sucked well from the beginning. His mother said she enjoyed breast feeding "because I like the person I feed." When Kasozi was six months old, supplementary solid foods were begun. His mother was guided in her choice of foods by a book written by Dr. Welbourn. There had been no feeding problems and no serious illnesses. Nevertheless, his mother was eager to receive whatever help we and the clinic could give her.

When Kasozi was two months old his mother began to train him to sit by supporting him with cloths wrapped around him. He seemed to be developing rapidly, and she hoped to train him to sit when very young because this would leave her freer to do her work. But it was not until he was four months old that he could sit unsupported. He crawled at six months and stood unsupported at ten months.

Elimination training was also begun very early—at one month of age. His mother recalled that he was about four months old when he stopped soiling the bed and about nine months old when he stopped wetting it. He had always slept in his mother's bed, but she hoped to be able to buy him a bed of his own before he was weaned. He was said to sleep well, but woke two or three times to be fed.

Ever since he was seven months old, when they moved to their new house, his mother had been driven by the necessity to work hard in the garden in order to raise food for the family. She was accustomed to breast feeding him in the morning and then to preparing food to last him the rest of the day. Before she went to the garden she took Kasozi to a neighbor who looked after him all day. At noon he *received* solid food. In late afternoon, when his mother finally returned from her work, she again gave him the breast. When they were together after her work he was fed on demand, but through the long hours of her absence he was not suckled. He was said to prefer solid food to the breast, however. He could feed himself with his fingers and could hold his own cup—from which he drank tea with milk in it.

Whenever his mother attempted to leave him alone in the house, even for a moment, he would cry and try to follow her. He always cried when left with the neighbor, although he was said to accept the neighbor's care after his mother had gone. The neighbor did all of the necessary things—feeding, bathing, "holding down," and putting him to bed for morning and afternoon naps. When his mother returned in the late afternoon, he would clap his hands and appear very glad to see her.

Kasozi was said to cry easily and frequently. He sometimes cried to be picked up, and he was easily frustrated and cried then also. His mother said that she did not pick him up every time he cried, but if the crying was prolonged, she did so and cuddled him until he was again calm. If he was crying because he was hurt or uncomfortable, she would give him the breast for comfort, but not if he was merely frustrated because he could not have something he wanted. "Beating" —that is, smacking him lightly on the arm with cupped hand—had begun when he started to crawl; he was smacked when he took anything that he might spoil or which might hurt him.

Kasozi was a very plump baby, his legs so fat that his ankles had deep creases. Indeed, he was so big that at the very first visit I confused him, for a moment, with his three-year-old sister.

When we visited at fifty-one weeks, Kasozi had a cold and snorted and wheezed as he breathed. He wore a rumpled blue dress and seemed untidy in comparison to Kristina, who was immaculate. He sat on his mother's lap, and soon began to grasp at his mother's dress in a determined manner, indicating his desire for the breast. She gave it to him and he suckled contentedly, pausing from time to time to look at us. Gradually he became drowsy. His mother began to move him from the breast, but he roused with a vigorous protest. He suckled a bit more and then went to sleep with the nipple still in his mouth; he was then taken away to bed.

His mother said that he had begun to walk about a week before but could manage only a few steps. She expected that he would be able to walk steadily within a month, at which time she planned to wean him. She sought advice about avoiding disturbance at weaning and at my request stated her plans; we reassured her, saying that her methods should keep disturbance at a minimum. She planned to drop the morning feeding first, then the evening feeding, and finally the nighttime feedings. She hoped to get him his own bed so that he would become accustomed to it before weaning and would not feel as rejected as he would if he were ousted from her bed at the same time as being refused the breast.

It was not until Kasozi was fifty-six weeks old that our next visit could be arranged. A few days previously his mother discontinued his daytime feedings. But within two days he developed a fever and refused to eat, so his mother resumed breast feeding. His fever remained.

His mother reported that one day recently, after he had been taken as usual to stay with the neighbor, he slipped out and found his way home. Finding the house locked and his mother gone, he cried alone until the neighbor came looking for him. His mother no longer felt that she could leave him as she had been doing and so she began to take him to the garden. He wanted a hoe to dig with, and she gave him a small hoe so that he could "help her."

During the entire visit he sat either near his mother or on her lap, and while on her lap he tried to get the breast. His mother refused him and he cried. She asked Kristina to fetch him a banana to eat, but he did not eat much of it. He was shy of Mrs. Kibuka, who conducted the visit alone that day, but accepted a piece of candy from her. He was said to dislike strangers. Despite his desire to be close to his mother, he was said to play well with his sister. He liked his uncle, the owner of the house—but very rarely saw his father.

His mother reported that he was now crying less than previously. It seems likely that this was a result of keeping him with her rather than leaving him with the neighbor. Nevertheless, he was still easily frustrated, and tended to have a tantrum whenever he was prevented from doing what he wanted to do or from having something he wished to have. His mother's policy was not to give him what he wanted when he cried for it, especially if it was food that the family was eating.

Shortly after this visit he was taken to the clinic. His fever had abated and despite it he had gained half a pound in a month. At fifty-eight weeks, however, he still had not regained his previous appetite, showing little enthusiasm for any food except porridge and milk. Later we discovered that the daytime feedings had been dropped the previous week; we had not been informed of this, despite the mother's promises to tell us in advance.

This was the second time that weaning had been attempted. Kasozi cried a great deal throughout the first day—more than he had the first time— and he clung to his mother more than before. Usually he was content to play outside with Kristina and other children, but after the weaning began he kept running in to his mother from time to time, as though he had remembered her and had had to come back to her as soon as he thought of her. His mother was struck by this behavior because it had not occurred nearly so often before weaning.

When Kasozi was fifty-nine weeks old he was finally weaned. We visited the following day. He had cried nearly all night; he woke four times and cried to be

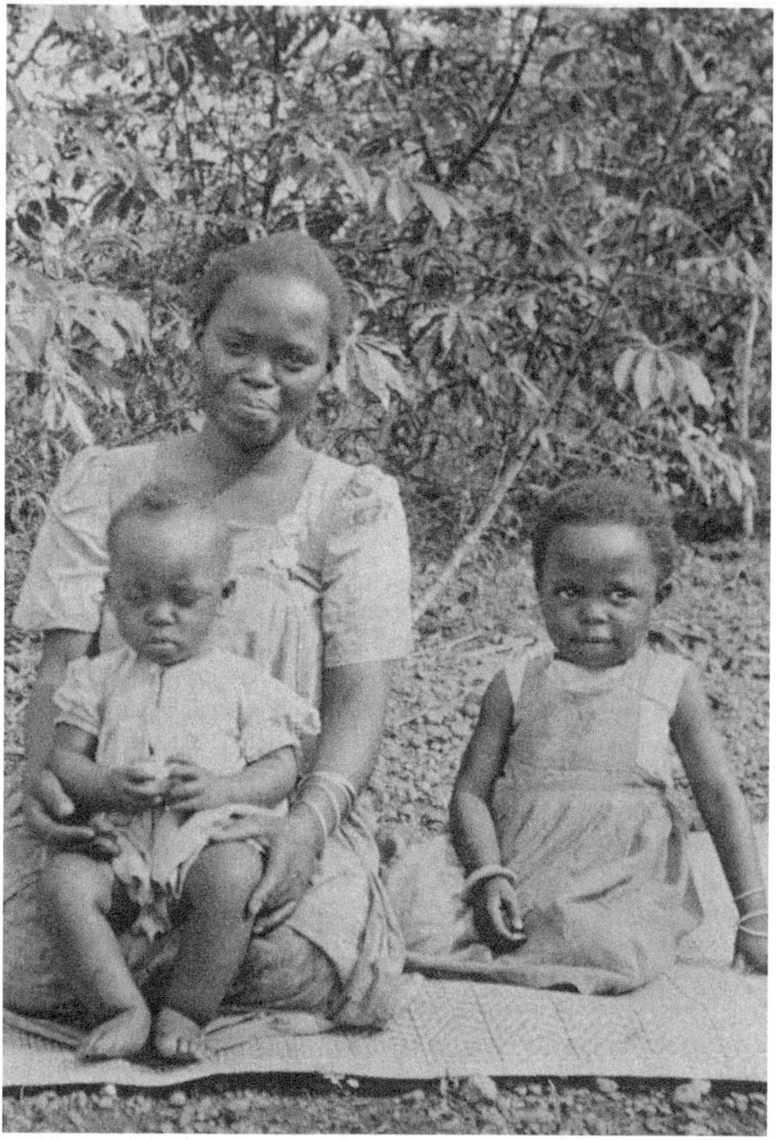

FIGURE 12 Kasozi at fifty-one weeks is a plump baby. He cries to be picked up and wants to be with his mother all the time. His sister, Kristina, is sitting properly, Ganda fashion.

fed, and the last time he stayed awake crying until it was nearly daylight. He refused the skim milk that his mother had prepared for him. She held him in her arms most of the night, rocking him and trying to comfort him, but he cried and threw himself about in a highly disturbed way.

The next day he wanted to be on her lap the whole time. He accepted milk and porridge but refused other food. He fell asleep twice but did not allow his mother to catch up on her sleep.

As soon as we arrived for the visit, Kasozi began to cry, seemingly from fear of me. His mother called him into the house, and he sat on her lap and watched me intently. Then he leaned back against his mother drowsily and finally went to sleep, and his mother put him to bed. She commented that he was resting up for another sleepless night.

Two days later we took him to the clinic. Because of his cold and continuous crying his nose was streaming. His mother said that he had slept soundly the second night of weaning but that he had cried most of the third night. During the day he also cried a lot. His mother was inclined to attribute his unhappiness to his cold and a slight fever rather than to weaning—and, of course, the circumstances were confounded.

Kasozi spent most of the fourth and fifth nights crying, but when we visited a week after he had been weaned—when he was sixty weeks old—he was said not to have cried on subsequent nights. Whenever he awoke at night his mother gave him a small amount of milk. She said that she intended to stop this practice when he recovered from his cold and regained his appetite. She reported that now whenever he saw her breast he covered it up. "He doesn't like it; he doesn't want to see it." His elimination control had not regressed; he had not wet the bed. He had begun to suck his fingers, however, which he had not done before weaning, but he would remove them from his mouth when told to do so. He still wanted to be with his mother all the time. She had tried to leave him with the neighbor as she used to do, but he protested so vigorously that she took him along with her to the garden.

When I greeted Kasozi upon arrival, he held out his hand from where he sat with his mother across the room. I held out a piece of candy, and he came to get it but immediately returned to his mother. He sat beside her with his head against her arm for most of the visit. He was encouraged by her to play with a key and a padlock, but he did not play for long.

A week later, and sixteen days after final weaning, Kasozi was said not to be crying nearly as much. Two weeks later we visited again briefly and found Kasozi with a cold. Despite the fact that the mother had joined the project for the sake of transportation to the clinic, she found that she was too busy to go, even when Kasozi was unwell.

Our last long visit took place when Kasozi was sixty-four weeks old. He was wearing a scarlet sunsuit and had bells around his ankles. He sat close to his mother. When I held out a piece of candy to him he started across the room for it, then stopped in his tracks and looked at me as though wondering whether it was safe to come closer. Mrs. Kibuka took the candy and offered it to him; he came for it and got very sticky eating it, sucking it, taking it out of his mouth to look at it, making it last a long time. His mother rose and went out of the house for a moment. Kasozi broke into a howl, scrambled to his feet, and followed her. When we took photographs Kasozi was quiet with his mother close to him. Back in the house he leaned against his mother and made contented noises. He spent most of our visit lolling back against her.

Nevertheless, his mother said that now, a month after final weaning, he did not need to be close to her all the time. He could play by himself. He could again be left with the neighbor while his mother worked in the garden. He was eating well and sleeping soundly. He wet his bed occasionally—perhaps once a week. He had stopped sucking his fingers. Whenever he saw his mother's breast, however, he still covered it up.

By this time he could understand a number of simple commands, including a request from his mother to fetch her some water. He called her *mama* and his uncle *taata* and also had a name for Kristina. When his mother threatened him with "I will beat you" he stopped whatever he had been doing. He was said to enjoy helping her while she was cooking, although she had to stop him from helping as soon as the fire was lit. He was said to enjoy digging holes in the ground, pounding peanuts, combing his hair, playing with paper and tins, and building things. None of these things did we witness, however, so constrained was he when we visited.

Gesell Testing

When Kasozi was fifteen months old, and shortly after our last visit, he was administered the Gesell Developmental Schedules by Dr. Géber. His test behavior was described as *dynamique* and his DQ was 109. The next year when Dr. Géber returned for retesting she found that the family had moved away.

Visits to the Clinic

Age wks.	*Weight lbs.*	*Comments*
48	20.7	
56	21.2	
58		cold

14

FOUR MORE MUSLIM BABIES

Alima, Namitala, Sulaimani, and Nakalema

The teacher in the Muslim school heard from the families described in the previous chapter about the transportation service we provided to the child welfare clinic. One day he approached us, imploring us to take his year-old son, Kitala, to the clinic with us, for he was ill. When his second wife bore a daughter, Alima, he sought to have his family participate in the research because he was impressed with its benefits. In enthusiasm he recruited the participation of relatives who lived near him, and soon Sulaimani and Nakalema were added to the sample. Finally, his first wife had a baby daughter, Namitala—the only baby born into the sample.

Alima and Namitala

The teacher's house was off the road that passed through the village, down a long, steep track that was too narrow for the car to pass. The house was set among handsome shade trees but was itself a small hut of wattle and daub, with a thatched roof, and was almost bare of furniture. Indeed, the only furnishings in the front room were two folding chairs, and it later became unclear to whom they belonged, for they were passed along from one family to another as we visited the cluster of families living at the end of the steep track. The ladies sat on mats on the floor, which were kept rolled up when not in use; these were taken from place to place as they were needed.

Our first visit was a very confusing one because of the many people there; besides ourselves there were at one point seven women and six babies, together with a number of older children who hovered in doorways and windows. The babies were fretful, and it was difficult to carry on a coordinated conversation.

DOI: 10.4324/9781003629337-17

We tried to focus our visit on Alima and her mother. The mother was a mere girl with delicate features and satiny light coffee-colored skin. She was the second wife, and this was her first baby. But it was the senior wife who controlled our visit and who gave the impression of controlling the junior wife and the whole household as well. She was very self-possessed and seemed not in the slightest degree awed by her European visitor. She talked freely and in a deep, husky voice. She wanted to serve us tea, but when she was deterred by Mrs. Kibuka, she rushed out to get us a huge basket full of pineapples and papaws. Thenceforward she was very generous with the produce from her garden, of which she was very proud.

The first wife was a big, vigorous woman, who usually seemed to be bursting with drive and energy. Her chief interest in life was her garden, which not only provided food for the household but also yielded cash crops. Growing such crops is considered a man's job, and in this sense the first wife was a career woman. Although most Ganda women spend a better part of the morning in the garden, she spent most of the day there. She seemed to have worked out an arrangement with the junior wife, relieving the latter of some of her share of the garden work, in return for which the junior wife took over most of the responsibility for keeping house, preparing food, and looking after the children.

Whether it was because of her preoccupation with the garden or because of an impatience with the role of mother, or both, the first wife regularly separated her children from herself at some time between weaning and the birth of a new baby. We met five of her children—two sons, five and a half and three and a half; a daughter, perhaps about seven, who lived with the maternal grandmother at the top of the steep track; a daughter aged two and a half, who lived with a paternal aunt; and Kitala, one and a half, who lived at home. Shortly after we began to visit, Kitala too was sent to live with his maternal grandmother. One day four of the five children were at home since the maternal grandmother had wanted to go away for a day. The mother seemed very proud of them, especially proud of the sons, and asked us to take a photograph of them clustered about her. Her maternal pride seemed at variance with her apparent lack of concern about any feelings of distress that they may have had (and which Kitala certainly displayed) at her sending them away to live with someone else. She seemed to feel that she fully discharged her responsibilities toward them by visiting twice a week and by having the children back if the maternal grandmother wished to be free of them for a day.

Because his school was nearby, we saw the father of this family more frequently than we saw most of the fathers of the babies in the sample. He was the only father whose initiative brought his family into the research sample. He seemed to have more active concern for the welfare of the children than did his first wife. This was particularly striking when we encountered him one day riding Kitala about on the handle bars of his bicycle. He was upset about Kitala's distress at separation and tried to keep him with him as much as possible, despite the fact that the child no longer lived at home. Indeed, he told us that he had tried to persuade his wife not to send Kitala away because he anticipated that it would be a very painful breach of ties.

When we visited this household we were often joined by the neighbors and their children and sometimes also by the older children who were no longer part of the household. A constant visitor was the paternal grandmother, a jolly old woman, who laughed uproariously at some of the strange things the European visitor did and said. It was she who kept the children in order, intervening if they were too lively, threatening to hit them. Indeed, if they did not respond to her command, "sit nicely," she would slap them. But she was obviously fond of the children and joked with them roughly, and they seemed to love it. It took many weeks to sort out just who were members of the household, who were members of the paternal grandmother's household nearby, and who were merely neighbors. It finally emerged that the household consisted of the father, his two wives, his son Kitala, a young paternal uncle, an eight-year-old boy of undetermined relationship, and the baby, Alima—and later, a second baby (the daughter of the first wife), Namitala.

Alima

Although we acceded to the father's request to give transportation to the clinic to Alima and her mother from the beginning, Alima was seven weeks old before we made our first visit to the family. She was still a tiny baby, delicate, light-colored, but with a great thatch of thick black hair. She had been born in hospital. It was four days before she suckled well, but then she did, and by the time we visited she was feeding avidly. Her mother fed her whenever she judged she was hungry, and, from what we observed, she responded to minimal signals from the baby; Alima did not have to cry to announce her hunger.

This young mother was perhaps overanxious. She was worried lest she did not have enough milk for the baby, and this was a persistent concern. She also was disturbed because the baby had bowel movements very rarely—only once a week. The mother was also alarmed because she thought the baby's tongue was "tied," and was not reassured either by my examination of it or by two previous examinations by Dr. Welbourn at the clinic. And now the baby had conjunctivitis.

Despite these concerns, Alima was judged to be healthy and was gaining about eight ounces a week. She fed well and awoke at night three times to be fed. She had baths three times a day, which she was said to enjoy, except for the midday bath in cold water. She took long naps and was not bothered by noise. For several weeks she slept with her mother at night, after which she slept in a crib in her mother's room.

When we visited at ten weeks there were again many people present, and again the first wife tended to dominate the interview. Kitala, her son, tried to make himself the center of attention, playing noisily, dancing around in the middle of the floor, and working his way into the foreground of every photograph we took. Alima's mother was quiet and demure but pleasant and a good informant whenever given an opportunity to talk. Alima sat propped up on the lap of her visiting half-sister. For a while I examined her locomotor function. She paid close attention to me as I did so. She seemed to be at about a twelve-weeks' level of development, except for a marked head lag when I pulled her into a sitting position. Later I noticed her sister holding her in a standing position; she maintained her weight on her feet, although she was steadied by her sister's hand around her legs.

Alima's mother said that she usually took Alima along when she went to work in the garden and put her down on a mat in the shade; but if she was working near the house she left her behind. The mother reported that Alima did not seem to differentiate between people at any distance but that she recognized her mother when close: "She can smell the difference." Despite her differential response to her mother, she nevertheless accepted being held by anyone—and she was held and "minded" by any of the older children who happened to be home.

Alima was twelve weeks old when next we visited. The chief purpose of this visit was to see Namitala, who was just eleven days old. A bed had been made for Namitala's mother—the first wife—in the front room. The father was at home to attend a funeral next door. Guests from the funeral kept dropping in, and there was much confusion. Alima was in the bedroom asleep when we arrived. Shortly thereafter her mother went to get her. She immediately wanted to demonstrate that Alima could sit alone. She placed the baby on the floor, carefully adjusting her feet so that the soles met in front of her and slumping her forward so that her hands were on the floor to balance her. Alima kept tipping over sideways, and her mother kept readjusting her position. Finally she sat alone for several moments, looking quite insecure and uncomfortable and crying. The next day at the clinic Alima weighed 9.8 pounds. This represented a gain of nearly a pound in two weeks.

Mrs. Kibuka visited when Alima was fifteen weeks old. She found the mother ill. She was huddled in the corner of the front room, clutching blankets to her, looking like a frail child. Alima was crying convulsively, and although her mother picked her up, she was not easily soothed. The mother not only felt miserable but also was very concerned about Alima; she said that her milk had failed because of her illness. Alima was hungry, but there was no other milk to give her, and so she had been given supplementary bottle feedings of weak tea with sugar. Although Alima usually cried very little, she was now very fussy because she was so hungry. Mrs. Kibuka held the baby for a while in order to relieve the mother who seemed weak and exhausted. The senior wife came in from the garden, and visitors arrived. After a while the visitors left, and the senior wife went back to the garden, giving Alima's mother Namitala to hold. The interview continued.

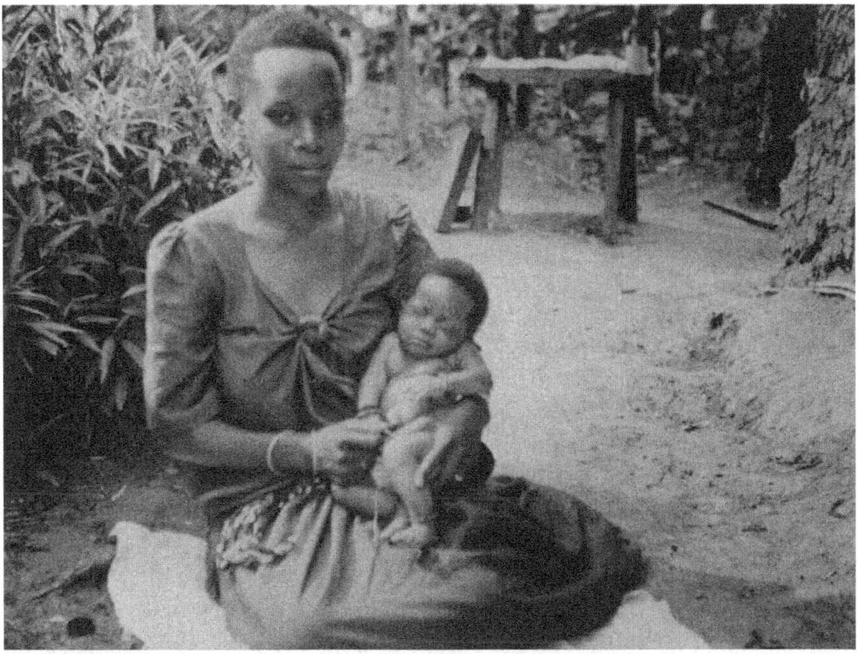

FIGURE 13 Alima (ten weeks) and her young mother.

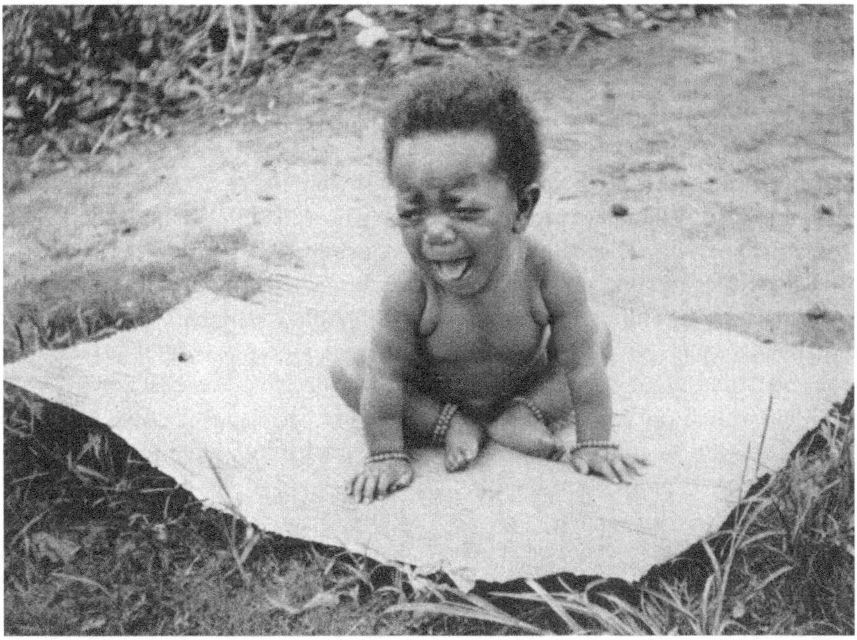

FIGURE 14 At twelve weeks Alima can sit alone, supported by her hands and legs—but she does not like it.

Alima's mother said that Alima had begun to show a differential response to her. She was used to being held by other people, but now if she was crying, she would not stop when picked up unless it was her mother who did so. "Now that she has started noticing me, she doesn't care about other people at all." She had begun to cry whenever her mother left the room, although she was never left alone in a room except when asleep. Although her mother sometimes left her in the house with other people or took her to be looked after by the paternal grandmother, usually she took the baby with her wherever she went, often carrying her in a sling on her back. Squash had been added to her diet on the decision of the paternal grandmother. We inquired about elimination training and were informed that holding down had begun "when she was very young," and that she now rarely wet the bed. During the visit, however, Alima wet Mrs. Kibuka as soon as she was taken onto her lap.

Mrs. Kibuka offered the mother some dried skim milk for the baby from a supply which had been left in the car. Unable to find anyone to send for it, the mother, despite her illness, walked up the long, steep track herself in order to get milk for the baby.

When we visited at eighteen weeks, Alima was asleep on a clutter of cloths in the front room. It was so dark in the house and the baby was so quiet that I did not notice her there for quite a while. Her mother was still concerned about insufficient breast milk. Although she had recovered from her illness, Ramadan had begun, and she blamed the fasting for the insufficient milk. Namitala had been left behind while her mother was in the garden. Soon she became fussy and did not stop crying even when Alima's mother picked her up. So, despite her insufficient milk, Alima's mother gave Namitala the breast. At this point Namitala's mother returned and exclaimed and laughed to see Namitala being suckled by the other woman. We were told that it was a very rare occurrence for a baby to be suckled by anyone other than his own mother.

Soon other visitors arrived. For a while there were, in addition to ourselves, five women, each with a baby, and three young boys. All the babies were hungry and fussed in a chorus of dissatisfaction. The women themselves seemed on edge, and for a while tempers ran high. But Alima's mother was gentle and pleasant as usual. The senior wife asked us to take more photographs, and both she and Alima's mother withdrew to dress themselves in their best clothes.

Meanwhile, Alima continued to sleep soundly. She had to be wakened when it was time for the photographs. She did not protest but whimpered when her mother tried to put a dress on her that was so tight at the neck that it could scarcely be forced over her head. During the rest of the visit she was held by various people, including me, and she accepted all of us. Twice she whimpered briefly and was taken by her mother and given the breast. Whenever she cried her mother said that she picked her up. If her mother was out of the room, however, Alima could at times be comforted by someone else—although we had been told three weeks earlier that she would stop crying only for her mother.

The implication was that she cried only when hungry or when removed from the breast before she was ready. A further implication was that she was given the breast whenever she fussed or cried, provided that her mother was present, which was usually the case. Her mother also reported that Alima smiled a lot, but our records made no special note of smiles.

Alima was twenty-six weeks old at the time of our last visit. She had been ill for a week with a cold accompanied by diarrhea and vomiting. Breast feedings had been supplemented with a little *matooke* and also with milk and tea given by nursing bottle. But the mother had discontinued the supplementary milk and tea since Alima had begun to vomit it up. Alima was held by her mother during the first part of our visit. In response to a series of vocalizations, which did not sound unhappy, her mother gave her the breast. After suckling for a while she was given to someone else to hold, and she accepted it. Then for a while she sat on the floor and played with a cup, rattling the small objects that had been placed in it. Once, placed prone, she crawled a bit but made little progress. Her mother said that crawling was just beginning. From time to time she sucked her thumb—something she had never done during our earlier visits.

Despite her illness she was said to cry infrequently. She did cry, however, whenever her mother left the room for a moment, leaving her alone or with one of the other children. She did not cry when left either with the first wife, Namitala's mother, or with her father, who was fond of her and held her a great deal. She did not accept the attentions of the other children and would cry if a child picked her up. Elimination training had been continuing. She had stopped soiling her bed until the diarrhea came; since then she had had several accidents. She let her mother know by crying when she wished to be held down. Occasionally she got angry, when hungry and not fed immediately, or when something she wanted was taken from her. She expressed her anger by crying, and her mother responded to it by picking her up and comforting her. On rare occasions her mother could not comfort her, and, exasperated, would "beat" her.

No very clear-cut vocalization had emerged yet—merely repeated syllables of the "ma-ma-ma-ma" variety. She did not vocalize in greeting but would express her pleasure in seeing a favorite person by smiling.

Visits to the Clinic

Age *wks.*	*Weight* *lbs.*	*Comments*
Birth	5.3	
3	6.6	
5	7.7	cough
9	9.0	conjunctivitis
11	9.8	mango worm

Namitala

Of course, in the meantime, we had been observing Namitala's development also. It was taken as a matter of course that we would do so as soon as she was born. When she was three days old we met her father, with Kitala on the handlebars of his bicycle, who informed us of her birth. The mother was staying with the maternal grandmother, in order to rest for a few days, and we visited her there. We expected to find her resting, but she was dressed and stooping over a tub outside the house, vigorously washing clothes. She assured us that this was the only work she was doing "these days." Alima's mother, meanwhile, was looking after the household and even prepared food for the senior wife and brought it up the hill to her.

Inside the hut we found Namitala lying on her mother's "bed" —which was a welter of cloths and blankets on the floor of the front room. Namitala was lying under the covers with a cloth over her face. She was asleep and scarcely roused when given to me to hold. She seemed a very large and well-developed newborn baby, with dark, rosy skin and profuse, black kinky hair. The mother told us that the birth had been quick and easy. She had intended to go to hospital but had too little warning that labor was imminent and went instead to the maternal grandmother for help.

A week later when we visited, Namitala and her mother were at home again. A bed was made up on the floor of the front room, and again the baby was lying in the bed, her head covered with a cloth. Her mother wanted us to take photographs. She picked Namitala up Ganda fashion, by seizing one arm above the elbow and swinging her up. Namitala did not seem disturbed by this seemingly rough treatment. The baby was said to be feeding well and sleeping most of the time.

Namitala developed rapidly. When she was eight weeks old she was so big and plump that I mistook her for Alima, who was four months old. She seemed very healthy, with glossy skin and thick black hair. During our visit she was held first by one of the boys and then by Alima's mother while her own mother worked in the garden. This was the occasion that Alima's mother offered her the breast when she fussed. She was fed again when her own mother returned. She was quiet for most of the rest of the visit, but toward the end she began to fret again—like all the other babies present. Her mother also complained of insufficient breast milk because of the Ramadan fast. She filled a nursing bottle with weak tea mixed with skim milk and gave it to Namitala, who sucked on it as contentedly as she had sucked on the breast. The mother said that she had been doing this throughout Ramadan. It was of interest that she did not provide Alima with a bottle at the same time—only her own baby.

The mother reported that she fed Namitala whenever she judged her to be hungry. Namitala was said to cry a lot; often she was given the breast when she cried, but not always. On the other hand, her mother was absent so much of the time that there must have been occasions when Namitala was hungry and went unfed. Her mother said that she usually held the baby for a while after feeding her, but if she was very busy, she put her down and went to work. The baby slept well at night, waking only once to be fed. She received no supplementary feeding, except for the bottle of tea and milk.

Both women said that Namitala had been sleeping very little during the day and that she had been crying a great deal. Since she was awake so much of the time, she was nearly always held by someone—by Alima's mother, by her own mother when she was there, or by one of the ubiquitous older children. She accepted being held by anyone and showed no signs of distinguishing between her own mother and Alima's. Although she could not sit unsupported, she sat on someone's lap leaning back, surveying the world with apparent interest. Her mother reported that she had begun to hold her down.

We next encountered Namitala when we met the mother on her way to catch the bus to attend the funeral of a relative in another village. She walked purposefully, with a bundle on her head and Namitala in a sling on her back. Namitala's head bounced about as her mother strode on.

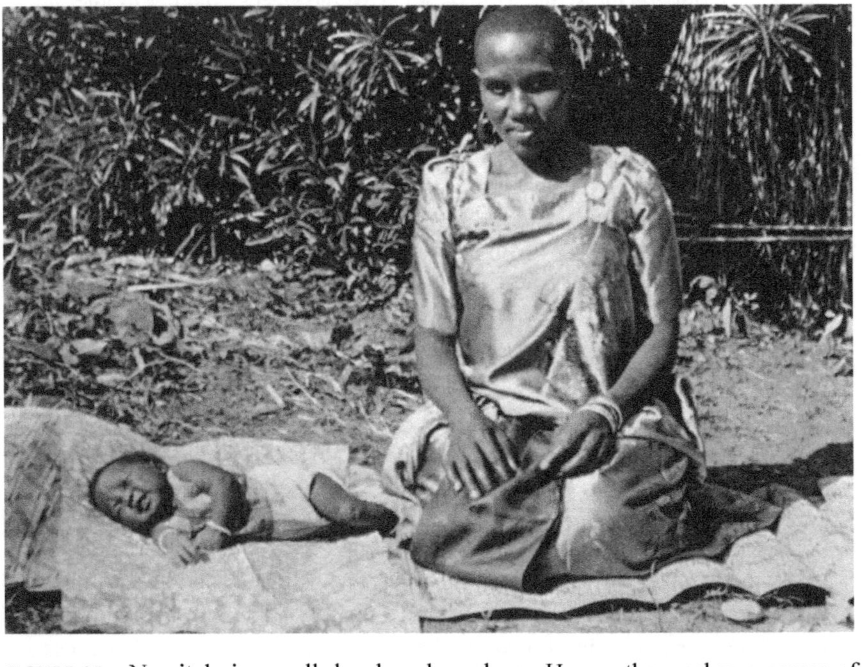

FIGURE 15 Namitala is a well-developed newborn. Her mother makes a career of her garden.

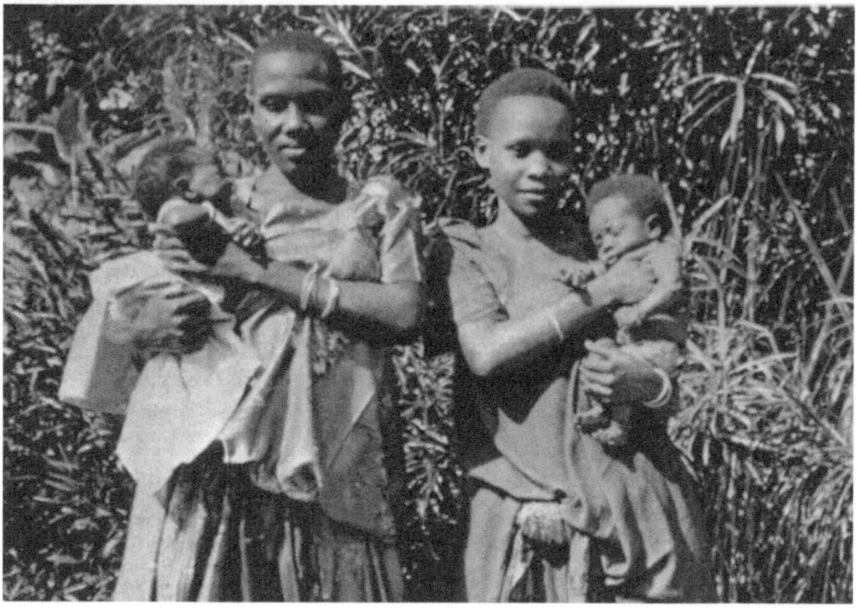

FIGURE 16 Two babies in one household. Namitala (eleven days) is on the left. Her mother is the senior wife. Alima (twelve weeks) and her mother are on the right.

When we went to visit her at twelve weeks, we saw her first at the house of a neighbor. She was naked and was being lugged about by a small boy. She looked well and accepted the boy's attention cheerfully. Back home she sat quietly, first on one lap and then on another. On her mother's lap she fussed a little but quieted without being fed, then went to sleep and was taken to bed, to a crib in her mother's room, Ramadan had ended; her mother's milk supply had improved. She was no longer chronically hungry and seldom cried. Now she was reported to be sleeping well during the day as well as at night.

Namitala was never left alone in the house. If neither her mother nor Alima's mother were available, there were always other children about who could be entrusted with the baby. Unlike Alima, however, she was sometimes left alone in a room while awake. She did not object to this and did not cry when her mother—or anyone else—left the room. Her mother usually left her behind while working in the garden. Most of the holding Namitala got from her mother was in the late afternoon after the garden work was finished and her mother "had time." We asked whether Namitala ever cried to be picked up and we were told that she sometimes did, but not very often. It was clear that she did not respond differentially to her mother and to her other caretakers.

A week later tragedy came to the family. Namitala's maternal grandfather was killed while riding his bicycle—hit by a car driven by a European from the Congo. All the people in the village were grief-stricken and were indignant about the circumstances of the accident. We were informed of the tragedy soon after it occurred. Soon we saw Namitala's mother walking briskly down the road with Namitala bobbing about on her back. Her face reflected classic grief and she lamented loudly, crying over and over again: *Kitalo nnyol* (What a disaster!) She mourned her father's death for some time and spent much time with her bereaved mother.

It was in the maternal grandmother's home that we made our last visit to Namitala. The house was full of women, all giving support to the widow. Under the circumstances, the mother was impatient about our inquiries concerning Namitala's development, but when she realized that this was our last visit she became cooperative.

Namitala was fifteen weeks old. When fourteen weeks old she had begun to sit alone. She continued to receive supplementary bottle feedings. There were still no signs that she discriminated her mother from anyone else: " She is the same with everyone." She cried very little—only when hungry or ill—and she never cried when her mother left the room. She was friendly with anyone who held her, even Europeans; she smiled at me and at another European when each of us held her.

When trying to assess this mother's excellence as an informant, my thoughts were rather at variance. On one hand, she was very friendly toward us, pressing gifts upon us, conscious of her role as hostess, and apparently concerned to give us the information we sought. Sometimes she responded to inquiries with detailed information given so rapidly that it was difficult to record it. When she talked about Namitala or about infant-care practices she talked freely and without apparent reserve. On the other hand, she was a difficult informant because she was always on the hop. Just when she seemed to be settled for an interview, she would jump up and rush away to do something—to get us a present, to prepare a bottle for the baby, or to attend to some unexplained duty elsewhere. Moreover, there were always other people present, and she was easily distracted into conversation with them about things not relevant to our inquiries. Her responsibilities in the garden, to other significant adults, to visitors, and as a hostess, seemed to preoccupy her to the extent that she found it difficult to find time to talk of her children. When she did respond to a direct question, however, she did so freely, elaborating her reply, and going on to volunteer details—at least until the next interruption.

Sulaimani

Sulaimani's mother was Alima's paternal aunt and lived nearby. She was present on the day when we arrived to start work with Alima. She was a second wife. The senior wife, a large and formidable woman considerably older than she, was childless. There had been two children before Sulaimani's birth, but they had not lived. The father was a farmer and therefore was at home much more than most of the fathers in our sample. We encountered him several times on our way to and from the cluster of families at the foot of the long steep track, but he never was present during one of our visits. He was always very cordial, however, and made us feel that he was pleased that his son was in the research sample and a recipient of the services we could give.

Sulaimani was not born in hospital. His mother had gone to hospital for her confinement, but the labor pains ceased, and she was discharged. She went to stay with a relative in Kampala. When labor began again, it progressed too quickly for her to manage to get back to the hospital. The baby was breast-fed and suckled well from the beginning. His mother fed him when she judged him to be hungry but did not offer the breast merely for comfort. Supplementary foods were begun at three months of age, starting with orange juice. He was said to have sat alone at three months of age. Elimination training began some time before that.

We first began to visit Sulaimani when he was twenty-five weeks old, although he had made several visits to the clinic before that. He wore a tiny pair of printed cotton trunks and had little bags of "medicine" slung across his naked torso. When we first arrived for our visit he sat quietly on the floor, looking about at us and chewing on a tin. Mrs. Kibuka held out her arms to invite him to come to her. He smiled and seemed eager to come. He accepted being held by her and cried when she put him down. She picked him up again, but he became restless sitting on her lap and began to fuss. Mrs. Kibuka handed him to his mother. He sat on his mother's lap, sometimes fussing, sometimes merely vocalizing. Finally he began to cry in earnest. The cry turned into a tempery scream. His mother tried to soothe him, talking to him and rocking him. There was a perfunctory quality to her soothing, and before long she slung him over her back and rocked him there. This treatment did not quiet him, however, so finally she gave him the breast—he immediately stopped crying and began to suckle.

His mother complained that he cried a lot. The crying was especially a problem when he was with his mother. With other people he was far less apt to cry. When his mother went to the garden or elsewhere, she had several different arrangements for his care. If she was working nearby, she left him in the house alone, but sometimes a young neighbor boy would baby-sit. He cried less when alone or with the boy than with his mother. Sometimes she left the baby with the maternal grandmother, but despite the fact that this woman seemed a favorite of the other children in the cluster of families, Sulaimani did not like her and tended to cry continuously when left with her. And he cried or fussed a great deal after his mother returned. His mother was concerned that he slept poorly. He was a very active child and did not seem to like to be put down to sleep. Even though the household was kept quiet for him, he cried when he was supposed to be napping, and when put down to sleep at night he fussed and did not sleep well.

Sulaimani was said to want to be with his mother all the time and to want to be held by her. He cried whenever she put him down. She would hold him in her arms until he fell asleep, but as soon as she put him down he woke and cried until she picked him up again. But, as we observed during our visit, he cried also while his mother held him. It appeared, even by twenty-five weeks, that a tense and insecure relationship had grown up between them. His mother had no confidence in being able to soothe him and was made anxious by his fussing. She did not offer the breast every time he cried, and yet she could find no other reliable method of quieting him.

He was a little over four months old when he joined the group visiting the clinic. He weighed 14.2 pounds on the occasion of his first visit. Two months later he had gained less than a pound. There were only minor illnesses that might have accounted for this slow gain.

At our first visit Sulaimani was just beginning to crawl, but he made little headway. Three weeks later, however, when he was twenty-eight weeks old, his crawling had become more effective—although it could be induced only by having his mother approach him after she had left him. His mother told us that his supplementary feedings included solids; she usually fed him these, but sometimes his father gave them to him. He was just beginning to feed himself with his fingers. Liquids were fed to him by means of a nursing bottle. He tried to hold the bottle but was not yet able to manage without help. He had learned not to soil his bed and was beginning to learn not to wet his bed.

Crying was still a problem. When left with other people he did not cry unless he was hungry, but when with his mother he cried to be picked up by her, and even after she had picked him up he usually continued to fuss; it seemed that nothing pleased him.

At this visit at twenty-eight weeks, Sulaimani was asleep when we arrived. His mother had been looking forward to having photographs taken. As soon as we arrived she wakened Sulaimani. He looked very sleepy. His face crumpled up and he soon began to cry. His mother had put him down on the floor beside her, but when he cried she took him on her lap and he quieted immediately. Soon she began to remove his pants, which were so tight she could scarcely get them off. She then handed him over to a young girl—a relative who was visiting for the afternoon—to take him outside and "hold him down." They disappeared around the corner of the house and almost immediately Sulaimani let out a howl. He continued to cry until he was returned to his mother. After holding him a moment, she put him down and left the room. He immediately howled again. She returned with a dress to put on him for the photograph and handed him to the young girl to dress. Sulaimani did not protest being handed over. The girl gave him back to his mother to put his pants on. This part of the dressing was fairly rough for it was difficult to squeeze him into his tight pants, but he did not protest.

We then went outside for the photographs; Sulaimani was held by his mother. Even while he sat on his mother's lap he made faces as if about to cry, so it was difficult to find a moment when his face was not crumpled up or his mouth open in a howl. Finally he quieted. I wished to photograph him by himself and suggested that his mother put him down on the mat. As soon as he was put down he screamed. I suggested that his mother give him something to distract him that might also induce him to crawl. His mother returned with a small tin of shoe polish and gave it to him. He fingered the tin and stopped crying. But when we took it away in order to use it as an incentive for crawling, he cried again and would not try to get it. I suggested, finally, that his mother come nearer. When she did, he crept toward her, and stopped crying as soon as she took him up.

When we settled down again for the visit the mother again discussed her concern about Sulaimani's crying so much. Soon she shifted her attention to Kitala, Namitala's brother. She criticized their mother for giving Kitala too much attention; she should just let him cry. Because of this comment, I wondered whether Sulaimani's mother was, in fact, giving him too little attention and asked when she held him. She replied that she held him when she was not working and that his father also held him and played with him sometimes. She said that she used to play with him more when he was younger, before he could sit alone. She reported that she never carried him on her back—only on her hip—and that no one else carried him. She did not make a practice of taking him to the garden with her; she either left him in the house alone or with someone else. During this interview the mother answered inquiries straightforwardly, and often, when talking about Sulaimani, her face would light up in a smile.

When Sulaimani was thirty-one weeks old his mother was supposed to have brought him to the house of Alima's and Namitala's family, but she arrived without him, saying he was sick with a cold. At the clinic a week later he was better and seemed to be gaining satisfactorily.

But when Sulaimani was thirty-five weeks old, on a similar occasion his mother did bring him. He sat for a while on someone else's lap, and then I invited him to mine. He sat quietly for a while but then cried when startled by an exclamation of mine. I returned him to his mother and gave him a piece of candy. He soon stopped fussing and squirmed down from his mother's lap. He began to creep about the floor. His dress hampered him, so his mother tied it up in a knot to keep it out of his way—and to keep it clean. He moved over to the doorway and with considerable effort got over the high doorstep. An older boy came into the house at this point, and as he passed, Sulaimani hit him hard for no apparent reason. As he stood in the doorway his mother told us that he had begun to stand at about thirty-two weeks of age. He was also able to cruise about, steadying himself against the wall.

His mother then took him and gave him the breast. After a short period of suckling we went outside to take photographs and Sulaimani was cheerful as long as his mother was close. He was left behind when we came in. I heard loud crying and, upon looking out, ascertained that it was Sulaimani. His mother was nowhere in sight. Very soon she returned and he stopped crying at once.

When Sulaimani was thirty-six weeks old and we were visiting Alima and Namitala, a messenger came to tell us that Sulaimani's mother was ill and could not see us. Alima's mother told us that the "illness" was injury. She had had a quarrel with the senior wife, who had beaten her very hard. Alima's mother urged us to visit her despite the message, which we did. We found Sulaimani's mother with a black eye but otherwise looking much as usual. Keeping up the fiction, however, she complained of malaria and asked for Daraprim, which we gave her.

Sulaimani was much more cheerful than he had ever been before when we visited. For a while he sat quietly on the floor. Then he began to creep around, with his green printed dress hitched up in a knot to give him freedom of movement. I gave him a piece of candy, and he messed about with it, sucking it, taking it in his hands, then putting it back in his mouth, spitting it onto the floor, then picking it up and putting it back in his mouth. Sometimes he offered the candy to his mother, holding out his sticky little hand and withdrawing it before she took the candy. After a while a man arrived to visit. He picked Sulaimani up, and he accepted this, staying contentedly on the man's lap for quite a while. The visitor gave him a coin, which he immediately put into his mouth. The visitor put him down on the floor; he sat quietly for a while, then yawned. Suddenly he stood up and reached his arms toward his mother in rather a rough gesture. She did not take him, so he sat for a while with his head in her lap. Then he became active, creeping toward the other room which was hidden from view by a curtain and separated by a doorstep at least a foot high. Sulaimani managed to get over the step. His mother brought him back. Soon she went into the other room for something and he followed her. At the end of the visit I picked him up and put him on my lap. He sat quietly for a moment without protest and then gave a slight squirm to indicate that he wanted down. He returned to his mother, but did not cling to her. During the visit he vocalized a lot, humming and making sibilant noises. At one point he wet on the floor. Without fuss his mother pulled a chair over the wet spot so that he could not get into it.

His behavior was in striking contrast to the fussy, clinging behavior that he had shown on all previous occasions. We were later informed that shortly after the violent quarrel the senior wife had gone away. It seems a reasonable hypothesis that her departure led to a relaxation of tension, and that this was somehow communicated to Sulaimani. Whether because the mother's practices changed or merely because she was more relaxed, Sulaimani's behavior was more secure.

His mother confirmed that recently he had been much less fussy. He cried only when directly frustrated. He now attempted to follow his mother everywhere she

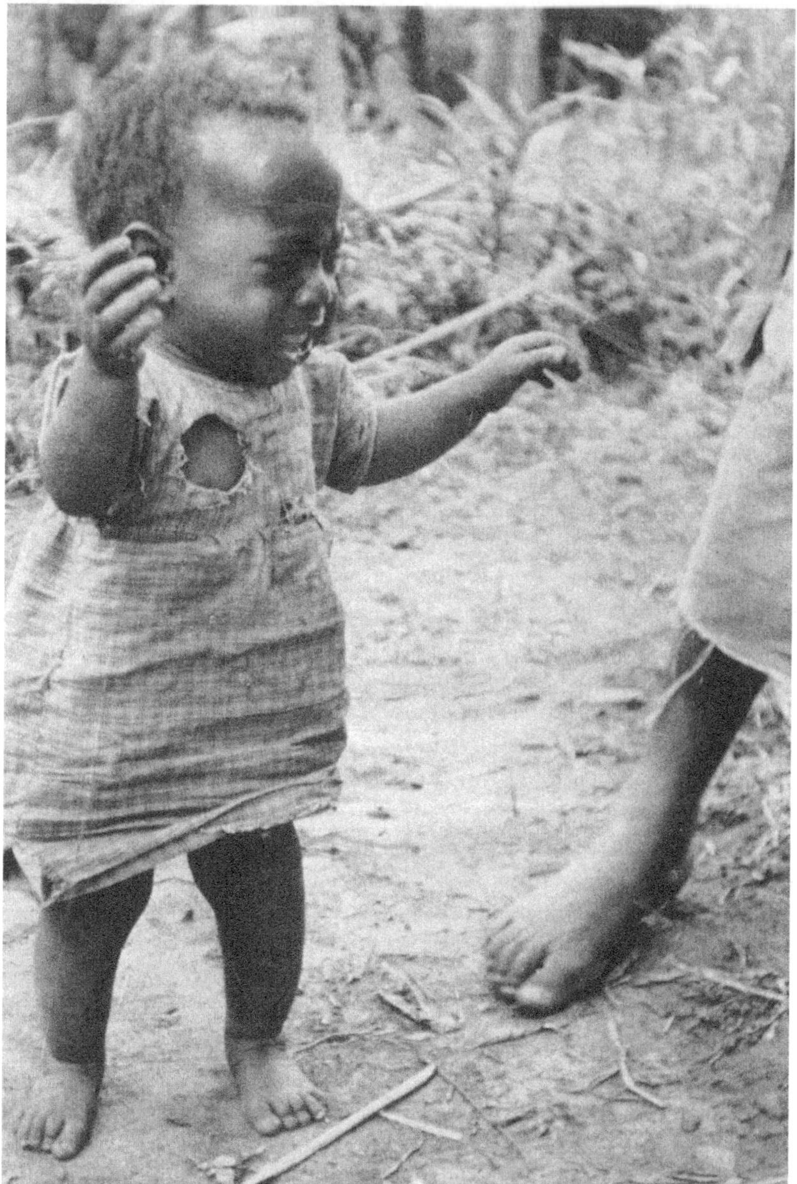

FIGURE 17 Sulaimani (thirty-five weeks) will not let his mother move away from him.

went. He was said to be very fond of his father and to prefer him to his mother, even when tired or ill. This preference seemed to have generalized to other men, and, indeed, he accepted the male visitor without any strangeness, although he was a complete stranger.

When he was thirty-eight weeks old Sulaimani became quite ill with fever, diarrhea, and vomiting. This was his first serious illness. He stopped creeping about and was reported to have been quite weak. He had appeared to be on the point of walking but had stopped trying when he became ill.

When we visited at forty weeks he was considerably better and was less fussy than he had been previously. He still wanted to be with his mother all the time, however, and cried and followed whenever she left the room. But when his father returned home he preferred father to mother and did not try to follow the mother when left with the father, unless he was hungry. He was also said to obey his father better than his mother. He still disliked the grandmother but had gotten to like children and to play well with them. He was said to be a bit shy with strangers, but after he had had a while to get used to the stranger he could be friendly. On the whole the mother was much relieved because the tense fussiness seemed to be a thing of the past.

Sulaimani liked—and had for some time—to imitate automobiles, even though these were rare in his experience. He moved objects around the floor with a "brrrr" noise to imitate the motor. His elimination training was progressing; sometimes he would go outside the house when he wanted to have a bowel movement or to wet; sometimes he did not. He no longer soiled his bed, but sometimes he wet it. He had been getting a wide variety of supplementary solid foods and by now he sometimes received supplementary bottle feedings of milk also.

When we arrived for this visit the mother was at the back of the house bathing. We glimpsed Sulaimani sitting on the ground near her. The mother brought him in with her when she came to greet us and set him on the ground for a moment. Sulaimani cried immediately when he was set down and stopped when his mother sat down and took him on her lap. Again she tried to put him on the ground; this time he screamed and did not stop even when she took him up again. He struggled and seemed on the verge of a real tantrum. I gave him a piece of candy and he quieted. His mother had some palm fibers nearby, used in weaving mats. Sulaimani wanted to play with these and removed some from the bundle. His mother obviously did not want him to have them, but when he threatened another tantrum she gave in and let him have them.

Mrs. Kibuka took him onto her lap. He sat there looking very insecure. She put him down and he began to play in a desultory fashion with a large tin container. Mrs. Kibuka pretended it was a drum. He watched but did not seem interested. He was quite inactive. When we took him out for photographs he was reluctant for his mother to leave him so that he could be photographed by himself. Finally it was accomplished. Back in the house, the mother left the room for a moment. Sulaimani did not notice her departure at first, but then he scuttled on hands and knees to the door and began to cry. It was true that he was less inexplicably fussy than before, but, nevertheless, he was more insecure in his behavior than were many of the others in the sample.

We inquired about discipline. His mother said that she "beat" him if he cried a lot—enough to annoy her. When she smacked him on the arm with her cupped hand, his response was to have a real tantrum and to try to hit his mother back.

He could understand several simple commands by this time— "Come!" "Stop!" "Go away!" "Give it to me!" and the like. He sometimes used *mama* and *taata* appropriately, but not always. He made repetitive sounds like "ooh-ooh-ooh-ooh" and tried to imitate sounds.

Our last visit, made one week later, was very brief since the mother was ill. Sulaimani seemed a bit more fussy than the last time, but when his mother gave him the breast he calmed and suckled.

Visits to the Clinic

Age *wks.*	*Weight* *lbs.*	*Comments*
15	14.2	
23	14.7	
25	14.9	scalp infection
27	15.0	cough
29	15.8	cough
33	16.6	

Nakalema

The families of Nakalema and Alima were bound by blood ties, although I was unable to establish the precise relationship. Nakalema's mother proved to be less cooperative than any of the other mothers in our sample. A series of events disrupted the regular schedule of our visits to this family and perhaps contributed to the less cooperative attitude; perhaps the mother participated in the research because of pressure exerted by Alima's father, who seemed the leader in this cluster of families.

The two families lived very close together; neither had enough land. The crowding was resolved by consolidating the two plots for one family while Nakalema's family found another plot some distance away. Although this provided more scope for the father, who was a farmer, the move was temporarily disorganizing. A new garden had to be started and a new house built. While this was being done Nakalema's mother took her elsewhere to live and was inaccessible to us. Two deaths also intervened to interrupt our schedule of visits—those of a grandchild of Nakalema's father and Alima's maternal grandmother.

It was difficult to establish just who belonged to the household because relatives and neighbors usually visited at the same time we did. Four children were eventually identified as Nakalema's brothers and sisters and appeared to live in the household. There may have been other children living away from home. A young man, identified as a paternal uncle, also seemed to be a member of the household.

Nakalema was twenty-four weeks old when our visits began. She was a healthy looking baby, with profuse black hair on the crown of her head, but with the hair lower on her head seeming to have worn off. She was naked except for beads around her waist and ankles and little bags of "medicine" tied around her back. She was asleep on a pile of old clothes in a corner of the dark room when we arrived and slept through most of our visit. When she woke she whimpered a little and rolled about on her bed. Her mother ignored her waking signals. Finally the grandmother, who was present for the visit, reached over, grasped one arm, and swung the baby over to her lap. Then Nakalema sat quietly and contentedly. There was, however, no interaction with her mother at all.

We obtained the following information about her earlier development. She was born at home, with the grandmother assisting in the delivery. She seemed healthy, and had suckled well from the beginning. Her mother said that she fed her whenever she was hungry, and, indeed, whenever she cried, for whatever reason. She had been receiving orange juice, porridge, *matooke*, bananas, and milk to supplement breast feeding; indeed, the mother expressed concern that her own milk supply had been failing. Her mother described her as greedy because she cried as soon as she saw food and before it was actually given to her. This greediness worried her mother. Nakalema slept with her mother, and woke two or three times at night to be fed. Apart from these feedings she slept soundly at night, but (despite her sound sleep during our visit) she was said to not sleep soundly during the day, waking at the slightest noise. She had three baths a day. "Holding down" was said to have begun when she was three months old, but she still wet and soiled her bed. She had had diarrhea for two months, and also had had a bout of malaria, both of which she had recovered from by twenty-four weeks of age.

When Nakalema was three months old her mother tried to train her to sit by wrapping cloths around her to support her; she could sit alone at four months. She could not yet crawl, although she could sit alone indefinitely and steadily.

Her mother complained that she cried a great deal. She cried whenever her mother put her down and whenever her mother left the room, regardless of whom she was left with. She was said to want to be with her mother all of the time. Usually her mother took her along to the garden and put her down on a mat while she worked. Sometimes she was left behind with other people, and she always objected to this.

When we visited at twenty-six weeks Nakalema was again asleep in the house. When she was brought outside to join the group who were sitting on the grass she was placed on a little mat close to her mother. She was very quiet, sitting up straight, looking around at the company, and occasionally fingering the grass. She began to fuss after a while, but nothing was done, and she stopped spontaneously after a few moments. I gave her an empty film cassette as a toy, and she manipulated it with apparent interest until another child quietly appropriated it. I approached her and she cried; I tried to pick her up, but she resisted. Her fear of me seemed to be because I was European, for she accepted being picked up by Mrs. Kibuka immediately afterward. She sat quietly on Mrs. Kibuka's lap, close to me. Toward the end of the visit she began to fuss again. While we made preparations to depart, her mother quietly put her to the breast and Nakalema settled down.

We did not see Nakalema again until she was thirty-five weeks old. One visit had been canceled because of a funeral, and then the family moved away for a while. Even when they moved back to the village the new house was only a temporary one—a small grass hut. The family seemed to be spending the afternoon out-of-doors. The mother was shelling beans. Three of Nakalema's siblings were present, as was the paternal uncle. Nakalema was sitting on a ragged cloth, not very near her mother. Chairs had been brought along for our use, and mine was placed near Nakalema. I picked her up and held her on my lap. She did not protest, although she was very quiet at first. Soon she began reaching to feel my face. I took out a piece of paper, and she grabbed at it persistently. Twice she put her lips to my throat, and I noticed later that she repeated this with her mother. I soon set her down on the ground because I wanted to take notes. She coughed, then yawned, then coughed again. Presently she began to cry and I handed her to her mother.

On her mother's lap she sat quietly for a while and then began to play with her mother's face. Then in a more purposeful way she grasped at her mother's dress in an apparent attempt to open it. Her mother discouraged her attempt to reach the breast. Soon Nakalema began to cry loudly, throwing herself back against her mother repeatedly. Her mother capitulated and gave her the breast. Nakalema sucked contentedly. She was through in a short time and accepted being put down on the grass beside her mother. She sat "blowing raspberries" and seeming quite happy. Saliva spluttered out—and all through the visit she was quite wet with saliva, for she slobbered a great deal. We did not see her put anything into her mouth, but her mother said that she always put playthings in her mouth.

The mother's delay in giving the breast was noteworthy because she had previously implied that she gave the breast very readily on demand—"and when

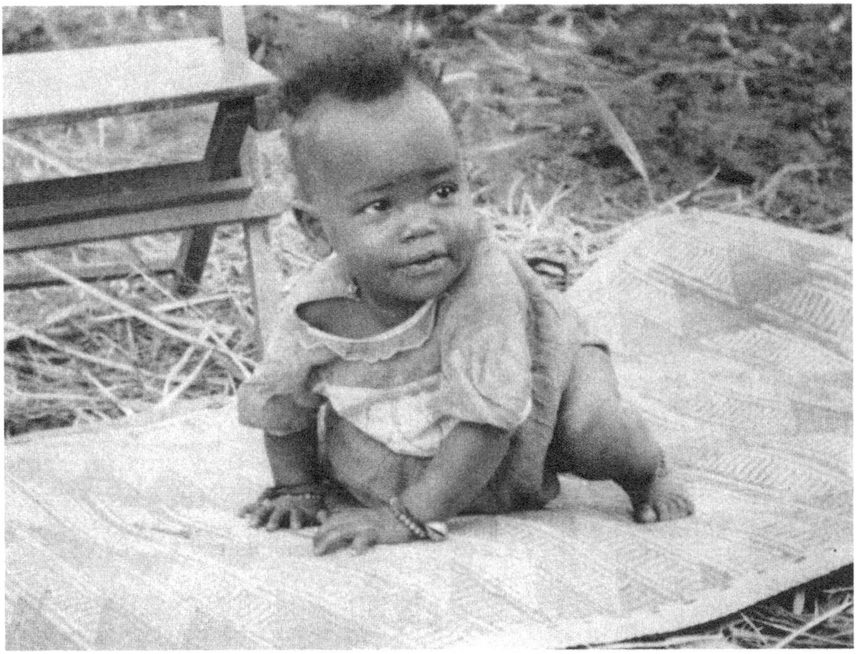

FIGURE 18 Nakalema at thirty-nine weeks is alone because her mother wanted to be photographed with her son, not with the baby.

she cries, for whatever reason." Perhaps she meant that she gave the breast when Nakalema cried hard. Her mother was surprised that Nakalema was so friendly with me, for she usually was not friendly with strangers.

Nakalema was just beginning to crawl, making very slow progress, pushing herself along with her hands. She cried and tried to follow her mother whenever she left the room.

We inquired about who looked after Nakalema. The other children helped but did not feed or bathe her. At times either the father or the paternal uncle helped to feed or bathe her, however. Sometimes she was left in the house alone, but only when asleep. She was rarely carried anywhere except by her mother; her mother sometimes carried her in arms, sometimes astride her hip, sometimes in a sling on her back. The mother said that she held her often and that the father and other children played with her often.

We had only one other visit with Nakalema—at thirty-nine weeks—and in the meantime another funeral had caused a cancellation. The family was still "camping"—sleeping in the little grass hut and spending most of the day outdoors. Meanwhile, construction of a new wattle-and-daub house had begun. The mother

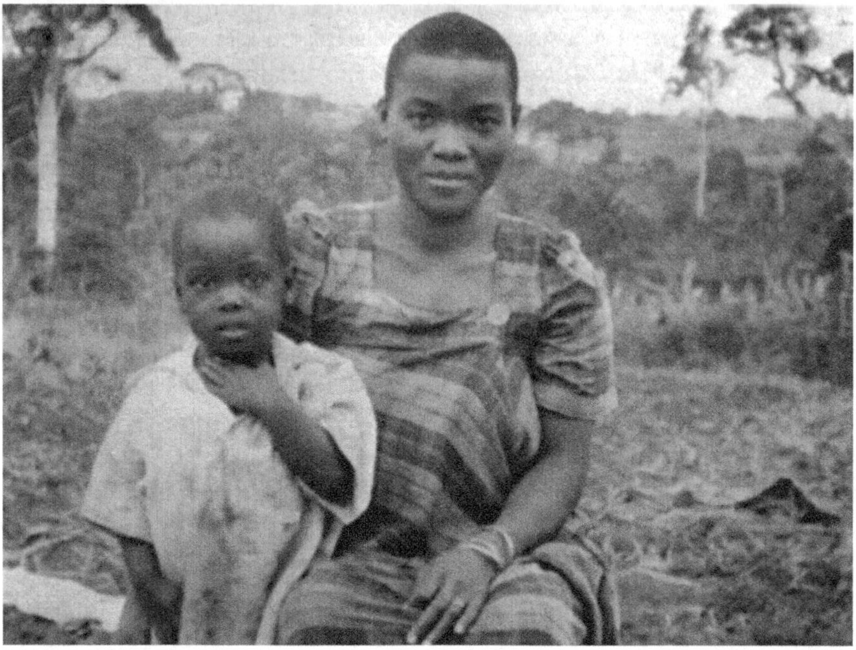

FIGURE 19 Here is Nakalema's mother with one of her sons.

complained of fever and huddled with a cloth aroung her like a shawl. It was an inopportune time for a visit, but there had been so many interruptions and I had so little information about Nakalema's development that I proceeded with questions. Before long the mother burst our irritably —"too many questions!" But when I explained that it was our last visit, she cooperated. She reminded us that we had promised to take photographs—and bustled about cleaning the children up and getting ready herself. She was concerned that she was not presentable for she had no brassiere on. This was solved by borrowing one from Sulaimani's mother, who was present during the visit. But when all was ready she refused to pose with Nakalema, saying that she already had one picture of herself with the baby. She wanted to be photographed with one of her sons. I got the overwhelming impression that she had a distinct preference for this boy.

Nakalema did not look very well. Her hair was matted and she had sores on her scalp and elsewhere on her body. Her mother had treated them but had run out of medicine. She was very dirty and this concerned her mother not at all. Even when she readied the children for the photographs she cleaned Nakalema minimally.

When we arrived for this visit we were placed so that we did not have a good view of the baby. My chair was placed facing the mother, and Mrs. Kibuka sat on a mat beside the mother. Nakalema was playing with the other children behind us and was not at all close to her mother. I turned to look at her from time to time. She spent most of the time sitting quietly, manipulating bits of grass and other things she found on the ground; she was rather inactive and apparently watched neither her mother nor us. Once I saw her clapping her hands as if rehearsing an interesting new activity—for there was no apparent stimulus for the action. Finally the older of her two sisters picked her up, presumably because her mother was just telling us how Nakalema protested being picked up by one of the children. The sister carried her over behind Mrs. Kibuka while Nakalema cried. She quieted for a moment as the sister held her and then began to cry again in earnest. The sister took her to her mother, who gave her the breast immediately. She quieted, suckled for a short time, and then her mother put her down. She was quiet for a moment and then cried again. This time the younger of her two sisters picked her up—a very small child, scarcely big enough to manage to pick up this nine-months-old baby. The child, attempting to be tender and maternal, tried to lift Nakalema up over her shoulder to pat her and soothe her. Nakalema screamed and struggled until finally she was released. Once on the ground again she gradually quieted. Later her mother picked her up and again she cried and struggled.

This baby seemed slower in her development than other babies of the same age in our sample and she also was said to cry a great deal. We were interested to find out whether there were any factors in her care or development that might account for these features. Of course, there had been a series of disrupting events, which, even though they may not have affected her directly, may have made the mother anxious or preoccupied with other things. Furthermore, on the occasion of this visit particularly it seemed that the mother was rejecting Nakalema somewhat; she certainly preferred one of the sons to any of the other children. And now the mother told us that Nakalema got ill often and repeated that she had had a prolonged period of diarrhea—this time it had lasted for three months and had been so serious that she had been taken to hospital for treatment. Moreover, Nakalema had vomited frequently—and still did so. This occurred expecially when she coughed. She would cry, then vomit, and then cough. Her mother did not seem at all concerned about this. When we inquired what she did, she replied: "I just leave her alone." On the other hand, the mother still insisted that she fed Nakalema on demand and for comfort—and, indeed, sometimes we had witnessed this. When we inquired whether she enjoyed breast feeding, she laughed, hid her face in her shawl, and said she liked it.

Nakalema could now creep on hands and knees, we were told, although we had never seen her do so. She had learned not to soil her bed, but she still wet the bed and soiled and wet in the house. She had not slept with her mother since about six months of age. She could understand her name and several simple commands "Come," "Stop," and "Go away." She could vocalize "da-da-da-da," but that was about all; she had no words.

She was said invariably to cry and to try to follow her mother whenever she left her side, even when there were other members of the family present. She behaved the same way with her father if he moved off leaving her alone; but if the mother left her with the father, she would cry and follow the mother. She was said to be fond of her father, however, and also of her paternal uncle. She had little interaction with her brothers and rejected the attention of her older sister. She was said to like the younger of her two sisters, but, as she demonstrated during our visit, she did not like to be picked up by her. Her mother now held her relatively little, except when feeding her. "Beating" had begun. Once her mother saw her fingering her genitals and smacked her fingers; it had not happened again. She also got smacked when she urinated and put her fingers in the puddle. On the other hand, Nakalema "beat" her mother when she got angry. When we inquired what made her angry, the mother replied, "When the girls pick her up, and whenever I go away anywhere; she wants to be with me the whole time."

15

FOUR BABIES FROM ACCULTURATED FAMILIES

WILLIAM, MARYAMU, AND THE YOUNGER TWINS, WASWA AND NAKATO

William was two months old when I first made his mother's acquaintance. This took place during my period of living in the village to learn the customs and language. Since it had been a tacit understanding with the chief that I would not begin the research until all the formal arrangements had been made, William was fourteen weeks old before regular visits began. Soon after this we asked the mother to suggest other possible participants, and some time later she introduced us to Maryamu's mother, who was the wife of William's paternal uncle.

While I was living in the village my attention was drawn to the birth of twins; I noticed a large number of people visiting the house of the shopkeeper who lived at the crossroads. The next day I paid my respects to the twins and their parents. But it was not until two months later that I could approach them with an invitation to participate in the research. This I accomplished through William's mother. It emerged that William's father was the brother of the twins' mother, and, indeed, she had lived with William's family for some years before marrying the shopkeeper and had left a daughter behind to be reared by William's mother.

William

William's mother was a handsome, light-skinned, fine-featured woman, with ten children ranging from William, the baby, to a twenty-year-old married daughter with a baby of her own. William's father was an assistant veterinary officer in government service and was subject to reposting from one locality to another. When first married he and his wife moved together from post to post, but as more and more children arrived, moves proved to be impracticable. They established a home base, where the mother made her garden and reared the family, and the

DOI: 10.4324/9781003629337-18

father visited as often as he could. While William was a baby, his father was too far away to come home, except infrequently.

Their house, although made of wattle and daub with a thatched roof, gave an impression of both grace and substance. Flowers grew in the front yard, and there was a graceful shade tree. Inside it was comfortable. There were simple but comfortable chairs. A woven reed ceiling lent coolness to the rooms. Family pictures covered the walls, and there was one colorful painting that one of the children had done at school. There were several little tables with cross-stitched covers. There was always a vase of flowers. When we came to visit we sat sometimes in the cool, dim living room, sometimes outside under the shade tree.

Our visits to this house had a characteristic pattern. After unhurried greetings and preliminary conversation, the children came in, one or two at a time, in a seemingly spontaneous way, and their mother spent a few moments presenting each child and mentioning something currently significant in the life of that particular child—an accomplishment, a special interest or talent, a prized article of new clothing, a special expedition or pleasure unique to that child. This inclusion of all the children was unusual, for most of the mothers we visited seemed to have their attention focused on the baby to the relative exclusion of the other children. Before long, however, this mother would fetch the baby, if he were not already present; the other children drifted away, and there would be peace in which to talk. This mother did not lose sight of the chief purpose of our visits and volunteered information about William, his development, and about her infant-care practices. Then, in due course, she served us a correct English tea with thinly sliced bread and butter and good homemade cakes—or sometimes for a special treat, Pepsi-Cola. Toward the end of the visit she often wished to discuss other concerns—techniques of dressmaking, patterns, her concern that one of the boys had failed to gain admission to the elite boarding school that seemed a condition for a successful career in Uganda, that another of the boys had a problem of bed-wetting, and so on.

This woman won our unstinted admiration for the competence and serenity with which she dealt with her large and complicated household. She grew all of their food. She made many of her children's clothes and had recently acquired a sewing machine to help with this task. She had time to devote to William, the baby, not only for routine care but for playful, intimate interchange. She treated each child as a person important in his own right—not only her own children but also her husband's little niece who lived with them. She had time to talk to us in an unhurried way.

For some years she had been a faithful attendant at Dr. Welbourn's child welfare clinic; she had been awarded a Red Cross certificate for completion of a course in practical child welfare. She was interested to learn as much as she could of European methods of child rearing, both to promote good health through proper nutrition and hygiene and to find more efficient methods that would help her to better organize her time.

She breast-fed all of her children but used a schedule as an aid to a planned daily routine. She was not rigid about the schedule and would feed the baby early if he seemed hungry—but, as she reported, the schedule seemed to help the baby to become hungry at predictably regular times. She found that the use of a potty was convenient, and this was begun with William when he was eleven weeks old. Instead of a baby carriage she used an iron wheelbarrow, in which William was nested amid snowy white cotton cloths. The wheel-barrow could be moved out to the garden while the mother worked or left under the shade tree in the front yard; thus he could sleep always within earshot of some responsible person. This mother did not believe in picking the baby up every time he cried. She played with him for a while after feeding, then put him down in his bed or in his wheel-barrow and expected him to settle down. But if he woke from sleeping with a cry, he was given immediate attention.

During our visit at fourteen weeks William sat on his mother's lap, supported by her body, facing us. He smiled at us occasionally. Gradually, however, he became restless. His mother gave him the breast and he fell asleep in her arms. The mother said that he still slept much of the time, that he cried but rarely, and usually settled down quietly after feeding without crying. The other children shared in the responsibility for him and seemed to enjoy doing so. Most of the responsibility fell to the seven-year-old brother, for the four-year-old and two-year-old were still too young to be of much help and the older children were at school most of the time. But all the children seemed fond of him and gave him a lot of affectionate attention. His father was said also to be very good with him.

On one of our visits when William was eighteen weeks old, he was given to me to hold. He sat supported on my lap, apparently nearly able to sit alone, and smiled at his mother across the room. He became increasingly restless, however, and gave me the impression of wanting to get to his mother, although he did not cry. Once back on his mother's lap he gave me a brilliant smile. On another visit when he was twenty-eight weeks old, he seemed much less baby-like. He watched us intently but did not smile. A week later he sucked his thumb through most of the visit, either sitting or standing supported on his mother's lap. Gradually he became more active and began to babble. He was handed over to Mrs. Kibuka, who seated him facing her. He looked down, averting his eyes, very quiet at first, and then began to suck his thumb again. When it was time to serve refreshments, the mother had William taken outside. After a while he let out a howl and his mother had him brought in again. He sat on his mother's lap, sucking his thumb, fussing intermittently. He went to sleep finally, leaning against his mother's shoulder, his thumb still in his mouth, and his mother carried him off to bed.

William was never left alone except when asleep, and then there was always someone close by. When awake he was always with someone, usually his mother but sometimes the other children. He was never left in the house by himself or with a stranger. As soon as he began to crawl, he tried to follow his mother whenever she left the room, setting up an immediate cry. At first his efforts to follow were in vain, but when his mother returned he would clap his hands and then put his arms up to her, as though asking to be picked up. He showed a marked preference for his mother, although he readily accepted the attention of his brothers and sisters. His father was home too infrequently for William to recognize him easily, but once they became reacquainted William showed excitement whenever he saw his father during the rest of his visit. His father was said to be very fond of him and to hold him often.

William could sit unsupported at twenty-two weeks of age, and at twenty-four weeks he began to crawl. By twenty-nine weeks he could stand, holding onto a chair or steadying himself against the wall. Soon after this he could pull himself up, and by thirty-two weeks I noticed that he could sit down again by himself. He cruised, holding onto the sides of his crib, and by now, of course, he was creeping on hands and knees rather than crawling.

By the time he was twenty-nine weeks old he had nearly achieved bowel control in the sense that he could give a specific vocal signal, and since nearly always someone was there to hear and heed, he had very few accidents.

Breast feeding was supplemented by orange or tomato juice, beginning at about three months of age. By the time he was thirty-two weeks old he was receiving all sorts of supplementary foods, including bean soup, eggs, porridge, and fruit. The solids were spoon fed and the liquids were given by cup. By thirty-eight weeks he was able to hold his own cup and to feed himself with his fingers.

At thirty-two weeks of age William had a setback in his development. He had a cold with a fever and seemed unhappy. His mother was concerned that he was not gaining weight. This illness continued, with ups and downs, for about three months. When we visited at thirty-two weeks he was somewhat subdued and quiet but he smiled frequently, particularly at his mother. He sat on his mother's lap, but when she wanted to get something to show us she put him down on the floor of the next room and left. William cried as soon as she left; his four-year-old brother picked him up and held him on his lap; William calmed and sucked his thumb. He spent much of the rest of the visit on the floor, creeping about, and for a while the other children were present and played nicely with him. Later, back on his mother's lap, he was fussy for a while and played with her dress; then he began to hit his mother and laughed. It seemed that he wanted to be fed, but she did not oblige him.

William's play at this age consisted largely of passing objects from one hand to another, rattling tins with pebbles inside them, and sometimes creeping about on the floor, pushing an object ahead of him. He also did some mouthing, and much vocalization to the playthings. He could understand *jjangu* (come).

By this age also, William showed a clear differentiation of the members of his own household from others. He was said not to like men other than his father. Women he accepted, but he did not seem really happy with them unless they had visited frequently enough for him to know them well.

On a visit when William was thirty-nine weeks old I was interested to observe that he could hold his own in a tussle with a two-year-old child. I did not see the beginning of the disagreement, but I saw William hitting the other child hard enough to make him cry and hit back. The mother thought that the difficulty was that the other child was a stranger and that otherwise William was not aggressive.

William's intermittent illness took a turn for the worse when he was forty-two weeks old; he had an attack of vomiting and diarrhea and his weight dropped from 18.8 to 18 pounds. When we visited him the next week he was still ill and was very subdued and clinging. His mother had planned to wean him at this age but decided to postpone this until he was twelve months old. Throughout the visit he sat on his mother's lap, leaning back against her breast and sucking his thumb. When we arrived Mrs. Kibuka approached him and he cringed, turning away. When his mother left the room for a moment she took him with her. I offered to pick him up as we were about to leave; he did not respond at all.

His motor development had been affected by his illness. He had begun to walk alone by about nine months of age, but by this time he no longer attempted to walk. He had acquired his first three words, however—*mama, taata, and jjajja.* He could understand simple commands like "go away," "stop doing that," "be quiet," and "give it to me." His mother had begun some discipline when he was about eight months old, tapping his hand when he was doing something that she didn't want him to do.

William's mother said that since he had been so ill he had wanted to be with her more than before. He protested her departure whenever she left him, seeming to become quite angry. The child with whom he was left would hold him and attempt to console him, and gradually he would calm down. He also become angry if the other children were playing with something he wanted and wouldn't give it to him; then he would not only cry but hit out as well. Sometimes his mother would give him comfort when he was angry; sometimes she let him cry.

William was forty-five weeks old when we paid our last visit. He sat on his mother's lap, friendly, laughing, and active. His mother said he was "so happy" to feel well again, and, indeed, it seemed so.

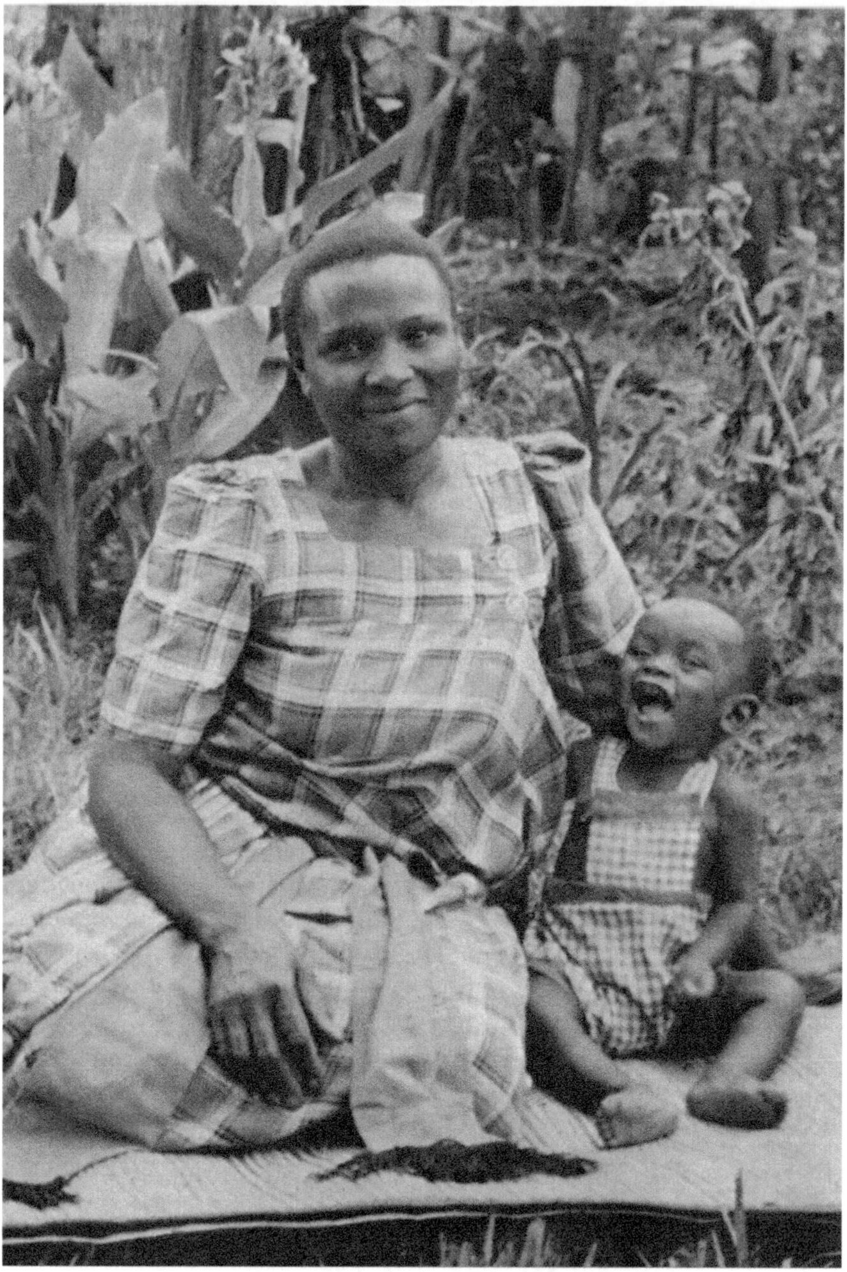

FIGURE 20 Here is William at thirty-seven weeks with his mother.

Gesell Testing

When William was forty-seven weeks old Dr. Géber administered the Gesell Developmental Schedules. His mother put him down on the floor close to her and he leaned against her. Throughout the test he obviously drew security from her, and responded little to the examiner. He either performed the tasks spontaneously, or he did so when his mother encouraged him. He looked at her from time to time; he leaned against her; and he climbed onto her knees to seek closer contact whenever he felt anxious for a moment. Three of the other children were present in the doorway. William seemed particularly oriented to one of them, occasionally showing him a test object or offering it to him. He appeared to be distracted by a stranger, who was merely sitting and observing. As the testing progressed he became more and more uneasy, as though he were asking himself why all the toys were presented only to him and not to his brother and why all the adults were looking at him.

Despite these moments of anxiety he was *dynamique* in the testing. He stood alone for a moment; he could walk a little when led with both hands held. He could say several words and tried to imitate the sound of others. He could make himself understood by pointing to what he wanted; he could touch himself to indicate his need to urinate. He communicated with others by vocalization. When given cubes, he manipulated them with one hand while clutching his mother's skirt with the other. He tried to make a tower but couldn't manage to let go of the cubes. He was not interested in the form board; he removed the blocks, inspected them, and showed them to his brother. He was interested in the ring, which he drew to him with the string and shook. He investigated the clapper of the bell, showed the bell to his mother, then rang it and laughed. In his excitement he climbed onto his mother's knees, then fell over backward and hit his head on the floor, but he did not cry. He laughed when he looked at the pictures in the book. He made a mark with a pencil and vocalized when he saw what he had done.

Meanwhile, his mother was very responsive to him; at the same time she was cordial to the visitors and was an excellent informant. Although she kept forbidding him to put things in his mouth, she impressed Dr. Géber as being very warm and as having an excellent relationship with the baby.

William's Developmental Quotient was 122. His best points were manual ability, language, and social behavior (127) and his weakest point was adaptivity (109). He was retested when he was two years old and again when he was three, receiving DQ's of 107 and 121 respectively.

Visits to the Clinic

Age *wks.*	*Weight* *lbs.*	*Comments*
29		
31	17.4	
33	18.1	
37	18.4	fever
39	18.8	
41	18.0	vomiting, diarrhea
43	18.5	fever

Maryamu

Maryamu's mother was a very pretty, well-dressed young woman. She had attended a Catholic secondary school for girls for three years, taking a domestic science course. She understood some English but was too shy to attempt to speak it with us. Her schooling showed up chiefly in her skillful needlework. She made her children's clothes by hand and they were beautiful.

The father was a mechanic who worked in Kampala and returned home every evening. There were two little girls in the family —Maryamu, aged thirty-three weeks, and Kasalina, who was scarcely more than nine months older. We did not meet the babies at first. A new house was being built, and the mother did not consider it appropriate for us to visit until the house had been finished. We interviewed her when we visited William's mother, and the babies were left behind with a "baby-sitter."

Meanwhile, she gave us the following information about Maryamu's development. She was born in hospital, and was healthy from the beginning. She was breast-fed according to a schedule, at first every three hours and then every four hours. Her mother had learned about scheduled feedings at school and went "by the clock." At night the schedule was put into abeyance, and the baby was fed if she woke, but this happened only once or twice a night, and by seven months of age she often slept through without waking. Supplementary foods were begun when she was five months old, and by this time she was receiving orange and tomato juice and porridge as well as extra milk. Sometimes her father fed her, for he got up very early in the morning to prepare breakfast and at times fed the children as well. After being fed in the morning, Maryamu was placed on a mat and left, either by herself or with her sister, or with a five-year-old boy who lived with the family, while the mother went to work in the garden.

Each of the girls had her own crib, both of which were in the parent's room. Elimination training had begun when Maryamu was six months old, and a potty was used. By thirty-three weeks of age she could signal her needs, so bowel movements were usually caught, but there were still many accidents, especially wettings.

At thirty-three weeks she was still unable to crawl, a fact which cast some doubt on the mother's report that she was able to sit unsupported at four months of age.

The new house was ready by the time Maryamu was thirty-eight weeks old, and we were received in it. It was a large wattle-and-daub house, with six rooms and a good roof. Maryamu was asleep, but Kasalina was asked to come into the living room to meet us. She was shy and had to be carried in protesting. Throughout the visit she sat with her back to me and sought much attention from her mother.

The mother conversed with us, smiling responsively and answering questions in a straightforward manner. But it was some time before we discovered that Maryamu had been weaned the week before. We had not asked to be given advance notice of weaning for it had not occurred to us that the baby might be weaned so early.

The mother said her milk supply had suddenly failed when Maryamu was thirty-six weeks old. Some time later the mother told us that the cause was another pregnancy. The same thing had happened with Kasalina, who was weaned at six months. The mother said she had been told that she could not become pregnant until menstruation was re-established, but now she realized that this information was incorrect. She was tired and felt that three pregnancies in such rapid succession were too much. Despite her fatigue, and despite the responsibilities of a household, a garden, and three preschool children to care for, she always appeared pleasant, calm, and unhurried, and was patient and gentle with the children.

Despite a great decrease in her mother's milk supply, Maryamu's weaning was not entirely abrupt. At thirty-six weeks of age her day-time feedings were stopped and she was given milk from a cup and the other foods that were already part of her diet. A week later the nighttime feedings were stopped.

For the first few days Maryamu protested the cessation of the daytime breast feedings and cried a great deal. She seemed uncertain about taking milk from a cup but before long took it readily. The first night that the breast was withheld she cried a lot. Her mother responded by holding her and comforting her. The second night she did not cry. Within a few days she slept through the night without waking. I noticed that she sucked her thumb most of the time we were there, but she was said to have done so since she was a tiny baby and no more than usual after weaning.

Maryamu woke in the middle of our visit, signaling her waking by crying. This was her way of announcing that her nap was over, and was, the mother said, the only occasion upon which she cried to be picked up. When brought out she was immediately given to Mrs. Kibuka to hold. She sat quietly. Soon she was handed to William's mother, who had accompanied us on the visit. By this time she was gurgling and active and appeared interested in manipulating things—although this interest did not keep her thumb out of her mouth for long. She was then placed prone on a mat. Her mother coaxed her to crawl by holding a brightly wrapped piece of candy just out of reach. Maryamu struggled to move herself forward, but in vain. Someone took the candy away, and she protested—the only protest she made throughout the visit.

She began to creep on hands and knees when she was forty-one weeks old and soon began to walk on all fours. She was very active during a visit we made when she was forty-six weeks old and she vocalized a lot with an "eee! eee!" sound, her voice falling on the first "eee!" and rising on the second. Her mother said that she was imitating a song she had heard the other children singing. She laughed a lot during the visit and smiled at us all. When her mother left the room Maryamu followed, not crying, but hurrying to keep up. Her mother said she had begun to follow as soon as she could crawl.

Weaning had had no apparent ill effects, for she was cheerful and gaining well. She had a good appetite and became very excited when she saw her cup, which she was now able to hold for herself, although she did not yet feed herself solid food.

This favorable response was still apparent at fifty weeks. Maryamu had acquired four teeth, which showed when she smiled, and she did frequently. When first brought out, dressed in a handmade, finely smocked dress and waterproof pants, she was quiet and sucked her thumb. When we took photographs she did not protest, even when left sitting on a mat by herself.

Her mother told us that she still followed, or attempted to do so, whenever her mother left her alone for a moment, crying only if she could not keep up. When left with her father, however, or even with her sister or the boy, she usually did not follow her mother. But she followed any of these familiar people if they went out leaving her alone. If left with anyone other than a member of the household, she protested. Whenever a member of the household appeared after an absence, she greeted them happily. Nevertheless, her mother was clearly her favorite person.

The mother said that she left the children together while she worked nearby in the garden. After work she held the baby for a while, as did the father when he came home in the evening. Only on rare occasions, when it was unavoidable, did she leave Maryamu with William's mother. These rare absences and the occasional frustration of wanting something she could not get—and now and then hunger— were her only reasons for crying.

By fifty weeks Maryamu could stand alone. She stood smiling at us with a biscuit in her hand. Occasionally she bobbed over into a squatting position but could regain an upright posture without help. She vocalized a lot and imitated sounds that I made. Then she burrowed her head in her mother's lap. She stood again, only to return to her burrowing. This was repeated over and over. Then she walked on all fours over to me, and was friendly when I took her onto my lap. When I put her down, she explored the room for a while, then returned to her mother and spent the rest of the visit scrambling over her.

Some slight illnesses followed, but her behavior did not seem affected and she continued to gain.

She began to walk shortly after fifty weeks of age, and by the time she was fifty-seven weeks old she was walking sturdily. She played with some toys Mrs. Kibuka had brought, ate cake, and went from one visitor to another in a friendly fashion. Twice she protested when I put her down after holding her, and once,

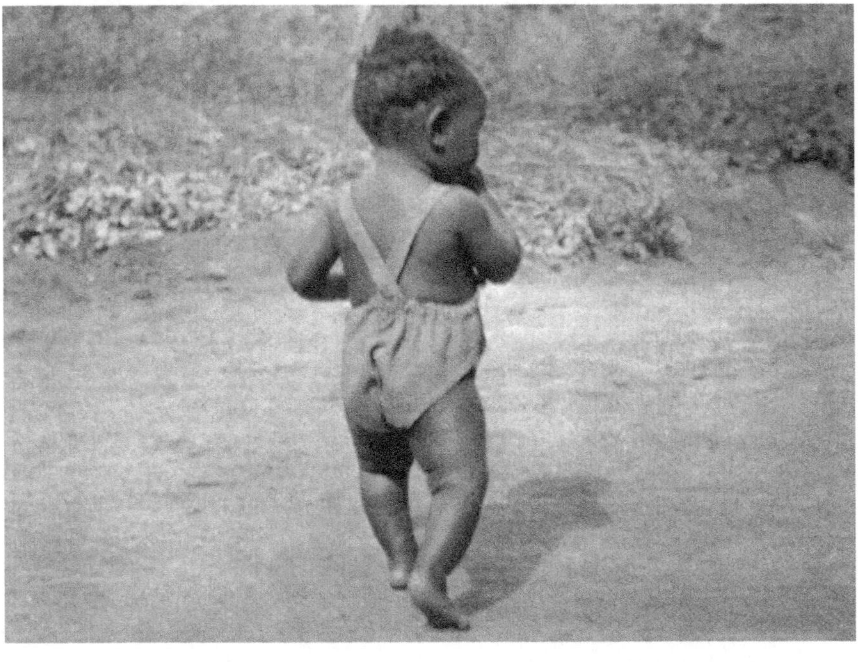

FIGURE 21 At fifty-seven weeks Maryamu is setting off to explore the world, walking sturdily.

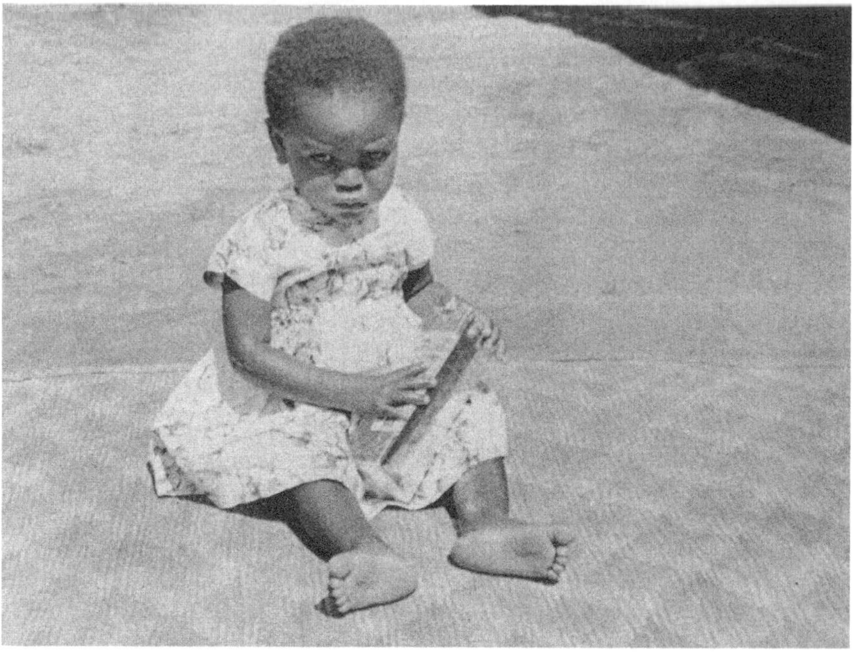

FIGURE 22 Maryamu's sister, Kasalina, has been a sad and clinging child ever since Maryamu was born.

in addition, she asked to be picked up by me. I handed her to her mother and she was content. Her mother did not find this behavior at all unusual. Maryamu was usually friendly with strangers, but she greeted her mother and father with special glee and still cried when her mother left her behind.

She continued to eat well and sucked her thumb as much as ever. Her vocabulary consisted of three words—*mama, taata,* and the name of the boy who lived there. She understood simple commands, as well as the words for cup, food, and milk. She imitated sounds and spoke jargon. She had stopped soiling the bed by fifty weeks of age, but she still wet it and had accidents in the house.

The mother did not worry about Maryamu but was troubled about Kasalina, who followed her everywhere she went, crying anxiously. She sometimes woke at night and cried for no apparent reason. She was almost two years old but clung to her mother much more than did Maryamu, especially when attention was being given to Maryamu. She was completely terrified when weighed and measured at the clinic and had to be held by her mother while the doctor examined her. She was so afraid of strangers and strange situations that her mother disliked taking her away from home. The implication was that she had behaved in this way since Maryamu's birth.

Gesell Testing

Maryamu was sixty-four weeks old when the Gesell Developmental Schedules were administered by Dr. Géber. When the visitors first arrived Maryamu was on her mother's lap; she looked at the examiner distrustfully and turned to her mother for security. It was decided to begin testing Kasalina, so Maryamu was handed to Mrs. Kibuka, on whose lap she remained throughout her sister's testing. She played with Mrs. Kibuka's purse and after a while she interacted with one of the observers. By the time it was her turn to be tested she had acquainted herself with the strangers and could attend to the test materials without being distracted by the new people. Indeed, although she remained close to her mother, she interacted more with the examiner during the testing. She was pleased to be given the test objects and to return them, and she was continually active and interested.

Her locomotion was well developed for her age (111). Although she ran stiffly, she walked well and seldom fell. She responded to the unfamiliar steps by climbing up them, and she could climb up onto a chair. She squatted while playing, keeping her balance. Her movements were quick and energetic. When presented with a football, she walked on it but did not manage to kick it. Her manual ability was average (100). She could pick up a little pellet between thumb and index finger; she could hold two cubes in one hand; she helped turn the pages of a book; she could throw a ball.

She managed to make a tower of the cubes on the third attempt, and she put the cubes into a cup when given it. Then taking the cup by the handle, she turned it over; when the cubes fell out she put them back into the cup. Then she put a small pellet into the bottle, shook it so that it rattled, turned the bottle over, saw the pellet fall out, and put it back into the bottle. She seized the string attached to the ring and drew it to her. She examined the clapper of the bell and rang the bell vigorously. She had a moment of negativism when the examiner tried to take the bell away while presenting the form board; but she quieted when the bell was given back. She did no more with the form board, however, than to pile the blocks up. Then she upset the board and began playing peek-a-boo with the examiner, hiding her face with the board, lowering the board, then hiding her face again, showing great pleasure in the game. She interrupted the test to ask her mother to "hold her down." She then turned some of the pages of the picture book, laughing and pointing at the pictures. She was more interested in the pencil and poked the paper with it—without scribbling, but excitedly. Although she looked more to the examiner than to her mother as someone with whom to share her play, she looked to her mother when she was surprised or when she needed assurance. The mother followed the testing with interest, was warm to Maryamu, and was always ready to help her. There seemed to be a good relationship between them.

Visits to the Clinic

Age *wks.*	*Weight* *lbs.*	*Comments*
39	17.0	
43	18.5	diarrhea
45	19.4	
49	20.1	fever (malaria)
57	21.4	cold
61		diarrhea

Maryamu's Developmental Quotient was 107. Her highest score was in social reactions (120) and her lowest in manual ability and language (100). When she was twenty-eight months old she was retested; this time she was apathetic and received a DQ of 99. When she was forty months old she was slow and received a DQ of 101.

The younger twins: Waswa and Nakato

My first glimpse of the twins was the day after the reception that had been held to celebrate their birth. I came to congratulate the parents on becoming *Nnalongo* and *Ssalongo*—mother and father of twins. I was received in the shade of a large temporary shelter that had been erected in the yard and loosely thatched with palm leaves. It looked like a marquee for a garden party. The twins, just two weeks old, were brought out one at a time for me to see and were placed in my arms. Prompted by a Ganda friend, I placed a coin in the hand of each to wish them prosperity. Their two-year-old sister stood in the background, looking forlorn, her dress dirty and her nose running.

Ssalongo, the shopkeeper, was a pleasantly sociable man. He was good with children and seemed to like company, as befitted his calling, for his shop, like an old-fashioned general store, appeared to be a meeting place where the villagers could linger and chat. Nnalongo was a well-dressed young woman, who usually served us a European-type tea when we visited, with thinly sliced bread and a thoroughly English cake. There was one other child of this marriage—the little girl whom we had seen looking forlorn at the birth festivities. Nnalongo had had another daughter by a previous husband; she lived permanently with William's family. Two girls of school age lived in the household, sent there by their parents to attend the nearby school, and earning their board by serving as nursemaids to the twins. The older of the girls appeared to be about eight; she was particularly fond of the babies and handled them warmly and gently.

The twins were born in hospital and had a combined weight of thirteen pounds. At first they were entirely breast-fed. Nnalongo did not adhere to a schedule but fed them "when they cried," feeding first the one who cried first. Up to the age of about two and a half months they cried frequently. After each was fed he was put down, but instead of falling asleep he stayed awake and soon cried again. Nnalongo picked him up and gave him the breast again. Nnalongo spoke of these early weeks as a nightmare filled with incessant demands from the twins. At night they did not cry as frequently as they did during the day, but when they did cry they were fed. Nnalongo became exhausted and resolved to begin a new regime. She refused to pick them up when they cried unless enough time had elapsed since the last feeding that she judged them to be hungry. Soon they adjusted themselves; at night they woke only once or twice to be fed, and during the day, although they slept little, they were said to cry infrequently and to be little trouble.

Nnalongo nevertheless worried that the twins were not receiving enough nourishment. She expressed this concern on the occasion of our first visit when the twins were thirteen weeks old and was not reassured when examinations at the clinic showed them to be gaining normally. When they were eighteen weeks old their gain had slowed down to an extent that the doctor advised supplementary milk and porridge. Although dried skim milk was available at cost, Nnalongo wished to try a much more expensive imported formula, which, as it turned out, the twins did not like. The mother at first tried to feed the porridge by spoon, but this was so tiresome that she made the mixture thin enough to be given by cup. Orange juice had been introduced before the first clinic visit, and papaw was added to the diet at five months. By the time the twins were thirty-two weeks old they were being given the breast once during the day and once again at bedtime. Night feedings had been dropped, and the twins slept through without waking. This reduction in the number of feedings was not intended as a step toward weaning: the mother believed that her milk supply was insufficient for more frequent feedings.

The twins had no serious illnesses, but after the age of twenty weeks they had frequent colds. They gained weight fairly steadily, nevertheless. At the last visit to the clinic when they were thirty-three weeks old, Waswa weighed 16.6 pounds and Nakato 13.8 pounds.

The twins were given fewer than the traditional number of baths—only one a day. "Holding down" was begun at four months and was done only after feedings. The twins slept in the parents' room, each in his own crib.

On the occasion of our first brief visit the twins were brought in for us to see, and just as were were leaving, the mother began to suckle one of them. This was the only time that the mother gave the breast in our presence. Indeed, it was the only time that she brought the twins to meet the visitors without special

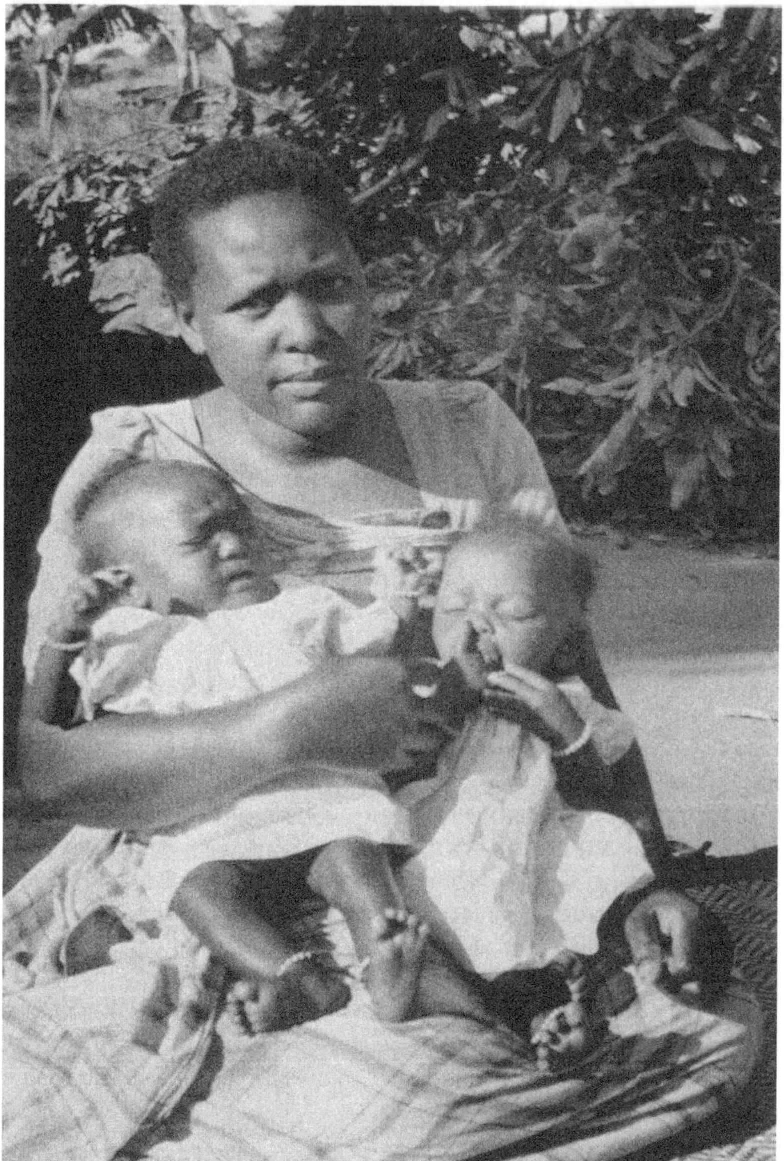

FIGURE 23 Nnalongo finds twins too much for her. The younger set of twins, Waswa and Nakato, are twenty-six weeks old here.

inducement. On two occasions when we suggested taking photographs, she fetched the twins; otherwise, she ignored them while we were there. Nnalongo always seemed glad to see us but was more concerned with entertaining us than with showing off the twins or talking about them. Usually we glimpsed the twins on arrival and on departure, either outside in the yard or in their father's shop. When in the yard they were lying on cushions, or, after twenty-three weeks of age, in a European-type "go cart"—the kind intended for an older baby sitting up and a tight squeeze for two babies. When school was out the two girls usually stayed close to the twins, but the mother did not hesitate to leave them outside by themselves. Indeed, she often left them in the house by themselves while she worked in the garden or went away for the afternoon. Ssalongo was, of course, nearby in the shop, but it was a quite separate building. During one of our visits the twins cried for a long time outside while their mother chatted with us imperturbably. Finally, the father went to investigate and the crying stopped. Once, when we dropped in unexpectedly, we found Nakato in the shop, being held by one of the customers. Ssalongo picked her up to bring her to us, and I noticed him nuzzle his face against her cheek, kissing her very tenderly.

We did not observe Nnalongo demonstrating affection for either twin. Indeed, she told us that she was much too busy to hold the babies except when feeding them. After feeding she handed them over to the girls, if they were home, or sometimes to the father.

The twins were somewhat slower in their development than other children in the sample. They were slow in sitting, and by twenty-one weeks the mother instituted "training," propping them with pillows for a while each morning, each child in his own crib. By twenty-three weeks they were said to be able to sit alone, but only momentarily and when placed carefully so that the soles of the feet were together and the body was leaning forward with the hands on the ground. Sometimes they lifted their heads up as though they wanted to sit, but they could not make it alone. At this age also they could hold their weight when held standing and enjoyed bouncing up and down. Waswa could retrieve a dropped plaything, but Nakato could not. Playthings were chewed rather than manipulated, and they also tried to chew their toes. They vocalized to their playthings, squealed when excited, and could imitate the sound of a motorcar.

By twenty-three weeks they usually obliged by urinating when "held down" but they both still soiled and wet the bed. Smearing of feces occurred occasionally, when they were not taken up immediately upon waking in the morning.

At our last long visit the twins were thirty-two weeks old, and, since we suggested taking photographs at the beginning of the visit, the twins were in evidence throughout. During the picture-taking Nakato cried most of the time. Nnalongo explained that she was fussy because she needed a nap but also said that she tended to cry when strangers were present. Waswa, on the other hand, was said to "like people." When we went inside the house Nnalongo carried

Waswa, and one of the girls carried Nakato. Nnalongo set Waswa down on the floor in order to take Nakato, and Waswa started to cry, although he soon quieted. A little later Nnalongo set Nakato down and left the room. Neither baby cried at her departure, although Nakato began to fuss before her mother returned. I held Waswa on my lap for a while, and then Mrs. Kibuka held him; he did not protest. He sucked his fingers almost constantly, and vocalized "da-da-da-da-da" for a while in a contented way. Nakato was said not to suck her thumb or fingers. We did not test her tolerance of strangers by holding her.

By this time both could sit well and were said to have begun to crawl at approximately thirty weeks of age. Nakato was said to be more efficient in crawling than Waswa, but neither crawled during our visit. There was a headless doll in the room, but the twins showed no interest in it nor in any other object. Nnalongo said that they put into their mouths everything they could pick up—playthings, grass, dirt, and so on. Sometimes they played with each other, pulling the doll back and forth, shouting. They also were described as enjoying things they could beat and make a noise with. They still soiled the bed and sometimes smeared, but, on the other hand, they could signal their needs, and sometimes the mother caught them in time.

Since we had observed no special sign of attachment of either twin to the mother, we inquired about this, as indeed we had inquired on previous visits. The mother confirmed that neither cried when she left the room. She said that they behaved toward her in the same way as they did toward the father and the girls. When they were twenty-three weeks old the twins had been described as greeting the mother by raising the head and vocalizing when she approached, but this was not a differential response, for they greeted others in the same way. Sometimes they cried to be picked up, and sometimes when put down, but neither response was differential, and this was still true at thirty-two weeks. The only evidence of attachment was confined to Nakato, who cried sometimes when a stranger came and who was more likely to cry if she was with the girls rather than with her mother or father.

I felt dissatisfied with the information we had gathered about the twins. We had made numerous visits, including five long visits of two hours or more, but we had had little opportunity to observe the twins themselves in interaction with their parents and with each other. Nnalongo volunteered little or no information about them, and although she responded to questions without apparent reluctance, she seemed unable to give us much detail about their development and soon turned the conversation to other things. I resolved to be more insistent in my last two visits, requesting that the babies be with us, and posing my questions more persistently. This resolve could not be realized, however, for tragedy intervened.

The twin's older sister, then two and a half years old, fell ill with fever. Within two days she was so ill that her mother carried her to a dispensary a few miles away. The nurse's aide in charge there could not help, and advised them to go to hospital. There were difficulties in obtaining transportation, but finally a car was rented. She was examined upon arrival at the hospital, but within an hour and before a bed was found for her, the child had died. Her mother carried her home on the bus, holding her as though she was sleeping. When we arrived for our next visit we found the family mourning and preparing for the burial. We came back a week later, but the shop was closed, and the house was full of visitors participating in the mourning.

Gesell Testing

Dr. Géber tested the twins when they were forty weeks old. The mother showed the visitors into the house and went to fetch Waswa. When she returned she settled him on her lap as she sat on the floor. At Mrs. Kibuka's request she placed him beside her on the floor; he immediately cried for a moment but stopped when the examiner rang a little bell. Thenceforward he was interested in the test objects. He seized the bell in his fist, rang it, and held it in his left hand throughout the test, relinquishing it only when he was given the mirror to look at. He was not interested in the form board. He could pick up the tiny pellet but did not attempt to get the ring by pulling the string; indeed, he took little interest in the ring, grasping it only when it was offered within his reach. He was attracted by the ball and crept after it, still holding the bell in his hand. He placed cubes in a cup and then took them out. When the cubes were put away he cried and turned to his mother but he stopped crying when the cubes were given back. At one point he turned to his mother to share his pleasure when he pulled himself up into a standing position, holding onto a large box. He stood without support for a moment, and he could walk when led with both hands held. He responded to his name but had no words yet. He did not communicate much with the examiner; once he offered her a toy but did not let it go; he did not smile at her.

His Developmental Quotient was 105. He was slower in language development (90) than in the other aspects of development. Dr. Géber found the mother very cooperative, but whenever Waswa failed a test item the mother excused him by saying that he had just awakened. Dr. Géber got the impression of a very good infant-mother relationship—an impression which did not match our view that Waswa had not become attached to her.

The mother then took Waswa out to his father, woke Nakato, and brought her in. Nakato accepted the test situation immediately and was described as more *dynamique* than Waswa. She was also more negativistic than he, protesting vigorously when an object was taken away from her or did not please her. She was more interested in the test objects than in the examiner. She was lively and spontaneous. She was more independent of her mother than her brother had been. She too could stand alone for a moment and walked when led or when holding onto something. She grasped the cubes immediately and banged them together.

She spontaneously put the cubes in and out of the cup when it was presented to her. She rang the bell more vigorously than Waswa had. She put the round block of the form board into her mouth immediately and sat sucking it. When this was taken away from her she cried and threw herself onto her mother's lap. The crying worked up into a regular tantrum. She could not be induced to continue with the testing, although she eventually calmed at her mother's breast. Her mother excused her on the grounds that she was hungry. Nevertheless, Dr. Géber judged her to have less frustration tolerance than her brother had. Dr. Géber returned another day eight weeks later to retest her. I have the details of her scores but not of the behavior.

Her Developmental Quotient was 119, and she was at about level on all the separate scales.

Visits to the Clinic

	Waswa		*Nakato*	
Age wks.	*Weight lbs.*	*Comments*	*Weight lbs.*	*Comments*
14	9.8		8.5	
16	10.5		9.5	
18	11.1		9.8	
20	11.8		10.6	cold
22	12.7		11.4	cold
24	13.0	cold	11.1	cold
26	13.3		12.0	
30	14.5		13.0	
32	16.6		13.8	

The twins were retested when twenty-two months old; they seemed frightened by the European strangers and were ill at ease; their DQ's were 93 and 92 respectively. When thirty-four months old they tested higher again—Waswa at 105, Nakato at 127. Then when four and a half years old their DQ's were lower again—99 and 97—but the test used was not well-suited for use with African children.

16

FIVE MORE BABIES FROM CHRISTIAN FAMILIES

Lusiya, Senvuma, Samwendi, Mutebe, and Kyimba

During the month of preliminaries in the village, Lusiya's father was a frequent visitor. He came ostensibly to help me learn Luganda but preferred to practice his own English. He asked me to give English lessons to his wife and to his two sisters who lived in the household. His wife was not well, so she rarely visited me, but the two sisters came often, bringing Lusiya and another baby, Senvuma, who had been born out of wedlock to one of the sisters. Lusiya's father was eager for his family to participate in the research once it began. Both of the mothers agreed, but just before we got under way Senvuma's mother had an opportunity to be married. Her husband did not want to rear the child of another man. Consequently, Senvuma was weaned abruptly at ten months of age and sent to live with relatives; his mother was married. We attempted to establish cooperative relations with Senvuma's foster family, but, as will be seen, this was not very successful. In the meantime, Lusiya's other paternal aunt was pregnant; when her baby, Samwendi, was born she agreed to participate in the research.

Word of our visits spread through the neighborhood, and one day when we were visiting Lusiya and Samwendi, Mutebe and his mother arrived as guests. Mutebe's mother was eager to participate, and we agreed, despite the fact that only three months remained. Mutebe was thirty-nine weeks old, and it was said that he was soon to be weaned. Wishing to add to our knowledge of responses to weaning, we were happy to include him, although, as it turned out, he was not weaned. Finally, Kyimba's mother, a neighbor of Mutebe's family sought to participate. Kyimba also was described as being near the age of weaning, so he was included. Later we found that a gentle deception had been practiced on us, that he had already been fully weaned before our observations began.

DOI: 10.4324/9781003629337-19

Lusiya

The household that Lusiya lived in was a complicated one. The father, aged twenty-six, was a farmer, and although all of the family were well-dressed, their house was even more sparsely furnished than most of the others we visited. The mother was a quiet, gentle twenty-one-year-old. Lusiya was her second child. The first child, a daughter (now three and a half) had been sent away when two years old to live with the maternal grandmother as soon as her mother realized that she was pregnant again. Instead of their own daughter, these parents were rearing a nine-year-old girl, who had been sent there to attend school. Since she had failed to gain admission to the school of their choice—a Catholic boarding school—she served as nursemaid to Lusiya.

The father's two sisters seemed to be much surer of their position in the household than did the mother. The younger, aged nineteen, was the mother of Senvuma. Lusiya's father gave every impression of pleasure in having his sisters live with him and he welcomed Senvuma. But neither Senvuma nor his mother had much of a part to play in Lusiya's life after she was eight months old. The elder paternal aunt, however, was very much a member of the household. She seemed fond of Lusiya, held her on her lap, and often put her face close to the baby's, nuzzling and giving little kisses. After Samwendi was born, however, she had considerably less to do with Lusiya.

Lusiya was born at home since no transportation was available to take her mother to hospital. She was breast-fed whenever her mother judged her to be hungry. If she was very much distressed, she might be given the breast for comfort, but not if her distress was minor. She slept with her mother, and was fed about three times during the night. By the time the project began, she was about thirty-eight weeks old and was receiving orange juice, papaw, sweet potato, and *matooke* as supplements. During the day she slept very little, and even at night she seemed wakeful. "Holding down" was begun at four months, and by thirty-eight weeks of age she no longer soiled the bed and very rarely wet it. She still had accidents in the house, however.

Her mother reported that she had begun to sit at five months of age, after a period of training during which she was tied upright in a large basin. She began to crawl at six months, to stand at seven months, and by thirty-eight weeks she was walking a little.

When we first visited Lusiya at thirty-eight weeks, she sat close to her mother. She grew increasingly restless and fingered her mother's dress in an apparent effort to get the breast. Her mother encouraged her to undo the buttons herself, but when Lusiya could not manage she was given the breast without further delay. She suckled for about five minutes and then sat contentedly for a while. She stood up several times, her feet wide apart. Although she was said to be able to take a few steps unassisted, she did not walk until the nine-year-old girl (named

Nighty because she was born at night) held her arms. Then, unobtrusively, she had a bowel movement on a mat. When her mother noticed this, she handed Lusiya to Nighty to take outside, and she herself cleaned up the mat without fuss or comment.

Lusiya looked much more robust than when I had seen her some weeks before. She still responded to me with a solemn, rather surprised expression and she looked at me frequently during the visit.

Lusiya seemed to have a good relationship with her mother. The mother, however, was not affectionately demonstrative with her as her aunt had been. Neither aunt was now giving her much attention, the younger being preoccupied with Senvuma and the elder being away. Lusiya was never left by herself in a room except while sleeping. When her mother worked in the garden she took Lusiya along, unless she was asleep; in that case either Nighty or the aunts were at home in case she woke up. Once in the garden, Lusiya was put down and given playthings while her mother worked nearby. Lusiya did not protest being put down under these circumstances. She was friendly with the aunts and with Nighty, all of whom took some part in caring for her, and sometimes she was very friendly with her father. But at night she wanted her mother, and no one else would do.

At thirty-nine weeks Lusiya was ill with a head cold, a severe cough, fever, vomiting, and diarrhea. She looked subdued at first, but then she became more active and finally was very active indeed. She walked on all fours. She stood facing the door for quite a while and kept reaching up toward the latch. She crept over to her mother and seemed to be trying to reach the breast. Her mother did not oblige her, so she crept about some more and played with a little metal box with a picture on the cover. Most of the time she wore a solemn expression, but once she smiled. Her mother felt that she was constrained in the presence of strangers.

Lusiya's mother reported that her daughter cried very rarely. Because of this, when she did cry, her mother thought there must be some special reason and picked her up to soothe her. It was said that she never became angry. She did occasionally hit out at Nighty or at her mother's breast, but this was not interpreted as anger.

On our next two visits the mother was absent and we found Lusiya in Nighty's charge. During the first of these visits Lusiya was subdued and listless; her nose was running from a heavy cold. The second time, Lusiya was crying when we arrived and she cried a great deal throughout the visit, even after her mother returned. She seemed to want the breast, but her mother did not offer it. At the end of the visit they walked to the car with us, Nighty carrying Lusiya, who was quite a load for her. Nighty seemed cheerful enough about her duties with the baby but was neither gentle nor tender. Our impression was that Lusiya did not care for her as a nursemaid.

We asked the mother about her plans to wean Lusiya and requested that she give us advance notice. But when we came to visit at fifty-one weeks, we found that the daytime feedings had been dropped five days previously. There was no special reason for weaning her at this time; it was just that she was "old enough." She had been receiving many solid foods by this time, and although all the daytime breast feedings had been dropped at once, Lusiya had not cried, and, indeed, there seemed to have been no change in her behavior. At night she still woke often and was given the breast. She was receiving milk by cup, and porridge, bread, and new vegetables had been added to her diet. In addition to the three meals with the family, she received fruit at mid-morning.

The mother said that Lusiya was not seeking the breast during the day. Indeed, she had been left with Nighty much of the time, except when her mother came to give her food. It was thought to facilitate the weaning process for her mother to stay away from her.

Lusiya looked well in a clean white dress, with diapers and waterproof pants on underneath; it was the first time we had seen her wearing either. Around each ankle she wore a string of bells and also an anklet of cowrie shells. She wore bracelets of beads on each wrist. At first, she watched us soberly, but later she began to run about in and out of the house, playing, her bells jingling. For a while she sat close to her mother, her head on her mother's lap, bouncing her bottom up and down, smiling at her mother, and babbling. Twice during the visit she got hold of something that she might damage, and it was taken away from her. Her mother had to tug to get it out of her grasp, but Lusiya did not cry, even though she obviously wanted to keep the attractive object. Once it was taken away, Lusiya immediately turned her attention toward something else.

She seemed to be close to her mother without being clinging or insecure. She followed her whenever she left the room, but did not cry. Her mother said that if she did not want Lusiya to follow she closed the door. Even then Lusiya would not cry but she banged on the door. When she was younger, her mother said, before she learned to walk, she cried to be picked up, but she no longer did so. When her mother returned after an absence, Lusiya would laugh, clap her hands, and then come to her as quickly as possible. She greeted her father in the same way when he returned after an absence. Her mother said that she did not warm up quickly to strangers, and, indeed, "she does not like people unless she has known them."

By the end of her first year she still did not speak any words but she obeyed simple commands. The command "stop" was enough to keep her from doing anything her mother did not want her to do. Her favorite play activity was to put small objects into containers—for example, coffee berries into a little box.

We visited the day before Lusiya's first birthday and found that the final weaning was to take place the next day—she would be exactly one year old.

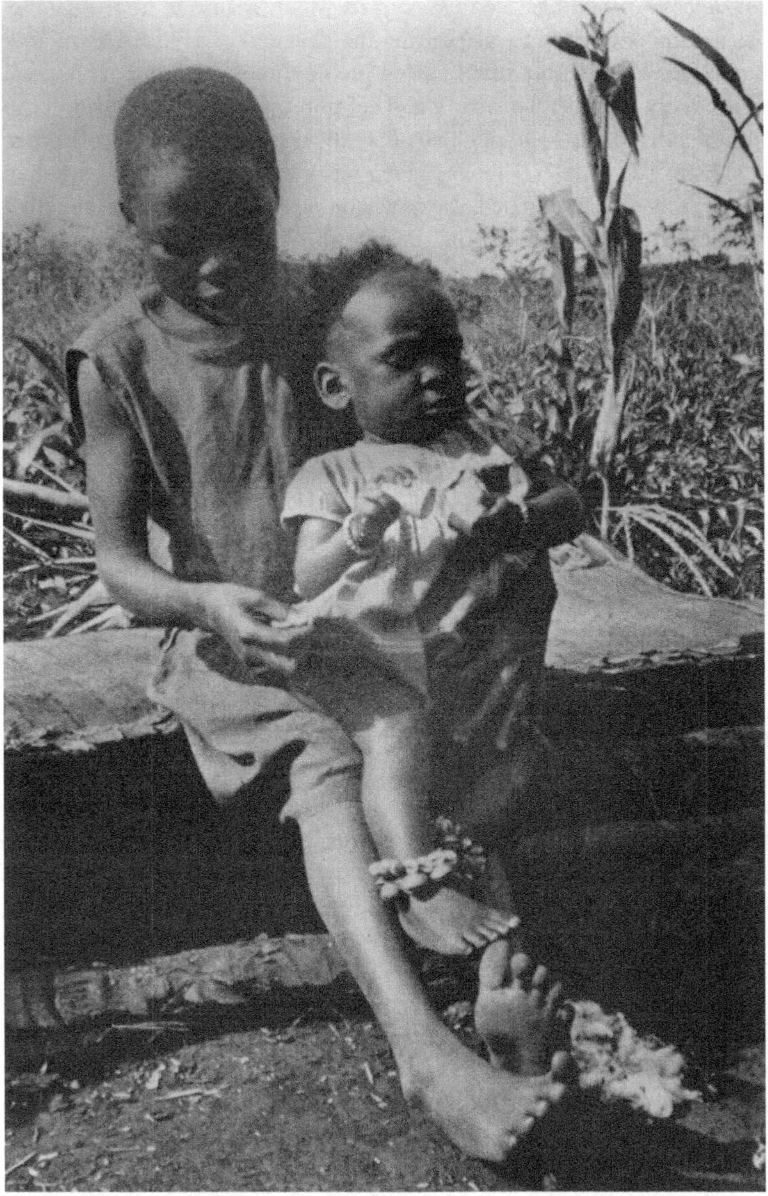

FIGURE 24 Here is Lusiya at twelve months, in the middle of weaning. Our impression was that she did not much care for Nighty, her nursemaid, with whom she was left increasingly often.

Six days later we came back to observe Lusiya's response to final weaning. Lusiya was asleep, and did not wake during the course of our visit. Her mother said that, although she had not cried during the daytime, she had cried a great deal at night, every night, since weaning. The mother's policy had been not to pick her up to comfort her—although she had always done so previously when Lusiya was distressed. Rather, she was given weak tea with milk by her father. Whenever the mother approached, Lusiya would strike out at her, directing her blows especially at the breast. But, despite this response when her mother appeared, when her mother was not in sight she cried inconsolably. For the first three nights there was great disturbance, but the fourth night was better, and Lusiya only woke twice.

During the day, her mother reported, she no longer tried to reach the breast, but she followed her mother more than before and demanded to be picked up and held more frequently. Otherwise, her behavior was said to be unchanged; she was eating well, sleeping well during her afternoon nap, and wetting no more frequently than before. She did not suck her thumb.

On the next visit to the clinic when Lusiya was fifty-three weeks old, she weighed 17.5 pounds and was judged to be well.

We visited briefly when she was fifty-five weeks old. She was impassive and showed less animation than we had observed before weaning. She accepted being held by a neighbor woman. When given back to her mother she squirmed away and walked about quite a bit, manipulating and chewing at a small box. She kept offering the box to people, snatching it away as one reached for it.

At fifty-nine weeks, seven weeks after final weaning, there was still disturbance. Every night she woke twice and cried, although she was no longer given anything to eat or drink. She wanted to be with her mother all the time. Her mother left her behind when she went to work in the garden, but when she returned Lusiya clung and could not be dissuaded from doing so. Indeed, throughout this brief visit Lusiya was close to her mother, either clinging to her, or sitting close to her on the floor, leaning back against her.

At a longer visit, four days later, the mother came in with Lusiya, put her down, and then went out again. Lusiya screamed until her mother returned. Then she sat with her head on her mother's lap for quite a while, and even when she sat up later, she did not budge from her mother's side. In contrast, just before weaning she had seemed a cheerful little girl, toddling about, busy with her play, and not needing to be close to her mother constantly. When we inquired about anger, the mother said that now she often became very angry. Whenever anything is taken away from her that she wants, she throws herself down on the floor in a tantrum. She did not hit anyone, however, and did not fight with other children. Soon after this I visited briefly and found Lusiya with Nighty; the mother was away. I tried to pick Lusiya up but she shrank away from me in an obvious gesture of refusal.

When Lusiya was fourteen months old she looked rather sad and subdued. I invited her to come to me, coaxing her with a piece of candy. She shrank away, then climbed onto her mother's lap. Later Mrs. Kibuka went over to try to pick her up, and again she shrank away. Throughout our visit she sat on her mother's lap, silent and impassive. The disturbed behavior continued. Lusiya clung to her mother whenever she was there and would not allow her to move away for a moment. On the other hand, now that the child no longer received the breast, her mother felt less obliged to stay at home and left her with Nighty more often than was the case before weaning. She had a good relationship with her father and with

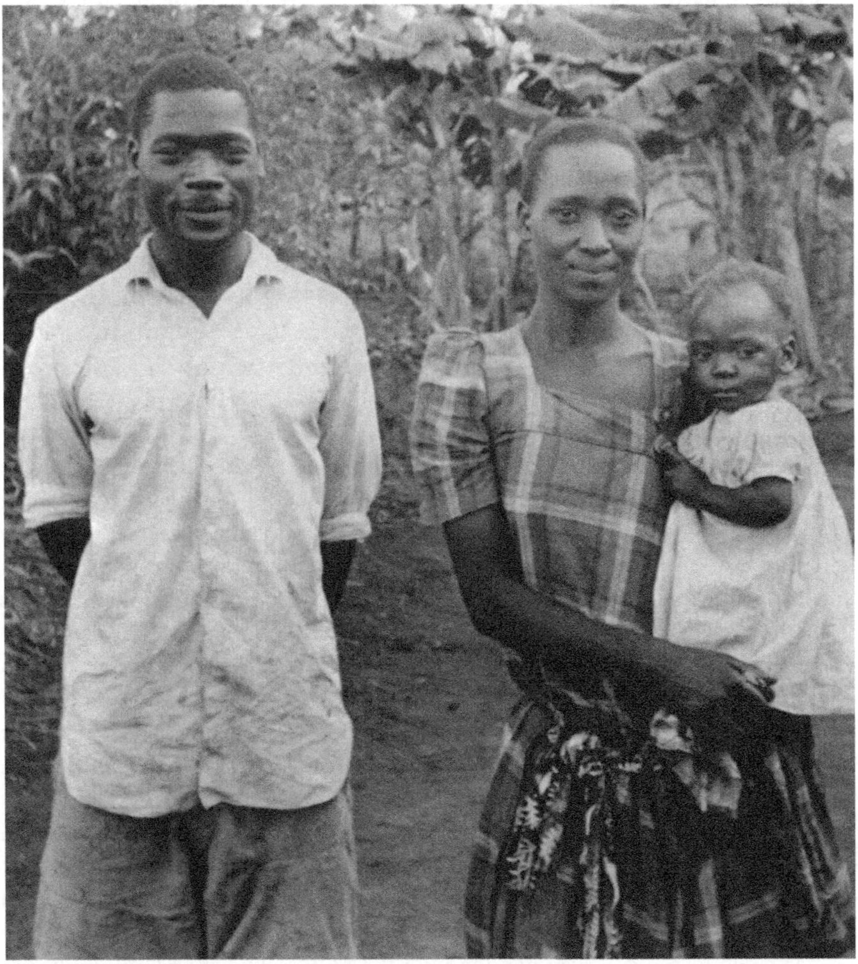

FIGURE 25 Here is Lusiya again, at fourteen months with her parents. She has been sad, subdued, and clinging since final weaning.

her paternal aunt, who was back in the household again, but she cried whenever her mother left her—even with these two familiar figures. Her behavior with us was said to be typical of her behavior with strangers. Recently her mother had been away on an overnight visit and when she returned Lusiya cried.

At our last visit two weeks later, Lusiya still wanted to be with her mother all the time. Whereas before weaning she was equally responsive to the father, except at night, now her preference was clearly for the mother. The chief time of day that the mother made a point of giving attention to Lusiya was after she had finished the preparations for a meal. Then, while the food was cooking, she gave Lusiya a bath and afterward sat and played with her.

Lusiya now was said to have a very good understanding of much that was said to her, although she still did not say more than two or three words herself. When she wanted something she pointed to it and did not need to say anything. Now that she was old enough to understand, her mother had begun to smack her when she got hold of something she should not have. This "beating" was viewed as training, "so that she will learn," rather than as punishment.

Lusiya was asleep when we arrived. After she wakened, she sat quietly near her mother, stared at the visitors, and made no response to our advances. The next day at the clinic, however, I sat beside her for a while and stroked her foot. Gradually she responded and played a game of taking her foot away, then pushing it back toward my hand.

Gesell Testing

Dr. Géber administered the Gesell Developmental Schedules when Lusiya was sixteen months old. Apparently she had recovered from her postweaning disturbance for she was reported to be active and interested in the testing and responsive to the examiner. She clung to her mother at first while staring curiously at the visitors, but when the test objects were presented to her she was immediately interested and left her mother's lap to play with them. She continued to be shy with the other visitors but she "talked" to the examiner and offered objects to her. Occasionally she turned to check on her mother's presence. Her manual movements were quick and precise. She showed spontaneous adaptive interest in the toys. She built a tower of four blocks and tried to add a fifth. She was especially interested in the form board, examining the blocks, and finally putting the round one in and out of the appropriate hole. She was delighted with the picture book, turned the pages, pointed to the pictures, exclaimed over them, and showed them to her mother and to the examiner. When given a pencil she took up the book to scribble in it, but when it was taken away from her she accepted the loss. She loved playing with the ball, rolling it and going after it. She vocalized jargon and was pleased when the examiner replied to her. She was astonished to see her image in the mirror but then smiled and patted it. She was able to walk by herself but was rather unsteady. She crawled up the steps but did not tackle them upright.

Her Development Quotient was 102. She was most advanced in manual ability (112) and least advanced in language (94) and locomotion (97).

When Dr. Géber returned for retesting the following year, she found Lusiya living with her aunt, presumably separated from her mother because of the birth of a baby brother. She looked sad and her DQ had fallen to 91. When she was three and a half she was still with her aunt and was unavailable for testing.

Visits to the Clinic

Age mos.	*Weight lbs.*	*Comments*
12.5	17.5	underweight, but well
14.5	19.0	coughing, vomiting

Senvuma

Senvuma was a robust, healthy, and active eight-month-old baby when I first saw him. His mother came to visit me several times a week during the time I lived in the village and she always brought Senvuma. Although other babies were passed around from lap to lap during visits, Senvuma was very much his mother's baby, looked after only by her, and scarcely ever given to anyone else to hold. He was at first very shy with me, but on repeated visits he became more responsive. He finally allowed me to hold him for a while and occasionally smiled at me. Most of the time he was active on the floor or on the steps of the veranda, close to his mother.

This was before the research project had begun. I was without an interpreter, and my knowledge of Luganda was too meager to enable me to converse with the mother about the baby or about her infant-care practices; but these frequent visits served to give me a vivid impression of both.

His mother offered him the breast frequently—at least once during each visit and often several times. If this offer came in response to a signal from Senvuma, the signal was imperceptible to me. He did not cry, nor did he become restless or fumble with her dress in any obvious search for the breast. The mother was nineteen years old and seemed entirely wrapped up in the child. She seemed more like a girl playing with her doll than a mother with her baby. She was tender and warm, but I sensed a certain irresponsibility in her attitude, and recorded this at the time, although I could not say what gave me this impression. Subsequent events bore it out.

The mother's brother, Lusiya's father, who was also a frequent visitor, told me that this young mother was unmarried. As he explained it, a friend of his came to visit them, and that was how she got the baby. Through Lusiya's father, my research plans were outlined, and it was agreed that Senvuma would be one of the babies in my sample.

On my first prearranged visit to their home with Mrs. Kibuka, I learned that Senvuma, then ten months old, had been weaned abruptly two days before and had been sent to live with relatives. His mother was soon to be married, but not to Senvuma's father. Her husband-to-be did not want to rear this child by another man. The only information we gained about the weaning was that he was weaned to a cup and given a pint of milk a day. We arranged to be taken to see Senvuma in his new home in order to observe his response to separation.

A week later our request was complied with, but instead of being escorted by one of the responsible adults who could introduce us to Senvuma's foster family, we were taken by Nighty, Lusiya's nine-year-old nursemaid. None of the adults were at home. Senvuma was being lugged about by a young girl, seemingly about Nighty's age, who had him on her hip. She was very shy and appeared reluctant to give information. Senvuma looked healthy enough, but very solemn. We asked if he cried much and the girl replied that he did not. We asked if he had cried a lot when he first came and she said yes. No other information was forthcoming.

It was two months before we were able to visit by appointment, and even then Senvuma's paternal grandmother, whom we were informed was his foster mother, was not there. A young woman was present, of whom we asked some questions about Senvuma, but it was slow going, for we had been unable to build up the kind of rapport with this family that would enable them to answer freely the difficult questions we wanted to ask.

The change in Senvuma himself was very striking. He was no longer the chubby, satin-skinned baby that I had seen before; his arms and legs were very thin and his belly distended. His feet seemed big on his thin legs. His hair was long and matted, quite unkempt, and there were several scabs on his scalp that looked like ringworm. He was dressed in a printed rayon dress and was very grubby. He had a cold, a cough that was said to be chronic, and he wheezed when he breathed.

He was very quiet throughout the visit, quite unlike the active baby who had played near his mother on my veranda in the village. For a while he sat near me on Mrs. Kibuka's lap and regarded me with great eyes but uttered no sound. Later he sat on the young woman's lap, leaning back against her quite passively, and finally he fell asleep.

I inquired about his initial response to separation and was told —contrary to the earlier report from the young girl—"He did not cry much, because he was brave." He was said to be happy, to eat well, to sleep well, and never to get angry. He was reported to have developed an attachment for his foster mother, and to cry and try to follow her whenever she left the room. He was said to be happy and active with other children of his own age. He had learned to walk since separation but was still tottery. His mother had visited him only once; Senvuma had not seemed to recognize her at all and had treated her as a stranger.

We were told that Senvuma's mother was unable to send any money to help support him and that the grandmother resented having to spend money to buy what he needed. He looked malnourished. We offered to bring a package of dried skim milk for him once a week and hoped that this would both help him and enable us to build a working relationship with the family.

Senvuma seemed apathetic and far from happy, so I was doubtful of the truth of much of what we had been told. Not knowing whether this apathetic behavior could be a response to us as strangers, a result of malnutrition, or a response to separation, we promised ourselves to keep an open mind and to see what we could observe on subsequent visits.

A week later we came with Senvuma's milk, but found that both he and his grandmother were away. Another woman, who was identified as the mistress of the house, greeted us but did not encourage us to stay. She did, however, accept our offer to take Senvuma to the next clinic.

When we picked Senvuma up at the appointed place to take him to the clinic, we were shocked to discover that they had sent him in the care of a girl much too young either to give any information about him to the doctor or to report the doctor's advice back to the foster family. Senvuma seemed entirely indifferent to the strange surroundings of the clinic. His face was expressionless. For a while the girl went off, leaving him alone in the midst of all the bustling strangers. He did not cry when she left him. I picked him up and carried him around for a while. He was quite unmoved and accepted me without responding to me. The doctor judged him to be in fairly good condition but urged us to see that he received more milk to drink and to give the family advice about feeding.

The next day we visited the home by appointment. As soon as the car stopped, a young girl, even younger than his nursemaid of the day before and scarcely big enough to hold Senvuma on her hip, popped up out of the bushes to inform us that no one was at home. As before, Senvuma was apathetic and very dirty. We left milk, cough medicine from the clinic, and a letter explaining what the doctor had said and requesting a visit the following week.

A week later Mrs. Kibuka took a packet of milk to the house in order to investigate the situation. She returned soon, accompanied by a third woman, who carried Senvuma in her arms. She told us that it was she who looked after Senvuma, not the grandmother. This was the first time we had seen Senvuma with his foster mother. He was all cleaned up and wore a pretty white silk smocked dress. He still seemed impassive, but, perhaps because he was cleaner, he looked less neglected and more relaxed. The following week we called again with another package of milk. Again Senvuma was with a nursemaid and the adults were out. This time he looked cleaner and perhaps a little happier than he had on previous occasions when with his child nursemaids.

A month later we made one more attempt to establish contact with Senvuma's family. This time we found at home the same young woman who had given us information on our first visit. She told us that Senvuma's foster mother was not his grandmother (who lived elsewhere) but his paternal aunt. This young woman was the daughter of the paternal aunt. She told us that it was the paternal aunt to whom Senvuma was chiefly attached, although she, our present informant, was responsible for much of his care. The paternal aunt, her mother, was away visiting much of the time and on the occasion of this call was away for a week. The young woman surprised us by welcoming us warmly; it was the first sign of friendliness we had been offered by the family.

Our informant told us that whenever Senvuma's foster mother, the paternal aunt, was at home, he wanted to be with her, but during her absences he attached himself to the daughter, our informant. "He does not like other people." she said. He could say *mama* and *taata* and used these words to refer to his aunt and uncle. His mother came again to visit, and this time Senvuma seemed to know her and was pleased to see her.

During our visit Senvuma sat either on the young woman's lap or near her. I tried to coax him to me with a piece of candy, but he would not come. The young woman helped him walk to the middle of the room. He stood there looking at me intently but did not approach. I went to him and offered him the candy. He was very hesitant in taking it. As we were about to leave, Mrs. Kibuka took Senvuma in her arms, walked out the door, and started up the path, to see how he would react to being taken away from his caretaker. He was entirely passive and made no protest.

A week later we were finally received by Senvuma's aunt, his foster mother. She did not seem pleased to see us, perhaps because she was dressed to go out. We gave her a package of milk and inquired whether Senvuma liked it. She said that he did not. Mrs. Kibuka suggested various ways of introducing it to his diet, but the woman did not appear interested.

Now that we finally had an opportunity to talk to the foster mother I persisted with questions, for I wanted to gain information about Senvuma's response to separation, even though it had taken place five months earlier and, therefore, neither complete nor reliable information could be expected. The foster mother said that Senvuma had cried all night the first night away from his mother. "He cried for the breast," she said. Nevertheless, he had seemed to "like" his foster mother from the beginning and he ate well. After the first night he slept well. Within three days he had begun to follow his foster mother, and he was still said to follow her about and to want to be near her. Whenever she returned after an absence "he is very happy." She described him as smiling a lot; I had not seen him smile since his separation. His foster mother pointed out that he was listless and unresponsive that day because he had a fever.

We were told that Senvuma's mother had visited him a few days before; he had looked at her with no sign of recognition. At this point in our visit our informant announced that she had planned to go visiting that afternoon, so our visit ended. Our offer to drive her was refused.

Senvuma looked much better cared for that day than he usually did. He sat on his foster mother's lap for a while. One of the young girls took him in her arms for a moment, but he made a slight protest at being taken from his foster mother. Then he was given to me to hold for a while; he was quiet and unresponsive. Again he was back on his foster mother's lap when the young girl picked him up rather roughly. This time he fussed. The girl, carrying Senvuma, accompanied us to the car; Senvuma made no protest this time at being taken away from his foster mother.

We caught our last glimpse of Senvuma a week later at the clinic —when he was fifteen months old. Again he was brought by the young girl, who was quite incapable of coping with clinic routine.

Despite the unsatisfactory nature of our contacts with this family, we did glean some information. First, it seems certain that Senvuma was distressed at the separation from his mother—and the concomitant weaning—although the phase of active protest was said not to have lasted long. Second, he was observed to have formed some attachment to his foster mother and to her daughter, although he did not protest their departures and his removals from them with any vigor. It was clear, furthermore, that he received much less attention from either of these substitute mothers than most of the babies in our sample did from their natural mothers, even those who had been weaned. Judging from our visits, the substitute mothers were frequently away from home, and Senvuma was cared for much of the time by the young girls, to whom he did not appear to be attached. Quite apart from Senvuma's neglected appearance, at fifteen months of age he was clearly more apathetic, inactive, and passive than any other child in our sample. His response to being left alone amid strangers at the clinic was entirely unlike that of a normal baby. His very absence of separation anxiety under these circumstances suggested a marked degree of detachment.

Samwendi

Samwendi's mother was not married to the baby's father, although she told me his name and said he was a clerk in another town. As had been the case with the sister's illegitimate child, Senvuma, it was clear that there was little or no sense of disgrace, and that the brother, Lusiya's father, welcomed their presence in the household.

Samwendi's mother was a rather impassive and uncommunicative young woman, who took great pains with her appearance. She dressed her hair in a neat but elaborate coiffure, with many little partings which divided her head into inch squares. The hair in each square was braided and then tucked in, so there was a puffy, waffled effect to the whole. Once, for a photograph, she combed her hair out so that it stood up straight, about a foot long. She said that she never wore it that way, and when I asked why she wanted to be photographed thus, she shrugged and said: *Njagala*—I want to; I like it. She usually dressed in a new *busuuti* for our visits, with rich-looking silk sashes, a pearl necklace, and a wristwatch, and the baby also was put into his finery for us to see. Despite this interest in externals, she seemed to be a loving and responsible mother, and she was a faithful attendant at the clinic.

It was Samwendi's mother who had been most enthusiastic about the English lessons. She had been through the fifth grade in a school in Kampala, where she had begun to learn English, and she wished to progress. I could get little out of her in general conversation, however, for there seemed little that she wished to communicate. Later, after the research project had begun, Mrs. Kibuka served as a bridge between us, but all of our talk had to do with the baby, and there was little that she wished to say about herself or about her feelings or hopes. She was a good informant about the baby, however. When I first began to visit the household to see Lusiya—the aunt was away "in the Maternity" to "get" a new baby—Samwendi. My first glimpse of him came when he was nine weeks old; he and his mother had returned to live in the household. His mother was asked to bring him out to show him to us. There was a long delay, after which his mother brought him out all dressed up, swathed in a fine, white, lacy wool shawl. He seemed well-nourished and had profuse, fine kinky hair of a glossy black color; there was a slight rash on his face. He was given to me to hold, but he was restless. I held him up over my shoulder for a while and he quieted, but then Mrs. Kibuka took him over. He was restless with her also, despite shifts of position, and finally he cried violently. He stopped crying as soon as his mother took him. It emerged that he and his mother were going to be away for two months, visiting relatives, but it was agreed that they would participate in the research when they returned.

Sam was breast-fed whenever he cried. Sometimes he was given the breast merely for comfort, when he could not possibly be hungry, in an attempt to stop his crying. He slept with his mother and woke to be fed three times at night. His mother said that she enjoyed breast feeding and also that she enjoyed holding him. Supplementary food had been added to his diet by the age of four months—orange juice, papaw, porridge, *matooke* mashed until very soft, and supplementary milk. "Holding down" began at about two months of age, after feedings.

When we saw him at seventeen weeks he was very plump and appeared healthy. Photographs were the first item at this visit, and for one, Sam sat alone unsupported, although he was a bit wobbly. This was the first time that he had sat alone. Back in the house, he sat on his mother's lap. After a bit he wet, and she stood him on the floor. He held his weight with only slight support. Back on her lap he began to fuss as though he wanted the breast. His mother agreed that he did but did not oblige him. She rocked him in her arms, then put him up over her shoulder and patted him vigorously. He gradually quieted and began to chew his fingers, getting most of one hand into his mouth. Finally he went to sleep, and his mother took him to bed for a nap. We never did observe this mother giving the breast, despite her repeated insistence that she gave him the breast for comfort. I can only assumc that she did not want to feed him in my presence, perhaps having learned that Europeans believe that breast feeding should be done in private.

Sam had a bad cold when he was taken to the clinic at nineteen weeks. Medicine was prescribed for him, to be given four times a day for three days. When we visited the next day, we found that the mother had been conscientious about giving the medicine—which many of the clinic mothers were not.

Sam, as usual, was all dressed up and was wearing diapers made of thin, non-absorbent cotton material. He sat on his mother's lap, sucking his thumb almost constantly, and, at first, watched us intently. Then he began to vocalize happily. His mother set him on the floor. He maintained an erect position very well and continued vocalizing. Later his mother lifted him back onto her lap, on her own initiative, and he gave her a brilliant smile. Mrs. Kibuka took him on her lap for a while, and he seemed content there; soon he was waving his arms and vocalizing cheerfully. At the end of the visit I took him, and again he was quite content. He cried only once during the visit. This was when he was taken outside for a photograph; he had been placed sitting on a slight slope, which made it difficult for him to keep his balance. Finally he toppled forward on his face and began to cry; he was quickly consoled when his mother picked him up.

His mother said that he ordinarily cried very little and only to announce that he was hungry. For the last few days he had been more fussy, however, because of his cold. He vocalized a lot, "talking" to his playthings and using vocalization to initiate social contact. His mother felt that he clearly "knew" her, although Lusiya's mother sometimes shared in his care and the nine-year-old girl, Nighty, sometimes helped to carry him. His mother usually left him behind when she went to work in the garden but she delayed her departure until he was fast asleep. Ordinarily he did not cry when she left him alone in a room briefly, but he made "a special noise" in lieu of crying. He was said to like people and to be content with whomever was holding him or looking after him—and, indeed, he accepted our attentions during the visit.

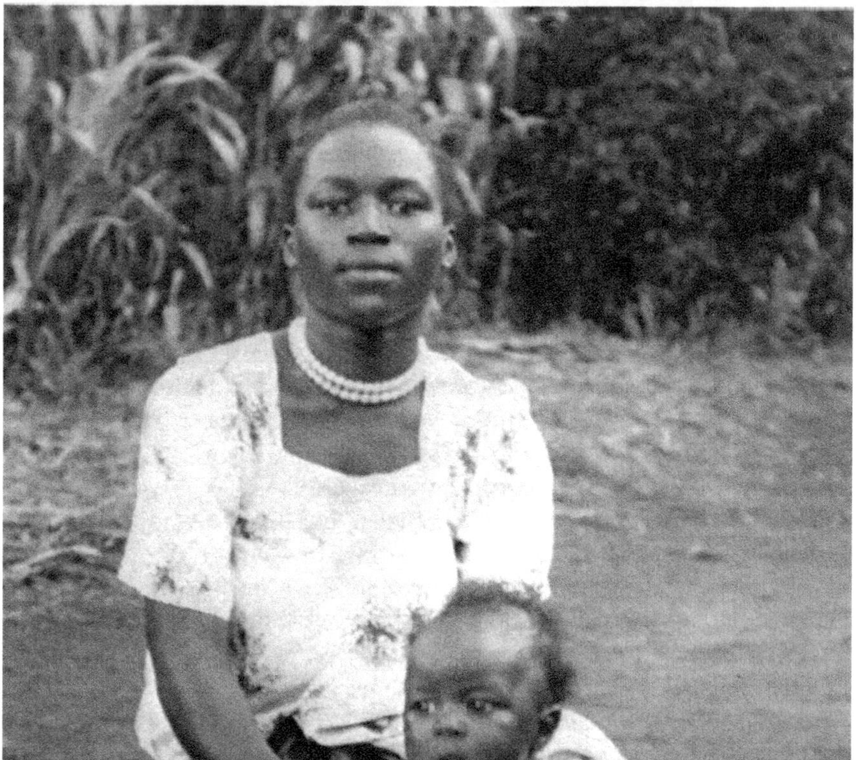

FIGURE 26 Samwendi with his elegant mother. At seventeen weeks he sits unsupported for the first time.

Further foods had been added to his diet—beans, bananas, and tomato juice. His mother said that she had added one new thing at a time. He received liquids from a cup, solids from a spoon. He was usually fed just before the adults had their meal.

At twenty-one weeks Sam slept throughout most of our visit. When his mother got him up, I noticed that he was wearing waterproof pants. He sat on Mrs. Kibuka's lap, sucking his thumb, and was responsive in a quiet sort of way. He gave me one unsolicited smile. He liked to play with empty powder tins. His mother said that she usually held him for an extended period after each feeding and sometimes on other occasions as well. Aggression had begun to emerge. If he was not fed quickly enough, he would cry and hit his mother's breast angrily.

It was not until he was twenty-four weeks old that Sam began to cry when his mother left the room, and then only if he were left alone or with people he did not know well. He accepted being left with Lusiya's mother, however, who indeed sometimes fed him or bathed him. He was said to be friendly with some strangers, but to cry at the approach of others. He had begun to grasp things and to hold them, although he had not yet begun to manipulate them with fine finger movements. He still soiled the bed and had not yet begun to crawl.

Visits to the Clinic

Age wks.	*Weight lbs.*	*Comments*
17		well-nourished
19		cold, cough
21	14.6	cough

Mutebe

Mutebe and his mother lived with the maternal grandparents, and the household included also a great-grandmother and Mutebe's two-and-a-half-year-old brother. The parents had separated. The father worked in Entebbe but occasionally visited. I did not discover whether he contributed to the support of his wife and children. The grandfather was relatively affluent, however, and contributed generously to their support. He was a dignified, white-haired gentleman, obviously respected in the community, who had been recently made head of his clan. He was obviously fond of his daughter and proud of her children. Both he and the grandmother had much interaction with Mutebe and his brother, although during most of the period of our visits the grandmother was away from home, reported to be visiting elsewhere while convalescing from an illness. The

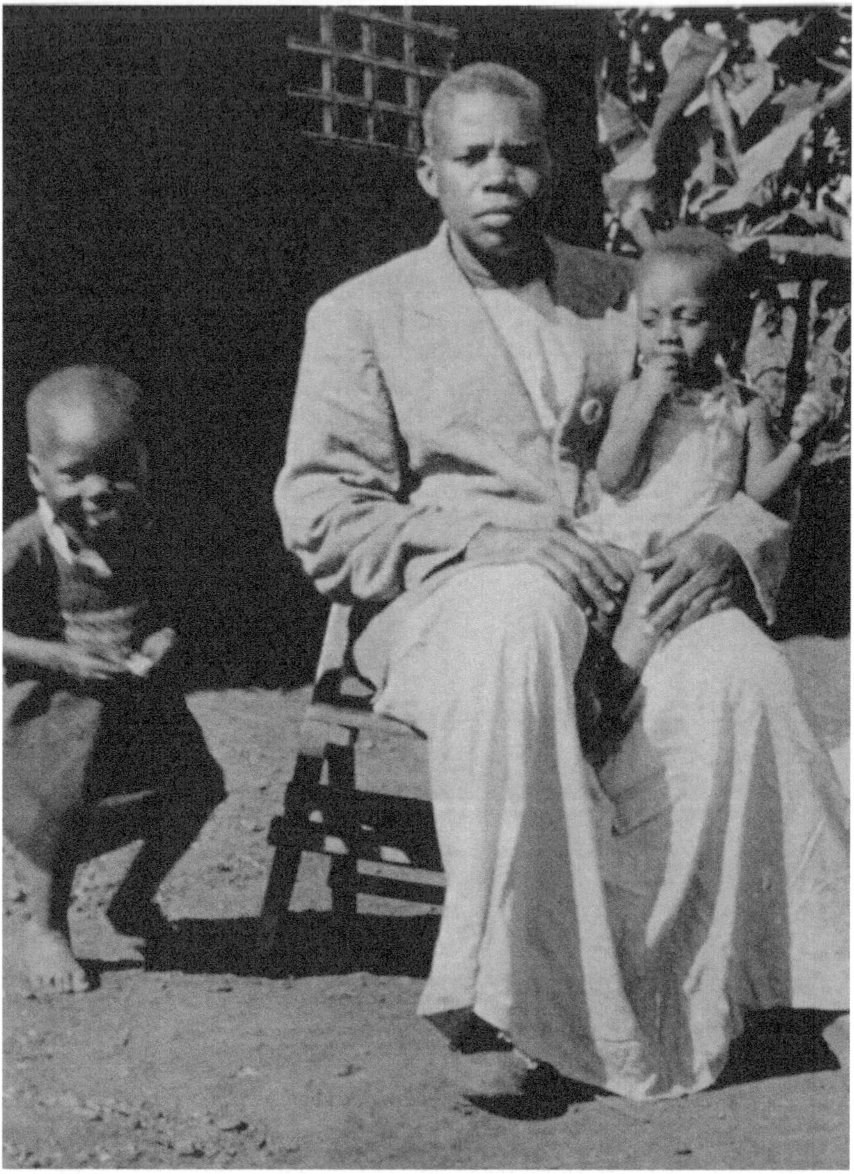

FIGURE 27 Mutebe's grandfather is a clan head and is dressed for the part, wearing a kanzu with a suit coat over it. Mutebe is attached to his grandfather. Mutebe's brother is excited to be having his picture taken.

great-grandmother was a vigorous old woman, who also took much interest in, and some responsibility for, the care of the children.

I was never sure how much property this family owned or controlled, but the path to their house was through an especially lush and pleasant landscape of gardens and fields. The house was an ordinary Ganda house of wattle and daub, but a much bigger house was being built nearby. It had an impressive, shiny, corrugated metal roof, and although the wattle framework was only partly filled in with daub, there was nicely finished woodwork, which was being painted green —the only paint that I can recall seeing on one of these village houses.

Mutebe at thirty-nine weeks was a handsome big baby, obviously very well-nourished. He was clothed in a smocked silk dress, beautifully handmade, and wore waterproof pants underneath. At our first regular visit two weeks later, we obtained information about his care and development.

He was born in hospital and was said to weigh 9.5 pounds at birth. He was not put to the breast until the third day, but from then on he sucked well. At three months of age he had such severe diarrhea that he had to be hospitalized for a week. His mother took him to the clinic fairly regularly, but, nevertheless, he had recurrent fever.

He had been breast-fed on demand, but not merely for comfort unless he cried very hard. His mother said that she had enjoyed the breast feeding at first, but now continued it only because it was good for him. Supplementary feedings of milk had been alternated with breast feedings since he was five months old. Solid foods had also been introduced so that by nine months he had quite a varied diet. Indeed, his mother had stopped feeding him porridge because he seemed to be getting too fat. He slept with his mother until he was six months old, and then his grandmother wanted him to sleep with her. After she became ill and was taken away to hospital, Mutebe resumed sleeping with his mother. He woke at night, demanding to be fed three or four times, but otherwise slept well. I did not think to inquire about night-feedings during the period that he slept with his grandmother. He had both morning and afternoon naps and slept soundly through all ordinary noise. He had two baths a day, at noon and at bedtime.

His mother judged that he was slow in motor development, and so when he was three months old she supported him by wrapping him in cloths in order to train him to sit; he did not sit alone, however, until he was five months old. He crawled at six months and could stand holding onto some support by seven months.

My inquiries about elimination training and control elicited rather confusing replies. His mother said that when it was time for a bowel movement he made a noise, in response to which an adult took him out so that he did not soil his bed. I inquired when he had begun this; the mother replied that “it was his nature” and that even when he was very young he very rarely soiled the bed. She said that she had started to “hold him down” at four months, but when I asked her at what times she did this she said that she did not do it consistently and that he wet everywhere. I assumed from this that he wet his bed, but his mother said that they managed to keep his bed fairly dry by vigilance—by taking him outside whenever he woke from sleep.

Although he had been chiefly cared for by his mother, his grandmother also helped—giving him some of his meals, and looking after him while the mother worked in the garden. The great-grandmother also helped care for him at times. He was quite accustomed to being left with his grandparents and did not cry when his mother went away. But if left by his mother either alone or with people less familiar to him, he usually cried and attempted to follow her.

When we visited at forty-one weeks we found Mutebe looking plump and handsome in a salmon-pink sunsuit. He spent the entire visit on his mother's lap, clinging to her and climbing over her. Once she left the room briefly and he cried frantically, although he did not follow her effectively. He calmed as soon as she returned. He seemed apprehensive of me, watching me warily from the shelter of his mother's arms. His mother thought he was afraid of me because I am "European"; he was ordinarily very active, creeping about and exploring.

When Mutebe was forty-four weeks old his mother reduced the daytime breast feedings to one only, although he was still given the breast three or four times at night. He protested the reduction of the daytime suckling. When he cried, his mother gave him milk to drink from a cup and he quieted down. Nevertheless, he cried much more than usual for several days after his mother began to withhold breast feedings.

The mother, who was a good informant, sketched out Mutebe's daily routine. In the morning he was not hungry, so his breakfast consisted only of tea with much milk in it. His mother then went to the garden to work, and now that the grandmother was absent, she took Mutebe along too, taking empty tins and other things for him to play with. After they returned to the house she gave him more tea. Then at lunch he ate with the adults—*matooke* with sauces of greens or peanuts, or bean soup. After lunch he played for quite a while and then had a nap. When he woke from his nap he was given the breast. Dinner was at six o'clock and consisted of *matooke* again.

His mother said that she still carried him on her back and that she approved of this method of carrying until the child is eighteen months old. She did not take him with her everywhere since he was accustomed to being left with his grandparents and cried very little during her absence. On the contrary, he seemed to enjoy being with them for they gave him much attention. But when his mother returned from an absence he gave her a fine welcome, crowing and clapping his hands and seeming pleased very to see her. His two-year-old brother played with him, but Mutebe did not seem appreciative and sometimes hit or bit him.

When we visited at forty-six weeks Mutebe had been asleep. When he was brought out he seemed very shy of us and clung to his mother. He sat on her

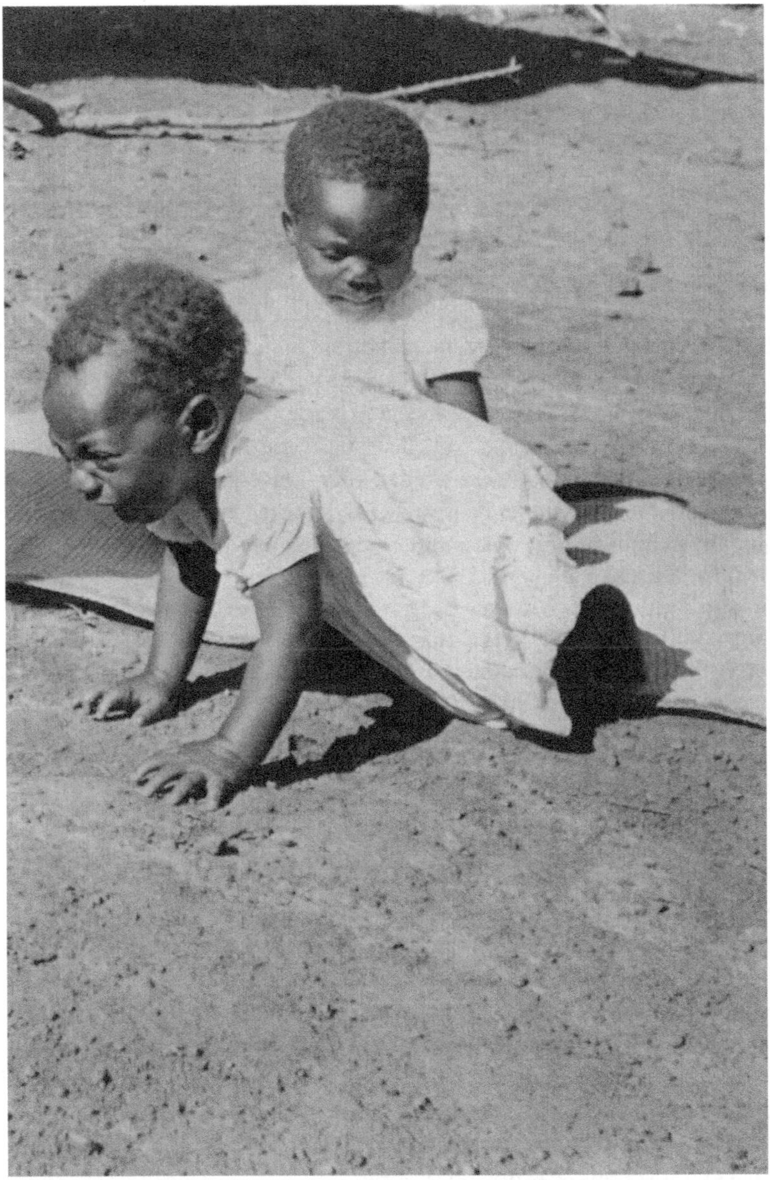

FIGURE 28 Mutebe at forty-six weeks cannot bear to have his mother put him down when strangers are present. He has a scar on his forehead from a bump. His two-and-a-half-year-old brother is in the background.

lap with his head against her breast until his mother dressed him up to have his photograph taken. His mother did not want to be included in the photograph and tried to arrange him on a mat, first with his brother and then alone, but Mutebe was very uncooperative, crying as soon as he let go of him. He seemed very frightened of me. Whenever I looked at him he cried and clung to his mother. I had to observe him out of the corner of my eye, not seeming to watch him. His mother thought that he had been frightened by a European during their stay in hospital when his brother was sick; besides, he had a cold and had just wakened. When we returned to the house he was very fussy and restless. His mother decided to give him the breast. He suckled quietly, seeming very absorbed. When he finished he remained quiet and seemed unafraid of me. He became sleepy and yawned several times. Just before we left I suggested that we try the photographs again, and this time he was quiet and accepted being left on the mat alone.

At forty-eight weeks we found Mutebe listless and feverish. He sat quietly on the mat near his mother, not paying much attention to anything but the candy I had given him. Toward the end of the visit I picked him up and held him on my lap; he did not protest. His mother accompanied us to the car, and my interpreter—a complete stranger—carried Mutebe; he accepted this throughout all of the long walk.

Mutebe had vocalized very little during our visits, but his mother reported that he could use the words for mother, father, and grandparent correctly and that he could identify certain animals correctly, saying *ennyonyi* for bird and *embuzi* for goat, and that he was capable even of a short sentence, such as "Look at the bird." He was still unable to stand alone or to walk—which seemed slow for one of these Ganda babies. He could cruise along the wall but had not attempted an independent step. He was so unusually tall that I thought that this might make it more difficult for him to stand alone.

His mother said that he cried very little. His crying was confined chiefly to occasions when he was especially hungry or when his mother left him alone or with an unfamiliar caretaker. Before his grandmother went away he cried also when she left him under similar circumstances. Sometimes he cried when he wanted to be picked up. He still hit his brother, and when his brother hit him back, Mutebe cried. But, on the whole, he was a very cheerful baby and cried infrequently.

When Mutebe was forty-nine weeks old he weighed in at 21.6 pounds at the clinic. He had a fever and was given Daraprim.

At fifty weeks Mutebe had not yet been finally weaned, although six weeks had elapsed since the daytime feedings had been reduced. His mother intended to wait until he was able to walk, and this had not yet occurred. Shortly after our last visit he had begun to stand, but then he developed a fever and stopped trying to stand. Just recently he had begun again. His mother wanted to discuss weaning, asking our advice as to how to undertake it so that it would be minimally distressing. She was considering sending him to live with the paternal aunt at weaning and wanted our advice about this.

She mentioned Mutebe's father for the first time since our initial visit. He came to visit often enough that Mutebe knew him and liked him.

We inquired specifically about "beatings." The mother said that she had first begun to "beat" Mutebe when she was attempting to train him to sit. When he grasped at the cloths that she had tied around him for support, she smacked his hands to deter him. Now she smacked him when he tried to hit his brother. These were the only occasions for discipline that she could recall.

We inquired about play, and his mother told us that he was very fond of playing with knives. She always took the knife away, for fear that he might cut himself.

At the first of this visit Mutebe was held by his mother. When she put him down he squealed briefly. She then sat down beside him and he quieted. He smiled at me when I offered him a piece of candy and was more friendly than he had been on previous visits. His mother got up to go out for a moment; on her way she picked Mutebe up and placed him on his grandfather's lap. Mutebe did not cry when she left; he seemed content with his grandfather. Later Mrs. Kibuka picked him up to hold him but he whimpered until she put him down again near his mother. She gave him her purse to play with. His brother wanted it too, and they struggled over it. Mutebe began to hit his brother. He was not crying and certainly was not in a tantrum. It was a determined, directed kind of hitting. Mrs. Kibuka settled the dispute by giving one her wallet and the other her compact. The mother showed Mutebe his image in the mirror of the compact. He seemed interested but made no marked response. Later in the visit I tried to get him to sit on my lap, but as I made a move to pull him toward me he squirmed away, moving closer to his mother. Then, from this safe point of vantage he smiled at me. We took photographs again and he did not cry.

We visited finally when Mutebe was nearly a year old. He was still not weaned since he could not yet walk. His mother was very worried about this retardation in his development because her first child had walked at eight months. The grandparents, when consulted, had advised that Mutebe not be weaned until he could walk—otherwise he would be weak and still further delayed in walking.

During the visit Mutebe was having a long nap. Finally his mother went to the bedroom to waken him. He was clinging to her when she brought him in. I asked to hold him, but when his mother began to hand him to me he cried immediately. She took him back and he spent the rest of the visit clinging to her.

Gesell Testing

When Mutebe was fifty-six weeks old the Gesell Developmental Schedules were administered by Dr. Marcelle Géber. Mutebe cried initially, when Dr. Géber arrived with her companions, and sought refuge on his mother's lap, but as soon as a set of cubes from the test materials was presented to him, he climbed down, began to manipulate the cubes actively, and showed a lively interest in the testing. Dr. Géber's report suggests that he showed much less anxiety with her than he had customarily shown with me when I visited. Whenever he was surprised or especially pleased in the course of the testing he communicated his feelings with smiles, laughter, exclamations, and a jargon-type vocalization, turning sometimes to his mother, but sometimes to Dr. Géber. He could make his wishes known. He was very interested in his mirror image and explored it. He was very active in his exploration of the test objects, trying to make use of their possibilities. He was enchanted when his locomotor ability was tested. He crept toward a large ball offered to him out of reach; he stood alone momentarily; he walked when led with both hands held and laughed with pleasure.

Dr. Géber commented that his mother was very cooperative in the testing, very interested in Mutebe's performance, ready to respond to his needs and to encourage him. Theirs seemed to be a good mother-child relationship.

Mutebe's Developmental Quotient was 102. In regard to the separate scales, he was most advanced in manual ability (108) and adaptivity (107) and least advanced in language comprehension (95) and social reactions (98).

When Mutebe was twenty-six months old he was retested. He was again active and happy during the testing and received a DQ of 109. The following year he could not be tested because he had been taken away by his father.

Visits to the Clinic

Age wks.	*Weight lbs.*
Birth	8.5
14	14.8
48	21.6

Kyimba

Kyimba's mother was an animated young woman with a ready laugh. On our first visit we also met the father, who was home for the day, on leave from his work as a clerk in a hospital in Kampala. He seemed a pleasant and intelligent young man and was eager for his family to participate. Kyimba was the couple's first baby. The paternal grandmother lived with them and, I felt, rather dominated the mother. They lived in a very tidy little house of wattle and daub, in the midst of an attractive garden. There was fragrant dried grass strewn on the floor, and clean mats to sit on, as well as two comfortable chairs for us.

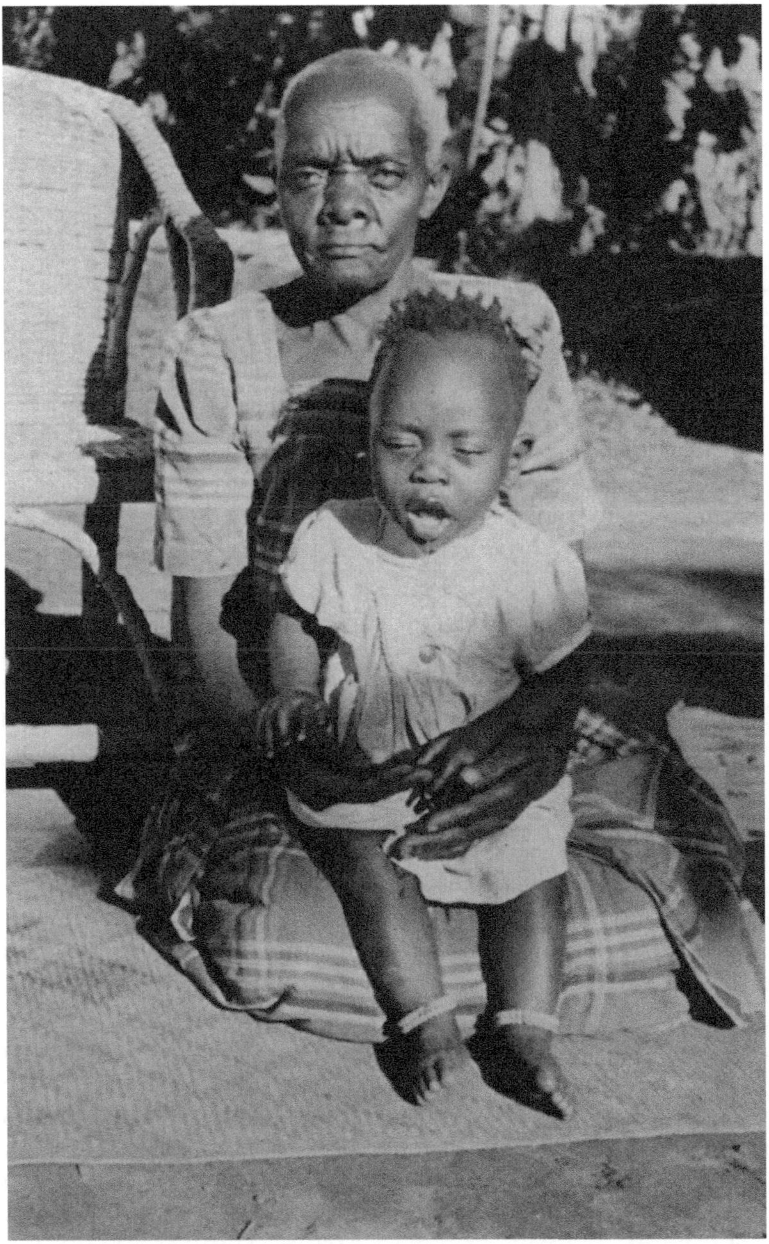

FIGURE 29 Kyimba at thirty-seven weeks with his grandmother. He is crying because he fell off the chair where she had previously posed him. He has been very fussy since weaning.

Kyimba was thirty-seven weeks old—bright, cheerful, and friendly. On our first brief visit we went outside to take photographs. The grandmother wanted to have the first picture taken of her and the baby. Kyimba's mother placed him on a chair while the grandmother posed herself on a mat beside him. She was so absorbed in posing herself that she did not notice him toppling over on his face. He let out a howl and could not be comforted; he cried the rest of the time we were there.

During this first visit we were explicit about the purposes of the research and made it clear that our sample consisted of babies who had not yet been weaned; we also made it clear that we were interested in observing the baby's response to the weaning process. When we learned a week later that Kyimba had already been fully weaned, we realized that we had been deceived, probably because of the family's eagerness to participate in the project. Kyimba had been finally weaned a month before—at the early age of thirty-four weeks. The mother was a good informant, answering questions readily and frankly and often elaborating information spontaneously. Moreover, the grandmother turned out to be knowledgeable of old Ganda customs and became one of our three informants on old customs.

Kyimba had been born in hospital, weighing seven pounds at birth. His mother said that he was given glucose for two days before being put to the breast. He sucked well at first, but for the next two days he did not and was put back on glucose. The mother felt that her flow of milk had been good throughout. He was fed on demand, and sometimes when there was something wrong and he was unhappy he was given the breast "to make him happy." At night he woke two or three times to be fed. Kyimba always sucked happily. His mother enjoyed breast feeding at first but found it a relief to wean him. Unlike the other babies in the sample, he was entirely breast-fed until weaned; no supplementary feedings of milk, juice, or solids had been given. He was described as a healthy baby who cried little and who had no illnesses beyond minor colds.

When he was two months old Kyimba was given a crib of his own to sleep in, but he was said to have refused to sleep in it; thus the mother allowed him to sleep in her bed until he was weaned. He was given three baths a day in the preweaning period, and this continued afterward. His mother began to train him in bowel control after he had learned to sit, but she made no effort to "hold him down" to prevent wetting. He was said to have learned not to soil the bed—chiefly because he made " noises" to alert his mother—and by thirty-seven months of age he usually went outside on his own initiative and rarely had an accident in the house. We inquired whether he handled his genitals and his mother replied that he often did and that she kept him dressed in pants in order to discourage this.

He began crawling at five months of age, even before he could sit unsupported. At twenty-eight weeks he began to stand, but he had not begun to walk when we first saw him at thirty-seven weeks.

The mother was certainly Kyimba's chief caretaker. She took him with her on all her expeditions, except when she went to work in the garden; then he was left behind with his grandmother. He began to follow his mother as soon as he could crawl, and he showed an obvious preference for her. He tended to cry whenever his mother left him, but he became accustomed to being left in the mornings with his grandmother. He seemed content to be left with her and cried and followed if she left the room, not invariably, but sometimes. His grandmother was fond of him, held him frequently, and he obviously responded with attachment. He had become attached also to his father, who was home every evening and held him, played with him and went for walks holding him in his arms. There were no other people familiar enough for him to have become friendly with them. As for other children, he usually bit them.

I suspect that the reason the mother weaned Kyimba so much earlier than is now customary in the neighborhood was that she realized she was again pregnant. She was not explicit about this, but her laughing embarrassment when questioned suggested this conclusion.

Weaning started at thirty-two weeks with the dropping of daytime feedings. Kyimba's mother said that he did not cry. She believed that this was because he was not hungry. She gave him lots of corn meal porridge with milk, feeding him with a spoon, and he accepted this readily. She also tried to give him milk from a cup, but he didn't like this. It is extraordinary that an abrupt change from breast feeding (with no supplements) to spoon feeding—although he was still breast-fed at night—caused so little disturbance, but this was the mother's report.

At thirty-four weeks nighttime feedings were stopped also. Kyimba cried throughout most of the first night. He seemed angry with his mother and hit her. At some time within a few days of final weaning—and our records do not make clear how soon this was—Kyimba began to sleep with his grandmother.

During our first long visit when Kyimba was thirty-eight weeks old, he fussed almost continuously. When his mother brought him into the front room, Mrs. Senvuma (who was substituting for Mrs. Kibuka that day) went to him, picked him up, and carried him to the side of the room where we were sitting. He shrieked so loudly that she returned him immediately to his mother. He sat on his mother's lap and continued to fuss—not loudly or continuously, but with constantly repeated, intermittent little cries. His mother rocked him, cuddled him, patted him—all in a somewhat vigorous way—but he did not calm down. At one point the crying went into a crescendo, and, crying loudly, Kyimba hit his mother quite hard. After this he quieted somewhat and continued fussing in a more subdued way while his mother bounced him about on her back and tried to carry on a conversation with us. Although her soothing efforts were vigorous, she was not rough, and, indeed, she showed him much tenderness, kissing his arm gently from time to time.

His mother said that he was crying a great deal and that his behavior during the visit was fairly typical. He wanted to be with his mother everywhere she went and he invariably cried and tried to follow if she left him for a moment. He usually fussed until she picked him up, and when held he often continued to fuss. When put down for a nap he would not stay in bed, he could be put to bed only if he had already fallen asleep. His mother attributed this unwonted crying to weaning and dissatisfaction with his feeding. Apparently he had been able to tolerate the new foods and the cessation of breast feeding during the day as long as he continued to have access to the breast at night. But in the four weeks since the night feedings were stopped he had been fussy and insecure.

At the clinic the following day Kyimba was again dressed in a fuschia-colored dress and pale blue waterproof pants. His mother wanted advice from Dr. Welbourn about his constant crying but she did not think to say, until prompted, that the problem had followed weaning. Dr. Welbourn prescribed a sedative to help him sleep at night and also recommended that he be given some of his milk from a nursing bottle to give him sucking satisfaction. His weight was 18.4 pounds and he seemed in good health.

A week later when Kyimba was forty weeks old, his mother said that the sedative had been effective. Kyimba, still sleeping with his grandmother, no longer cried at night, and even if he woke he settled down quickly and went back to sleep. She said that he had begun to be even more attached to his grandmother than before. She even said that he preferred his grandmother, but upon further inquiry it emerged that he still showed preference for his mother by crying and following when she left him with the grandmother—although sometimes he seemed content to be left. Although the nights were more peaceful, he still tended to be fussy during the day and frequently cried to be picked up.

As soon as we arrived his mother told us proudly that Kyimba could now walk! He could, however, take only two or three steps before falling down. His grandmother had begun to "hold him down" to teach him not to wet in the house. He had made no progress in response to this training, but, on the other hand, his bowel control had not lapsed under the stress of weaning.

He was receiving corn meal porridge and milk for breakfast. At lunch and dinner he got some of the adult food, chiefly *matooke.* He enjoyed cooked sweet bananas but rejected papaw. He did not suck his thumb, but since weaning he had shown an increased tendency to put into his mouth everything that he got hold of.

During our visit Kyimba clambered over his grandmother rather than his mother. When we showed her the photographs we had brought, Kyimba grabbed at one, but he did not cry when she took it away from him. Then his grandmother left the room. Kyimba did not cry but sat contentedly near his mother and played with a pineapple. For a while he squatted in front of his mother and looked up at her, but then he began to play with a bottle that he had found on the floor. He lolled back against his mother and began sucking at the cork of the bottle. Then he began to make persistent efforts to go out of the house. He kept creeping toward the door, but his mother caught his leg and pulled him back each time he started off. He accepted this frustration without protest; finally his mother allowed him to go. He stayed outside by himself for quite a while. When he had come back inside I picked him up and held him on my lap. He sat quietly — but tensely and uneasily. When I put him down on the floor he cried briefly—I thought with relief—and scuttled to his mother.

At forty-two weeks not much change was reported. Kyimba was still fussing more than his mother thought normal during the day, but at night he was quiet. His preference for his mother continued, but next to her he preferred his grandmother. He was said to become very angry sometimes, crying and throwing himself about, but he no longer hit his mother as he had done at the time of weaning. The outbursts of anger occurred chiefly when he demanded food, while his mother was still in the process of preparing it and could not yet give it to him. His mother said that she did not punish angry outbursts but rather tried to calm him by bouncing him about on her back or by cuddling him in her arms.

It was interesting to find that he did not say *mama* or *taata* but used the word *jjajja* correctly to refer to his grandmother. He was said to be able to give the simplest of greetings. He understood some simple commands; he responded to *jjangu* (come here!) but not to the words for "stop!" or "go away!" He was said to like to play with water especially, splashing it all over himself. He also wanted to play with fire, and his mother had to be careful while cooking. Her chief concern, however, was that he tended to eat everything that he picked up, so she followed him about to keep a close eye on him.

Kyimba sat on his mother's lap throughout our visit. He was very quiet and sat for a long time with his eyelids drooping before he finally fell asleep.

Our visit at forty-three weeks was primarily devoted to inquiring about old Ganda customs from the grandmother. Kyimba sat near his mother while we talked. He became increasingly fussy but did not make much noise about it. His mother rocked him until he quieted, and then he sat sucking his thumb. He was not friendly with us, and his mother confirmed that he was generally unfriendly with strangers.

Visit to the Clinic

Age wks.	*Weight lbs.*
38	18.4

17

THREE BABIES FROM RELATIVELY AFFLUENT FAMILIES

Paulo, Petero, and Magalita

Paulo's mother was the only woman in her village who agreed to participate in the research. Although the chief who introduced us seemed cordial and cooperative, we suspected that he was covertly distrustful of our purposes and had conveyed his misgivings to the families whom he approached on our behalf. This woman's motivation to participate must have been especially strong for her to stand out against the rest of the village, and even she was very cautious at first. The fathers of Paulo and Petero were friends, and it seemed that it was the influence of Paulo's family that brought Petero into the sample, although it had been tactfully arranged that the chief should effect the introduction to Petero's mother.

Magalita lived fairly close to Petero's family, and the parents of these children knew each other, although they were not close friends. Magalita came to our attention through her three-year-old sister, who was suffering from a chronically itchy foot. Dr. Welbourn, unable to find any organic foundation for the trouble, referred her to me in the hope that I might find some psychological reason for it and be able to help the child. Our visit to the family for this purpose resulted in their participation in the research, with the focus on Magalita, who was forty-two weeks old.

Paulo

Paulo's mother had two special reasons for wanting to participate in the research. She wanted help with the eldest child in the family, a daughter, who was epileptic and retarded in development. And she was lonely. Her husband's work took him away from home, permitting him to visit only once a month. Moreover, she was

DOI: 10.4324/9781003629337-20

Soga, not Ganda, and was the only Soga in the community except for her young brother who lived in the household. She had not been able to make close friends in the village. Perhaps the fact that she had more education than the others increased the distance. She had been a school teacher before her marriage—presumably at a primary level for she did not speak English. She enjoyed our visits; she always received us cordially and was an excellent informant.

Paulo's father was a surveyor. He had graduated from the Catholic secondary school at Kisubi and had gone on from there for special training in Entebbe. He spoke good English. Although he was absent when we arranged to meet his family, he was very pleased that his wife had decided to participate and gave us a fine welcome on our first encounter. He was delighted to find that I was a psychologist, for he had read several popular books on psychology and felt that the field offered much help to people. He was also pleased to find that I was Canadian, for he had come to love and respect several Canadian White Fathers while at school. He seemed to be a devout Catholic, and, indeed, I wondered whether his eagerness to participate in the research might be diminished when he discovered that I was not Catholic—but it was not.

The mother was restricted by her three children. Paulo was twenty-nine weeks old when we first began to visit. Tereza, although five and a half, required much help because of her disability. There was spasticity on the right side of her body and she could not use the fingers of her right hand; she walked clumsily; severely retarded, she was excitable, irresponsible, and had weak control. Kasalina, who was two and a half, seemed insecure and clinging. She demanded much attention from her mother, and did not want to be parted from her for a minute. She was shy of strangers, and especially shy of me.

Although the house in which this family lived was of wattle and daub, it was larger than most of the village houses. There was money for a few luxuries. The mother did some garden work but was helped by two men who were employed to look after the raising of cash crops—these included coffee and peanuts.

Paulo was born in hospital, weighing 7.5 pounds. He was vigorous and healthy from the beginning. He was fed on demand and sometimes given the breast merely for comfort. His mother had used a four-hour schedule for her other babies, but she was too busy now to be able to adhere to a schedule; she found it easier to feed him on demand. At night he slept in his own crib and woke three or four times to be fed. Orange juice was begun early, and from about twenty-four weeks of age he was given supplementary foods. "Holding down" began at four months of age. He did not sit alone until he was six months old; his mother tried to speed up this development by tying him upright in a large basin. He began to crawl shortly after he could sit.

Paulo was looked after entirely by his mother. She took him with her wherever she went—even to the garden while she worked there—carrying him in a sling on her back. On the few occasions when he was left with other people he cried.

His sisters did not help with him—one being too young, the other disabled—and he cried whenever his mother left him with them. He had not learned to know his father, who was home so infrequently. He was described as a happy baby who cried very little.

Paulo was asleep under a crocheted coverlet when we arrived for our first visit. After a while his mother wakened him and held him on her lap. He sat quietly at first but gradually became more active. His mother gave him to me to hold. He did not protest, but he was very active on my lap, occasionally throwing himself back in my arms and arching his back. He seemed very strong. Since he was restless and oriented toward his mother, I gave him back to her. Soon she took him to the door—still inside the house, but away from the mats on the floor—and held him down. Paulo obliged by urinating on the earthen floor. Then she returned to her mat and put him down beside her. He began to creep about the floor actively. For a while he played with a big stick, banging it on the floor vigorously.

A week later when Paulo was thirty weeks old, he spent most of the time playing actively on the floor, playing with the lid of a biscuit box, interested in looking at his reflection in the shiny metal inside the lid, manipulating an empty roller for adhesive tape, putting it in and out of its container, and also banging the roller against the lid very noisily. He looked fat and healthy and was naked except for strings of beads around his waist and ankles. For a while he was given to Mrs. Kibuka to hold. He seemed content on her lap until his mother left the room for a minute. Paulo immediately let out a yell that continued until his mother returned. Toward the end of the visit he became increasingly restless, climbing over his mother and clawing at her dress as if he wanted to get the breast. His mother agreed that he was hungry but tried to distract him by patting him and bouncing him about. He began to give rhythmic little whimpers and persisted in his efforts to reach the breast. Since it seemed obvious that the mother did not wish to feed him in our presence, we terminated the visit.

During the brief visit when Paulo was forty-one weeks old, he wanted to stay close to his mother, either on her lap or on the floor beside her. His mother tried to hand him to me to hold, but he protested vigorously, and she did not force the issue. He did not cry, however, when his mother went out for a few moments to cut some sugar cane for us. While she was away, the maternal uncle came into the house. Paulo scuttled quickly across the room to meet him and crowed with glee as his uncle picked him up. A little later he squealed in protest when his uncle began to put him down, so the uncle came out into the yard with Paulo in his arms as we said our farewells. His mother told us later that he was very fond of his uncle but would not let any other person pick him up. During this visit we noticed Paulo raising himself up on his feet as though to stand, although he kept his hands on the ground. A day or so later he began to stand alone.

At forty-two weeks Paulo stuck even closer to his mother, perhaps because he was feeling miserable with a bad cold, a hard cough, and occasional vomiting. Throughout the first half of our visit he sat on his mother's lap, squirming restlessly and saying "ma-ma-ma-ma" over and over again but without actually fussing. He was free to leave her lap and move away, as indeed he did later, but despite his restlessness he remained on her lap. After a while he stood up on her lap and made smacking sounds with his lips, apparently enjoying the feel and the sound of this activity rather than signaling hunger. His two sisters, who had been sitting nearby, got up and left the house. Paulo scrambled down from his mother's lap and crept to the doorway, following them. He stood up, holding onto the door jamb, and continued to make smacking sounds. He was holding a little string of colored celluloid balls, which rattled as he jiggled them. He played with them happily for a while. And then he became more active; he crept about, rattled his toy, and seemed happy and noisy. Occasionally he smiled across the room at his mother. He started to wet, and immediately his mother rushed him outside and held him down around the corner of the house. The girls came back inside, but twice more they left the house and Paulo crawled out after them, only to have his mother retrieve him. For a while he played with Kasalina, but he and Tereza paid little attention to each other.

His mother told us that he could feed himself with his fingers and wanted to do it himself, brushing away help. He tried to hold a cup himself but spilled his milk without his mother's help. During the day he rarely demanded the breast—perhaps only twice—presumably because he was so well fed with supplementary foods. But at night he still woke to be fed three or four times. His mother thought that the reason he woke so frequently was that he insisted on sleeping on his face; but no matter how often she turned him onto his back he would flip back over into his favored position. We inquired about elimination control. The mother said that Paulo had learned not to soil the bed but still soiled in the house and had not yet learned bladder control. She did not believe that bladder control could be established until after weaning, when the child's intake of liquids is reduced. She expressed great disapproval of the custom of holding a child down in the house so that the floor is wetted—although some weeks previously we had noticed her holding Paulo down in the house.

We inquired about relationships. Paulo was obviously attached to his mother, and had attachments also to his uncle and to Kasalina, whom he followed. He also was said to follow a two-year-old neighbor boy when he came over to play. He did not seem attached to Tereza. When his father came home to visit, Paulo was unresponsive to him for about three days, after which he began to warm up. At the end of our visit Mrs. Kibuka, who was holding Paulo, carried him in her arms to the car and got in with him, saying, "I think I will take this lovely baby along with me." Paulo did not protest, but Kasalina became very upset; she ran to her mother, hung onto her skirts, and whimpered.

A week later when Paulo was forty-three weeks old, his mother became so ill that she had to go to hospital. She arranged for the girls to be looked after by another family but took Paulo with her. He was kept in a small crib close to his mother's bed. When we visited two days after their admission, we found Paulo quiet and subdued. Mrs. Kibuka picked him up and held him; when she put him back into his crib he caught onto her and would not let her go. So she gave Paulo to his mother; soon he was nursing at the breast. The following week we visited again, after they had returned home, and drove them to another village to pick up the girls to bring them home. During the fifty-mile drive Paulo was in fine fettle. He was in the front seat between his mother and me; he crawled around, investigated everything, and vocalized cheerfully and continuously. His mother said that he had been equally active in hospital, which had been very tiring for her when she was ill. The following week we called to inquire whether they wanted to go to the clinic the next day. Paulo was outside when we drove up in the car. When he saw us he crowed with glee and crept over on all fours with great speed. We suspected that it was the car rather than us which aroused his enthusiasm.

At forty-six weeks Paulo began the visit on his mother's lap and kept throwing himself back against her. Presently he began to creep about the floor exploring; occasionally he stopped in a squatting position. Later, he played in the doorway, making several short excursions outside. Each time his mother called him back, and if he did not come, she went out to get him. She said that she liked to keep him in sight always. Back in the house he played intently with two bottle caps. After a while his mother picked him up, intending to give him to Mrs. Kibuka to hold. Seeming to anticipat her intention, Paulo began to struggle and scream, hitting at his mother, but since she was holding him face out he could not reach her with his blows. Resisting his protest, the mother placed him on Mrs. Kibuka's lap where he continued to scream until he was put down.

His mother told us that he usually played actively when he was with her and that he was quite ready to make excursions away from her. But whenever she left him he cried the entire time she was gone, regardless of with whom she left him. He sometimes cried to be picked up by her. She did, in fact, hold him a lot, but when other people tried to hold him he would bite them. He also hit and bit the children when they tried to take something away from him that he wanted to keep. His mother did not punish him for these temper displays but, rather, tried to calm him by holding him and soothing him. Apart from these instances, he cried very rarely and seemed a happy child.

By this time he could understand his own name and several simple commands. He was reported to say *mama* appropriately, but, he had no other words. He did imitate noises, however, and whenever anyone in the household read aloud Paulo would make a continuous "reading" sound in accompaniment.

At forty-seven weeks Mrs. Kibuka made a brief unannounced visit. To her surprise Paulo came to her directly. She picked him up and held him, and he seemed quite content. There was another visitor present, and, of course, the girls were there. Mrs. Kibuka began to play with the children, making noises which the children imitated. The mother left the room for a while and Paulo did not protest. Rather, he continued in the game, and like his sisters imitated the noises and laughed merrily.

But at fifty weeks of age Paulo would not come to Mrs. Kibuka when she coaxed him and he cried when she picked him up. During all of this visit he stuck close to his mother and sat on her lap most of the time. For a while he suckled at the breast. His mother left the room briefly and he cried bitterly while she was gone. A visitor came for a while and took Paulo onto her lap. He did not cry but squirmed off soon and went to his mother. His mother complained that it was very difficult for her to get her work done because Paulo refused to be left with other people. It had been rainy and wet all week—too wet for him to be outside—so she had stayed at home with him, neglecting her garden work. During this visit he demonstrated his new accomplishment; walking had begun at forty-eight weeks and he could now walk halfway across the room before he toppled.

By fifty-three weeks Paulo could walk well but still seemed to prefer creeping when he wanted to get about quickly. He was dressed in a plaid sunsuit and had bells around his ankles. After we had seated ourselves inside, Paulo crept out toward the car. He was said to be very interested in cars and to imitate their sound with a "vvvvvvv" sound. I had to go out to the car to get something and brought Paulo back with me. He did not protest at all when I picked him up and brought him back to his mother. He sat beside her burying his face in her lap. Then he climbed up onto her lap and tried to open her dress, fussing when his first efforts were unsuccessful. He persisted and finally succeeded in opening the dress. His mother then gave him the breast. He suckled while squirming about actively on her lap, not really tucked into a nursing position. After having one breast for a while, he was offered the other. It was the longest period of breast feeding that we had witnessed with this mother and child.

We then went outside for photographs. The yard was spread with peanuts drying in the sun. These did not hamper Paulo, who crept about actively, making persistent efforts to get as far as the car before he was brought back. When we returned to the house he remained outside and did not come when his mother called him. She went out to get him. He kicked his feet and crept off quickly but he did not cry when she picked him up and brought him inside. Once inside, he sat beside his mother, hiding his face in her lap. He began a fussy squealing, which was not exactly crying. His mother bounced him about to quiet him, but unsuccessfully. She then suggested that I give him a piece of candy— which I had not offered him previously because on earlier visits his mother had always declined on his behalf. As soon as he had the candy he quieted down. Once his mother went out of the room for a moment and he did not seem to notice. Soon he went outside again and presently wet on the ground. He began to play with the moist patch, but one of his sisters noticed this and told his mother, who went out to get him and brought him back inside. Inside again, he was restless and rather fussy. When we got up to go the whole family came out to the car with us. The mother handed Paulo to me through the car window, suggesting that I take him with me. Paulo did not protest; he was quiet and subdued and did not take his previous active interest in the interior of the car. I started the car and began to maneuver it for a turn. Paulo tolerated this for quite a while and then made a slight movement of protest. I immediately handed him to his mother. Kasalina, meanwhile, was screaming and clinging to her mother, very upset.

During our interview nothing new emerged except that when called, Paulo now answered "mmm" in the conventional way; and he had been much friendlier with his father when he last visited than he had ever been before.

Our next visit occurred when Paulo was thirteen months old. He was outside by himself when we arrived. He became quite excited when he saw us and ran to get his mother—literally ran. I could not judge from the distance whether he was frightened or merely excited. During the visit he sat near his mother and played on the floor. Once his mother got up and went outside to get us a gift. Paulo began to scream. His uncle picked him up, but Paulo continued to scream until his mother returned and took him on her lap. After a while his mother went out to the garden again. Paulo sat crying on his uncle's lap and would not be consoled. Two weeks later he seemed more cheerful. He was walking well and did a lot of active exploring. I gave him a plastic cup and saucer, which he clutched for the rest of the visit. For a while he sat contentedly on Mrs. Kibuka's lap. He seemed friendlier than usual, responding to our overtures. His mother did not leave the room during our visit, however, and she said he still cried whenever she left. Occasionally he would be content to be left briefly with his sisters, but more usually not. His mother told us that she had started to "beat" him, sometimes giving him a smack on the bottom and sometimes tapping his arm gently with her cupped hand. Recently he had begun to hit and bite his sisters, without provocation and "like a game." His mother decided that it was time for discipline to begin.

Several times over a period of months the mother had suggested that perhaps I would like to have Paulo since I admired him so much. At first I thought she was joking, but I gradually began to realize that she was serious. Finally she explicitly proposed that I should take Paulo back to Canada with me and raise him as my own child; I could give him so many advantages which they could not give him, and Canada had so many more opportunities than Uganda. Moreover, I clearly loved him and would be good to him.

Paulo's father has written me annual letters ever since I left Uganda, keeping me posted about the entire family. At the time of his last letter Paulo was eleven

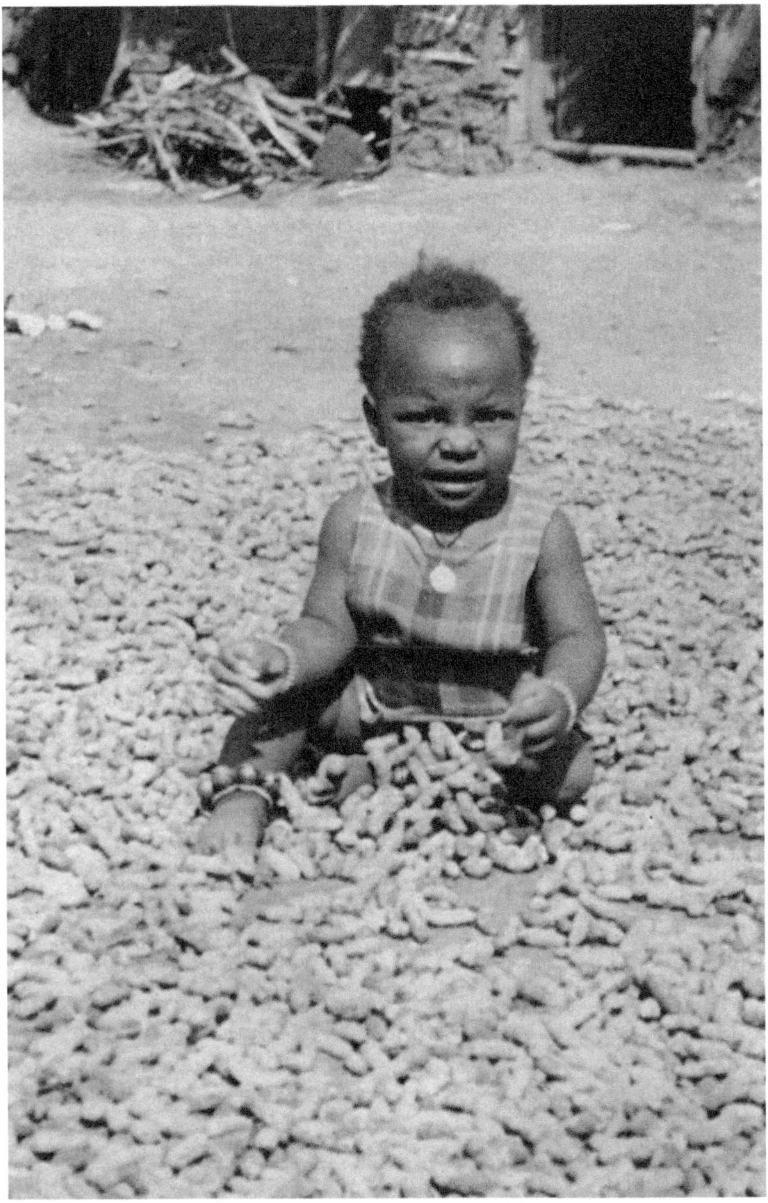

FIGURE 30 At fifty-three weeks Paulo loves to explore his world. Here he is playing with the peanuts which have been spread out in the yard to dry.

and a half years old and had successfully finished six years of primary school; he was about to enter secondary school at Kisubi where his father had been educated. "Your little Paulo has now grown up" said his father.

Gesell Testing

Paulo was sixty weeks old when Dr. Géber administered the Gesell Developmental Schedules. He was on his mother's lap at the beginning, but when the test objects were presented to him he crawled toward them, leaving his mother. He accepted the test objects, handling them and holding them to himself for a long time. He seemed insecure during the testing and handled his genitals as well as the test objects. He did not use his mother as a secure base. She in turn did not encourage him, perhaps feeling that she should not, although she was very interested in his performance. He avoided looking at the examiner, and although he seemed to profit from her encouragement, he did not communicate with her. Although capable of pointing to things he wanted, he did not do so during the testing. It was not until the very end of the test that he smiled at the examiner. He was capable of using several words but did not do so during the test. He was observed to walk well and to run stiffly. He could mount a chair but refused to try to climb the steps which were part of the test equipment—of course, he had never encountered steps before. His equilibrium was good when he was squatting playing and when going in and over the doorsill.

His Developmental Quoitient was 114. He was most advanced in locomotion (128) and manual ability (128) and tested least advanced in social reactions (100) and language (107).

After his testing was finished, his sisters were tested. Paulo became very active when attention was withdrawn from him, and, to judge from Dr. Géber's report, he then behaved in much the same way as we had observed him to behave in our visits.

When twenty-seven months old Paulo was retested; his DQ had fallen to 100. But when he was retested at thirty-nine months, the DQ had gone up again, to 117.

Visits to the Clinic

Age wks.	*Weight lbs.*
Birth	7.5
29	18.6
31	19.5
49	21.3

Petero

Petero's father, like Paulo's, was a surveyor. The household seemed even more obviously comfortably fixed than Paulo's. The house was of cement block, with a red tile roof, and it contained European-style furniture. The father owned a car, which enabled him to get home on Wednesdays as well as on weekends, even though he was posted elsewhere.

The mother was pleasant, cooperative, and very much taken up with her five children, who ranged in age from a boy seven years old to Petero, who was nine weeks old. The second and third children were girls, and the fourth another boy. The children seemed to us to be polite, outgoing, and spontaneous, but their mother perceived them as noisy and disobedient.

Petero had been born in hospital, but according to his mother he had been "born weak" and was much less active and slower to develop than the other children had been. He was breast-fed on demand— "whenever he cries"— including two or three times at night. His mother said that she could not possibly keep to a feeding schedule since she was alone, and had all the other children to look after. Our first brief visit took place when Petero was nine weeks old. His mother held him on her lap. He began to whimper a little, and his mother gave him the breast. Immediately after the feeding was over he had a bowel movement. His mother exclaimed and held him away from her so that he would not soil her dress. She reached into a shopping bag that she had nearby, drew out a roll of toilet paper, and proceeded to clean the baby up. She then removed the cloth that had been wrapped around him, bundled it and the toilet paper out of sight, and sent one of the children to get a fresh cloth. While this was going on Petero cried. Then the mother held him up against her shoulder, stroking him, and he soon calmed.

At eleven weeks we visited again, for a longer time. As soon as we arrived Petero was given to me to hold on my lap. He protested being handed over to me by his mother but stopped crying immediately when she took him back. Soon she put him down in his crib, which was placed in the living room. Again, he cried as soon as she released him. She took him up again, and he continued to cry; he finally reached toward her breast, making it clear what he wanted. I inquired how long it had been since the last feeding, and his mother said with surprising precision: "Two hours and ten minutes." He suckled eagerly and was given both breasts. Finally he fell asleep at the breast and was put down in his crib where he slept soundly. His mother said that he slept most of the day and that he cried little. She said that she was the only one who took care of him, except that the oldest girl helped a little, although she could not do much for him since she was not yet six years old. When the mother worked in the garden she took Petero along and put him down on an old mattress in the shade. She nearly always had him in sight and never was out of earshot.

Petero was eighteen weeks old when we next saw him. In the meantime, his mother had been ill. She felt weak, had abdominal pains, and had been twice to hospital for treatment. And now Petero was ill with diarrhea. He was brought out wrapped in a cloth, and cloths were handed to Mrs. Kibuka to cover her lap while she held him. His mother brought a white smocked silk dress, which Mrs. Kibuka put on him. He looked thin and delicate—but cheerful. He was content to lie prone on her lap. His arms and legs were active, and he grunted and vocalized a great deal. A week later at the clinic he still had diarrhea, but the doctor found him in good health otherwise. He weighed 12 pounds.

When we visited at twenty weeks Petero sat on his mother's lap, leaning back against her and smiling at us from time to time. After a while he was given to Mrs. Kibuka to hold. He leaned back against her but jerked his arms and legs around and made little noises that became increasingly unhappy in tone. Since he seemed about to cry he was given back to his mother. She held him in a standing position on her lap.

His mother said that he could not yet sit alone, although when lying supine he sometimes raised his head as though he would like to sit up. This mother was one of the few in our sample who sat on a chair. I had never seen her put Petero on the floor; he was always either held by her or placed in his crib. "Holding down" had just begun—after feedings and only during the day.

His mother said that she sometimes left him in a room by himself, but only if she was working in an adjoining room. He accepted being left thus but perhaps only because his mother talked to him from a distance. He seemed to be dependent on this vocal contact and did much vocalizing in response. Indeed, he and his mother would "talk" to each other from room to room, alternating vocalizations. Face-to-face, also, he responded vocally to his mother when she talked to him. Sometimes he cried to be picked up. Sometimes his mother responded by picking him up and holding him, but sometimes she left him to go to sleep. Under these circumstances he usually began to suck his fingers and before long settled down to sleep.

At twenty-four weeks I found Petero lying on a mat in the living room when I arrived—it was the first time I had seen him on the floor. He was making happy squealing noises, lying supine. He stared at me steadily, although he had to roll up his eyes and look at me upside down. Occasionally he smiled. I took him on my lap for a while. He was responsive to my attentions and was active on my lap, doing a lot of kicking. I handed him back to his mother, and then he was put back down on the floor. He began to vocalize happily, but after a while he became very noisy lying there on his back. His mother took him up and laid him prone across her lap and he quieted down. He seemed a very young baby—slower in his development than most of the others in our sample. He was still entirely breast-fed. He still received three baths a day. The older children enjoyed playing with him and were occasionally allowed to hold him, but they did not help with his care otherwise. He was never left with them unless the mother was nearby and could hear what was going on. When she left him he had begun to cry—although previously he had been content to be left. Although he cried when she left, he soon settled down and accepted the children's attentions. The mother did not let the children carry him, and when she worked in the garden she took him along with her as before. He had no playthings—his mother said that he was too young for them. The following week at the clinic Petero was found to weigh only 13.7 pounds—to have gained only 9 ounces in a month. The doctor was concerned that he was not gaining more rapidly and urged his mother to bring him to the clinic more regularly. The doctor also suggested supplementary solid foods, and after these were begun Petero gained more rapidly, although he remained underweight. Meanwhile the mother, herself, was in poor health, and the other children had assorted illnesses.

At thirty weeks we found all the children ill with a fever and diarrhea, including the baby. Petero had not yet begun to sit, although his mother had begun to train him by wrapping cloths around him to give him support. His mother had concluded that her milk was insufficient to nourish him and had supplemented breast feedings with milk from a nursing bottle. He much preferred the breast, and objected to the bottle. His mother also had been feeding him solid foods — mashed sweet potatoes with sauce, or *matooke*, or squash, feeding him bits with her fingers. He tended to reject these foods, so breast milk was still his main source of nourishment. He did not take the same initiative as many other babies in our sample in seeking the breast. He never tried to open his mother's dress. His mother said that she still held him a great deal. He cried very little—only when hungry or, occasionally, when the children were too noisy. When he cried his mother gave him the breast. He no longer accepted the attentions of the other children. His mother felt that this was because he was ill. He cried whenever his mother left him now. He did not "know" his father, although he was home on weekends and once during the week. At the clinic the following week he was found to have lost a little weight; he weighed 14.4 pounds.

When we visited at thirty-two weeks we found that Petero had been very ill. He was battling a fever, diarrhea, and vomiting. His mother took him to Kampala to see the clinic doctor, but she was absent, so they returned to the village. Petero became worse, shivering and finally fainting. In panic his mother again took him to Kampala, this time to hospital. He received treatment but was very ill during the night; the next day he was given some "medicine" but remained very ill. The mother felt that he was being neglected, and, against advice, took the baby out of hospital to an Indian doctor in private practice, who gave injections and glucose. His mother was still very worried about him and indignant about the hospital. By the time we visited he had improved somewhat. He was at his mother's breast when we arrived. Occasionally he stopped sucking to whimper, then sucked again. As he sucked he played gently with the buttons on his mother's dress. He looked thin and weak and cried when his position was altered, apparently from abdominal pain. After the breast feeding his mother fed him glucose with a large spoon. Of nearly every spoonful quite a lot trickled down the side of his face, and the mother scooped it up again with the spoon. The glucose feeding was not helped by the fact that Petero looked steadily at me, turning his head so that it was not easy to feed him. We called during the next week; Petero was said to be improving, although he still looked peaked and weak.

At thirty-four weeks he was much better and was very active during the visit. His mother told us that he had just learned to sit. We took photographs, wanting Petero to show off his new accomplishment. His mother tried to place him as she wished. He sat leaning forward but did not topple. His mother said that he had begun to sit earlier but then had stopped when he was so ill.

When we returned to the house he refused to sit alone. He stood near his mother, supported by her. He jiggled around, lifting his feet and putting them down again, quite active, and occasionally smiling up at his mother. He then got up onto his mother's lap and scrambled over her, vocalizing continuously, and occasionally smiling across the room at us. His vocalization was repetitive—"da-da-da-da" and "eh-eh-eh-eh." He responded when we said his name. His mother said he also responded to the command *sirika* (hush).

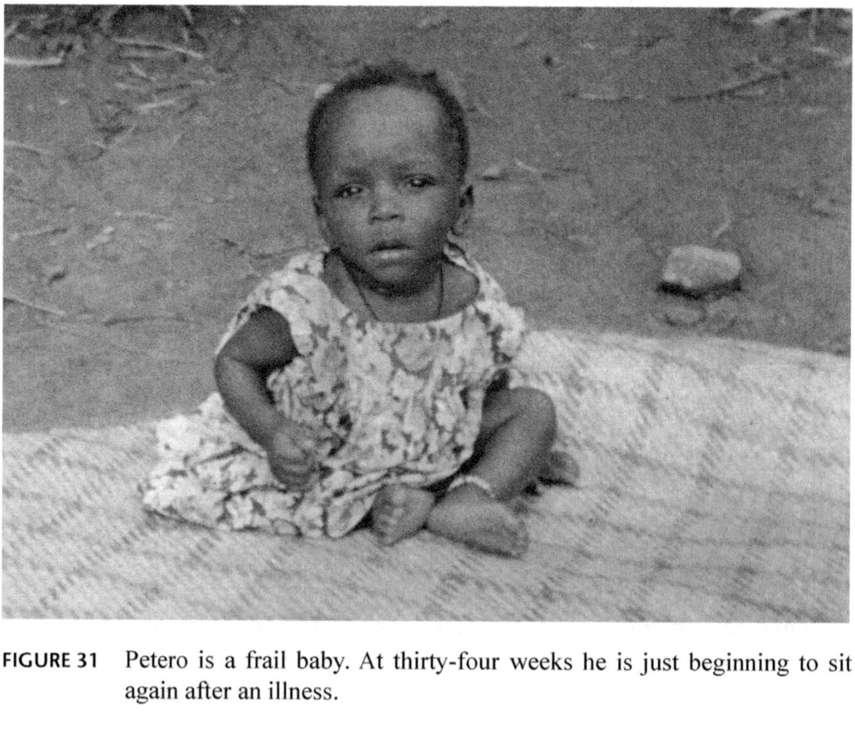

FIGURE 31 Petero is a frail baby. At thirty-four weeks he is just beginning to sit again after an illness.

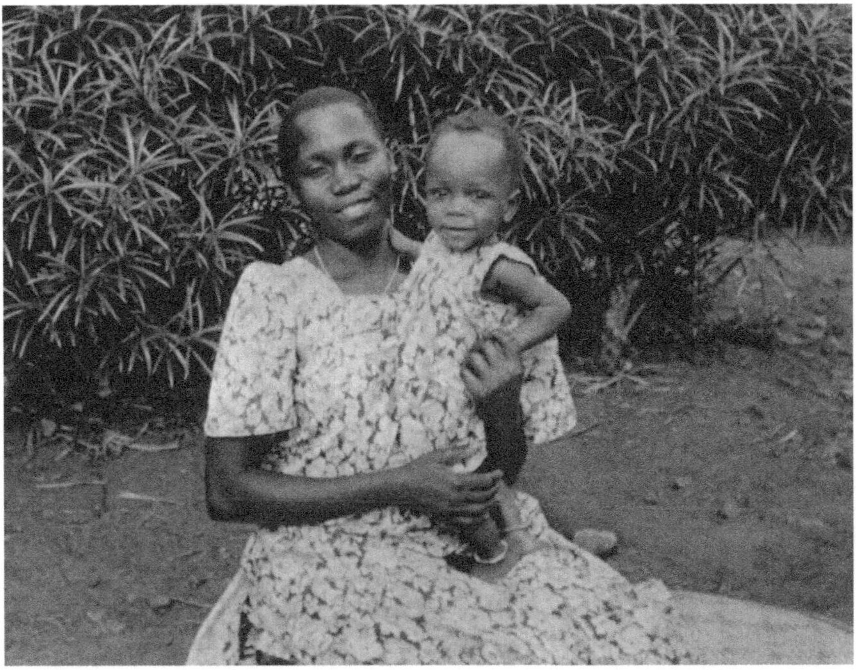

FIGURE 32 Petero felt much more secure after his mother picked him up.

For a while he lay on his back on his mother's lap, looking very much the little baby, cooing and kicking his feet and waving his hands. He struggled to his feet again and began to suck his hand. He leaned his head toward his mother, burying his face in the angle between her neck and shoulder, and in this position he continued to jig around. This he did for some time; then he placed his face on his mother's supporting hand and bit it gently. He then wet and his mother changed his dress. Again she tried to make him sit. He made a sound between a laugh and a cry, and refused. Finally his mother gave him the breast and he suckled. After the feeding I took him onto my lap for a while. He accepted this and was active, scrambling around but somehow behaving less intimately than he did with his mother.

His mother said that he accepted strangers, and adults generally, without fear as long as she was present. He was said now to 'like" his father but not to like his brothers and sisters. But whenever his mother left him, even to go out of the room for a moment, he cried. When she returned he always stopped crying and was "very happy" to see her. His mother sometimes left him to cry, but if he did not settle down readily, she returned to hold him and give him the breast. As long as his mother was present he was cheerful and active.

His mother said that he had recently stopped soiling his bed, but he still frequently wet his bed, and he still soiled and wet in the house.

Gesell Testing

When Petero was nine months old he was administered the Gesell Developmental Schedules. His behavior was *dynamique* and his DQ 108. Next year when Dr. Géber returned for retesting his mother refused to have it done.

Visits to the Clinic

Age *wks.*	*Weight* *lbs.*
20	12.0
24	13.7
30	14.7
32	14.4

Magalita

Magalita was the fifth child in the family. The eldest boy and girl were away at boarding school and another boy was in the local school. A three-year-old sister—the one with the itchy foot—was at home. The father, whom we met only briefly, had a clerical job in Kampala. The paternal grandmother was a member of the household —a forceful old woman who walked with a crutch—one leg having been amputated—but who nevertheless did her share of the garden work. There was another household nearby which included two grown sons of the father by another marriage, a twelve-year-old school girl, and an adolescent daughter who died shortly after our contact with the family began.

Magalita's mother was gentle and soft-spoken. She seemed chronically fatigued, complained of feeling weak, and during most of our contact with her she was actually ill. Nevertheless, she was cooperative and an excellent informant.

Magalita herself was slimmer than other babies of her age in our sample. During our first visit at forty-two weeks she sat beside her mother or on her lap. Although quiet, she was quite active, playing vigorously with her doll, and at one point she managed to get her toes to her mouth and chewed them. Once she lost her balance and fell over backward, bumping her head hard against the wall. She began to howl, and her mother took her in her arms and comforted her. She soon stopped crying and began to suck her thumb.

Magalita was born in hospital and weighed 7 pounds 4 ounces. She was described as a tall baby, and still seemed more tall and slim than plump and vigorous. Her mother hemorrhaged badly after delivery and was very weak, but Magalita thrived at first. Her mother said that she had had insufficient milk from the beginning and attributed this to her hemorrhage. She fed the baby on demand at first but introduced supplementary solids at three months, and gradually fell into a schedule. She had been a regular visitor to Dr. Welbourn's clinic. Her milk, scanty from the beginning, seemed really to begin to fail. She stopped Magalita's daytime feedings, intending to conserve her milk for nighttime feedings. Dr. Welbourn explained to her that she needed to feed the baby at times throughout the day in order to stimulate the flow of milk, so daytime feedings were reinstituted. Supplementary milk was given as well. At first the mother used a bottle, but she found it too troublesome to sterilize bottles and used a cup instead. At the time our visits began, the mother breast-fed the baby at 8:00 a.m., noon, 4:00 p.m., and once during the night. Solid foods were given at family mealtimes. Magalita could feed herself with her fingers, but her feedings were supervised either by her mother or by her half-sister (when she was at home). Just how much reality basis there was for the mother's feeling that her milk had always been insufficient, I do not know, but she always felt that this was so; consequently, she never felt that she could afford to "waste" milk to comfort the baby when distressed and only fed her "when she was hungry." Magalita had always sucked well, and she also took readily to the solid foods. She did not, however, like milk. She sucked her thumb a lot.

Magalita thrived until she was two months old. Then she succumbed to diarrhea. From then on the diarrhea was recurrent, and it was often accompanied by fever and a cough. When she was forty-three weeks old she weighed 15.6 pounds; a month later she weighed only 15.5 pounds. The mother's concern about her health and physical development seemed justified.

Nevertheless, according to her mother's report, her earlier motor development had not been retarded. On the contrary, she sat at three months, crawled at six months, and stood alone at eight months. She was said to have learned not to soil her bed at six months, but she still wet the bed. The sounds that she made "when she wants to be held down" served as signals to the mother.

Although the mother was responsible for most of Magalita's care, and, indeed, held her a lot, other people helped—in preparing solid food, feeding, and other care as well. Perhaps because she was not well, she cried a lot, and always had. She could not tolerate being apart from her mother unless she was left with one of her favorite people. When I inquired who her "favorite people" were, I was told that Magalita was most attached to her mother, her father, her twelve-year-old half-sister (who is usually at school), and one of her grown half-brothers. Magalita was highly differential in her attachments. She rejected her grandmother, seemingly being afraid of her. She was not especially interested in her brothers or half-brothers—except for her one favorite. She seemed to enjoy playing with her three-year-old sister but often hit her.

At forty-six weeks Magalita slept through our visit. At forty-nine weeks she sat quietly for a while, sucking her thumb. After a while she started to cry, for no reason apparent to us. Her mother picked her up and took her outside for a moment, presumably to "hold her down." When they returned, Magalita sat on her mother's lap, snuggled in, her head on her mother's breast, sucking her thumb and seeming very much the little baby. Later in the week, at the clinic, she again sucked her thumb the whole time. She still had diarrhea and was not gaining well. At one point her mother put her down and disappeared for a moment; Magalita cried bitterly until she returned. When we visited again at fifty-one weeks we found Magalita quite ill. Her mother had taken her to Kampala for treatment, but no improvement had yet been noted. Her three-year-old sister was even sicker, and it was she who sat on her mother's lap throughout the visit; she was so ill and weak that she could no longer even crawl.

Just before her first birthday Magalita was found to have lost another ounce, and had a fever and a cough. When we arrived the next day to visit, her mother announced proudly that she had begun to walk. She could walk only three of four steps, and then she fell, and she still seemed a little afraid to try. Her walking had started before she became ill this last time, and then the illness interfered with it; then when she began to feel better she started again.

Near the beginning of this visit we suggested photographs. Magalita looked very fetching in a green and white checked dress with a very full skirt. She had a piquant little face, but the photography made her very unhappy. Her mother took out tables and chairs and placed Magalita on a table. Magalita was so frightened that she wet the tablecloth. She cried and was handed to her adult half-brother to be comforted. Back in the house, she first sat on her mother's lap and then got down on the floor, but buried her head in her mother's lap and wiggled her bottom back and forth in the air. Then she climbed up again onto her mother's lap and sat there sucking her thumb quietly. Presently she began to play, seeming quite happy, vocalizing, and kicking her legs about. There was a two-year-old child present; at one point Magalita reached for her in a friendly fashion, but getting no response she began to play with her mother's face. Her favorite half-sister suddenly entered, returning from school for a visit. Magalita greeted her with a squeal of delight, laughed, and quickly crept toward her. Just as we were about to leave she began to fuss. Her mother carried her out of the house, accompanying us. She glimpsed her favorite big brother and crowed with delight. While we were saying our farewells at the car she wet on her mother, who was holding her. Her mother put her down on the ground, and she began to scream. We left while she was still screaming.

Next week at the clinic Magalita clung to her mother. At one point her mother put her down and left her with me; Magalita cried anxiously until her mother returned; she would not let me comfort her. Her mother wiped her nose when she

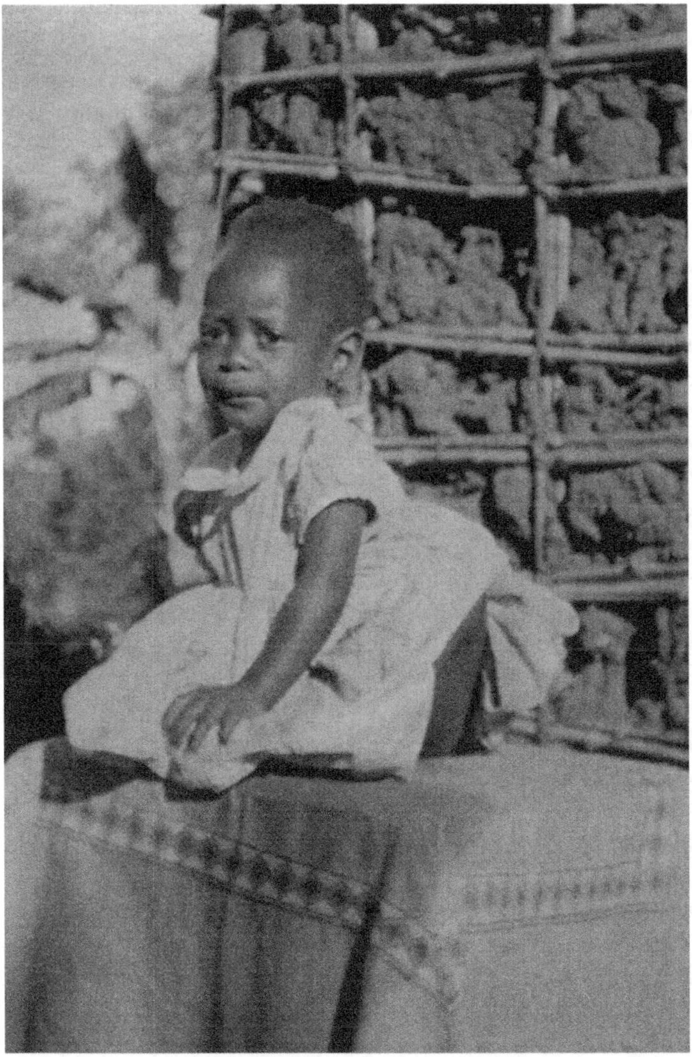

FIGURE 33 Magalita at fifty-two weeks was so frightened when put down on the table to be photographed that she wet the tablecloth.

returned and set her on her lap; Magalita quieted and looked up at her mother's face. She was given a guava to play with and sucked at it for a long time with much salivation. Finally she dropped it and sucked her thumb instead. At one point I noticed her in close interaction with her mother; she pointed to something on the ground, then her mother pointed too, and they discussed it intimately. When she was examined by the nurse she cried at first and then sucked her thumb. She had an earache, which was treated, and she had gained only one ounce—still weighing 15.5 pounds.

A week later she was still ill—with the fever and diarrhea. She was said to be weak, and she looked weak. This was a long visit, during which her mother gave us much interview information.

She still got two baths a day, although when she was a little baby she had received three. She did not like her baths and cried, although previously she had enjoyed them. She cried only when her mother bathed her and not when the other children helped by bathing her. Before she became so weak and ill, her mother said, she could go outside on her own initiative to wet or to have a bowel movement, but now she did not do so. At night when her mother heard her becoming restless, she took her up to "hold her down." Ordinarily, therefore, she had achieved good control of elimination. She slept with her mother for the first four months and then in her own bed in her mother's room.

She was better developed in speech than in locomotion or manipulation. She could say *kiki* (what is it) and *kiri wa* (where is it). She also used the words *taata* and *mama* appropriately. She was fascinated with eyes and poked her finger into people's eyes asking *kiki?* She understood quite a number of simple commands, including "sit down!" She made sounds while playing, especially imitating the sound of an automobile. She made sounds in imitation of the gramaphone. Recently the family had acquired a radio. This puzzled Magalita who pointed to it whenever it was turned on and asked *kiki?*

She was still very attached to her mother. Whenever left alone in a room by her mother she cried and followed, and her mother usually responded by picking her up. She was described as being very fond of her father, who gave her much attention. He was tolerant of fussiness. When Magalita was tired she would sometimes cry and throw herself about, and, when her father was at home, he would pick her up and soothe her. She was so fond of her half-sister that she gave her mother the impression that she preferred her to anyone—despite the fact that she was rarely at home. And she still showed distinct preference for her grown half-brother. Since becoming ill she had returned to her earlier overwhelming preference for her mother, however, and wanted to be held by her all the time. She was not friendly with strangers but was more tolerant of them than she had been for a while.

When I asked who held her most often, her mother replied that she held her, mainly after lunch and dinner. The three other people who held her happened to be her three other favorite people.

During this interview at fifty-four weeks, Magalita sat on her mother's lap sucking her thumb. Sometimes she put her head down on her mother's shoulder; sometimes she merely leaned back against her. She seemed sleepy, but several times her mother put her down to sleep on a bundle of cloths nearby, and each time she cried. Once her mother carried her to the bedroom after she seemed to have fallen fast asleep, but she woke and whimpered and her mother brought her back.

At thirteen months Magalita had recovered from her illness and had gained a few ounces. A few days later we were told that she had just been weaned, but we did not have an opportunity to visit to get full details; we merely learned that she was crying a great deal.

Gesell Testing

When Magalita was still thirteen months old she was given the Gesell Developmental Schedules. She was reported by Dr. Géber to have been interested in the test and to have received a DQ of 104. When twenty-six months old, on retesting, her DQ was again 104, and again she was said to have been interested. When thirty-nine months old, however, she was described as insecure, and her DQ was 97. Dr. Géber returned when Magalita was five, but she had gone to live with her grandmother.

Visits to the Clinic

Age *wks.*	*Weight* *lbs.*	*Comments*
44	15.6	diarrhea
50	15.5	diarrhea
52	15.4	fever, cough
54	15.5	earache
56	16.0	

18

AN EXCEPTIONAL CHILD

Sembajwe

Sembajwe stood out as an exception in our sample for several reasons. First, his mother was highly idiosyncratic in her methods of infant care and child rearing, following neither traditional customs nor European ways nor practices used by the other women in the village, Secondly, and perhaps to avoid being interfered with, this woman held herself apart and participated little in the rounds of visiting in the village. And, of course, Sembajwe was an exception in regard to age. He was nineteen months old when we first visited him. But he was not yet weaned, and the *muluka* chief had obviously gone to much trouble to persuade the mother to participate.

At the time of our first visit the mother had dressed up to receive us. She wore a pretty *busuuti*, white with a delicate floral pattern, and had powdered her face heavily, which gave a startlingly gray appearance to her very dark skin. Also present was a ten-year-old boy, her brother, who was visiting her for a while, and two other house guests—a woman with an eight-month-old baby. Both the visitor and the boy were powdered also, and the air was heavy with perfume.

The house was a small hut of wattle and daub with an extraordinary roof. There were two sheets of corrugated metal, which did not meet in the middle, and which were weighted down with big stones. In the middle, not covered by the sheets, was an underroof of rusty metal plates. The living room was smaller than that of the other homes we had visited. It contained three chairs, a table with a cross-stitched cloth, a vase of flowers, and an alarm clock. The house was bright, clean, cheerful, and cluttered.

The father was said to be an itinerant merchant who sold cloth; he was unable to return home every night. Sembajwe was the first child of this marriage, which, the mother later told us proudly, was a legal marriage. Thus, the household

DOI: 10.4324/9781003629337-21

consisted only of these three—although there were house guests at the time we visited, and later on the mother's four-year-old sister came to visit them.

Sembajwe was dressed as a little boy rather than as a baby and was so big and fat that he seemed to be bursting out of his clothes. He wore bells around his ankles, which jingled as he walked; he walked sturdily, placing each foot down with a firm jolt. He had rather an angry expression on his face. During the second half of our first brief visit his mother gave him the breast—in response to no signal that I could observe. He suckled eagerly, sitting on his mother's lap but not supported by her, and managed the breast by himself.

At our second visit, despite the fact that we had carefully explained our purposes the week before, the mother seemed suspicious. She sensed some criticism in our questions about Ganda customs that differed from European customs, for she laughed uneasily before answering, although her answers seemed straightforward enough. She asked whether we were willing to give help and advice about feeding and child rearing. I said we would give what help we could about health, but if it were a matter of custom, I would not give any advice, unless it was about something that especially worried her. I pointed out that customs differed from one country to another and I emphasized that some Ganda customs might well be better than ours. For example, in my country it was the custom to wean babies sooner than Sembajwe would be weaned, but some experts believed it would be better if breast feeding continued longer than was our custom. I said I was very interested to see how well Ganda babies with longer breast feeding were developing and I congratulated her on Sembajwe's health and development. She seemed totally reassured and accepted us.

Subsequently, however, there seemed to be some ambivalence in her attitude. She never took advantage of transportation to the clinic, and sometimes she was not at home when we called by prearrangement. When we caught her at home, she was both cordial and a good informant, giving us much spontaneous detail about Sembajwe's behavior. It emerged that she differed considerably both from Europeans and from her neighbors in her child-rearing practices. I was impressed with her thoughtfulness in deciding what practices she would adopt and the understanding of Sembajwe's needs that was reflected in them. But, since she was a deviant, she probably felt apprehensive that we or the clinic staff would criticize her methods.

We were told that Sembajwe had been born in hospital and weighed 10 pounds at birth. He was fed entirely by breast until about four or five months of age whenever he seemed hungry and, indeed, for comfort whenever he cried. He was fed at night if he woke and cried, but by this time he sometimes slept through without a feeding. Other foods were introduced gradually, and he now had quite an extensive diet. He had always slept in his own bed but in his mother's room. He took an afternoon nap, but his morning naps had stopped when he was eighteen months old. He was said to be much too busy with his own affairs to sleep in the morning.

This mother did not attempt to train Sembajwe not to soil or wet the bed. Unlike other Ganda mothers she did not " hold him down." She said, proudly, that he had learned by himself. He had stopped soiling the bed at six to eight months of age and was said never to have soiled elsewhere in the house. Even as a small infant he was able to make sounds that indicated that he wanted to have a bowel movement, and she took him to "a special place." After he could crawl he went there by himself. If he wet the bed, she changed the sheet. He was improving in keeping dry, although he had not yet learned that he should never wet the bed. Despite the mother's pride in Sembajwe's accomplishments, she seemed uneasy when we questioned her about elimination control, so we did not press her toward further clarification.

When he was two or three months old his mother trained him to sit by digging a hole in the ground and placing him in it for ten minutes a day, supported by mats and blankets. After two weeks of this he could sit alone. He began to crawl at six months of age, and walked at eight or nine months.

As soon as he began to crawl he followed his mother wherever she went, from one room to another. No one else shared in taking care of him, and she took him with her when she went to work in the garden nearby. He cried very little throughout the first eighteen months of life, but by the time we first saw him he was crying a great deal, seeming to want the breast much of the time.

He had always been a big baby and had developed well despite having been ill with malaria quite often. Now he seemed to be getting it less frequently. Recently he had had an attack of dysentery, and the mother kept emphasizing that before it he had been even stronger and fatter than now.

When we came for our second visit a week later, Sembajwe was standing in the middle of the room. He stared at me steadily with an unfriendly expression. While we talked with his mother he stood about and occasionally walked about with his bells jingling. His ten-year-old uncle, who was still visiting, took him on his lap for a while and made a fuss over him. He sucked his thumb throughout most of the visit. He also played with an old bed spring. After a while he went to his mother, who was sitting on a chair, and held onto her knee. Visitors arrived. The nine-month-old baby, who was also a house guest, went to the mother and held onto her other knee. Sembajwe apparently did not want to share his mother and demanded to be taken up onto her lap. Once there, he reached inside her dress to get the breast. He did not smile once throughout the whole visit.

His mother said that she had begun to teach him politeness by training him to sit down when she said *tuula wansi.* She also was training him to come back when she called, whenever he started to walk away on his own. He was said to understand some other commands and to be able to talk a little. He could call his mother, and when we waved good-bye at the end of the visit, he waved and said *aba* (contraction of *weeraba*); this must have been a new word, judging by the exclamations of his mother and the other ladies.

We found the mother at home only once in the course of the next five visits. Once we found that she was away for the day, but the father was at home. He was cordial and informed us that weaning had begun for Sembajwe—that he was no longer given the breast during the day. This was when he was twenty-one months old. Much later, we found out that he was upset and difficult for about two or three weeks after the daytime feedings had been dropped. He wanted to be near his mother all the time and kept trying to reach the breast. She usually had an afternoon nap, but he would not let her sleep. His mother told him repeatedly that she was not going to give him the breast, and he seemed to understand what she said. And, although he was fussy and demanding, he did not seem angry with her. He had already been given quite a variety of solid foods and was using a cup for liquids, but now he ate less than usual and refused milk so determinedly that his mother had to force him to drink it. He slept well at night, however, and woke only once for the breast. He wet the bed more than usual—he was not yet "trained" at all. His mother said that during this period she worked with him holding onto her skirts constantly.

Another time we visited, only to find that the mother had had to go to hospital, suffering from abdominal pains. She had taken Sembajwe with her. Later we found out that he had been finally weaned while there, when he was twenty-two months old.

About two weeks after final weaning, we found the mother at home. She told us that Sembajwe cried all night when he was first refused the breast. She explained to him that she was not going to give him the breast any more and held him close, which seemed to comfort him. The second night, and thereafter, he did not fuss for the breast. She gave him milk to drink at bedtime, and although he woke up once or twice during the night, he went promptly to sleep again.

To the mother, the most striking thing was that Sembajwe had stopped wetting the bed, suddenly, at final weaning. And despite the lack of formal training, he suddenly gained complete bladder control, going outside by himself whenever he needed to urinate.

The mother was very pleased also that after the first night of final weaning he had been much more cheerful and independent than previously. He no longer fussed and cried easily. He no longer demanded the breast. His mother could now go away for a while, leaving him behind, and he seemed content.

We too found the change in Sembajwe very striking. Before, he had seemed surly and very dependent upon his mother, as if he resented having to share her with anyone. He scowled at us whenever we directed our attention toward him. But on this visit after weaning, it was entirely different. His face appeared ready to light up with a smile whenever anyone looked his way. He came to us readily, either on our invitation or at his mother's bidding. He was very responsive to his mother, but had acquired a sturdy independence.

When we first arrived Sembajwe was in the garden with his mother. After our call they came toward us, Sembajwe walking sturdily with his ankle bells jingling. His mother stopped, but Sembajwe continued toward us. Mrs. Kibuka gave him a package of tea, which we had brought as a little gift. He took it to his mother and then indicated that he wanted to keep it himself. He wandered about, trying to pick the package open, active and busy. His mother went to get us some eggs as a gift. She wrapped them in a paper, gave them to Sembajwe, instructing him to give them to us. He picked up the eggs, then remembered that he had left the tea behind, went back for it, picked it up with his free hand and came over to us, offering us first the tea and then the eggs with a charming smile. When we left he accompanied us to the car with his mother. We gave him a piece of candy and he smiled his thanks. His mother prompted him to say thank you, and he mumbled something. He skillfully undid the paper wrapping and popped the candy into his mouth.

At one point during the visit the mother said, quite cheerfully, that she was not feeling very well and could not enjoy her food. We guessed that she might be pregnant and twitted her about it. She giggled and did not deny it. We concluded that this was the reason then Sembajwe had been weaned at this particular time.

At another visit when Sembajwe was twenty-three months old, he was very friendly, responding to overtures with an almost adult, knowledgeable smile. He sat near his mother and listened to our conversation. His four-year-old aunt, who was visiting, took him on her lap for a while, although he was nearly as big as she. Then his mother took him on her lap, and he lay back against her, looking blissfully happy and drowsy. He finally went to sleep and was taken out of the room.

On this occasion the mother was expansive, obviously proud of Sembajwe and telling of his accomplishments. She described how he liked to clap his hands and dance. When the father was at home in the evening, they would play the gramophone, drink beer, and talk and laugh. Sembajwe would enter into the fun; he would have some beer with his parents and then clap his hands and dance around happily. Mrs. Kibuka was horrified that a child that young would be given beer, but the mother assured us that he only had small amounts. Besides, she said, she believed in eating well and drinking beer is good for the health.

Sembajwe's talking had spurted, she told us. He had quite a number of single words. He called everyone by name, even guests. He understood everything that was said to him, and even listened attentively to his father's talk with his friends. He knew where his mother kept everything. If, when in one room, she sent him to another to fetch something for her, he could be trusted to return promptly with the correct article and then would kneel down in the polite Ganda fashion to offer it to her.

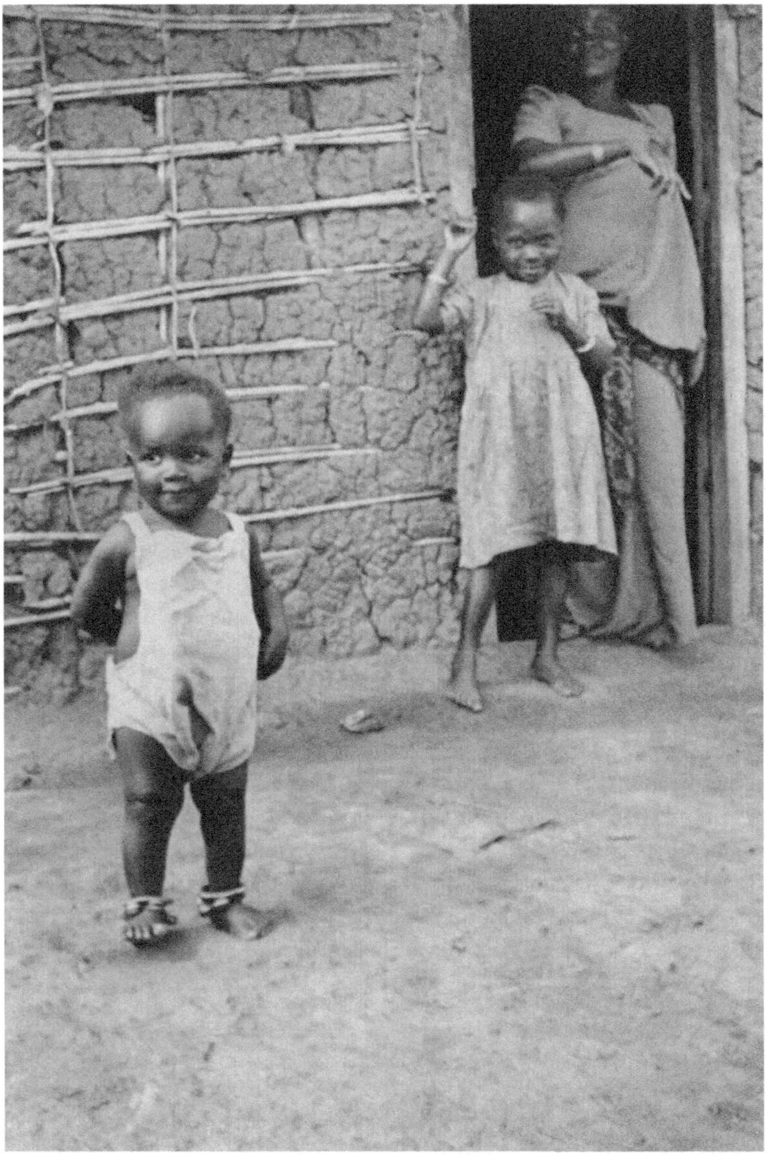

FIGURE 34 Sembajwe at twenty-three months is quite grown up after weaning. His proud mother and young aunt are in the background.

Our last visit occurred just after Sembajwe's second birthday. The mother was in the garden when we arrived. Sembajwe was standing just outside the kitchen where his little aunt was washing dishes. He seemed shy at first, but when I offered him a piece of candy he came, took the candy in a determined fashion, and moved off. He was wearing a sunsuit and looked quite plump. When his mother appeared in the distance, Sembajwe ran to meet her, but he did not cling. When he reached her he turned and accompanied her to the house in an adult way.

We proposed taking photographs. His mother changed him into a shirt and short pants that buttoned onto the shirt—both quite grubby. She could scarcely button his shirt over his chest and fat tummy. He put up with being dressed, despite obvious discomfort, but rebelled and hit his mother when she tried to brush his hair. She was tactful about his refusal, talked to him nicely, and handed him the brush so that he could do it himself, but he threw the brush on the floor. Finally she picked him up on her lap and brushed his hair without further friction. He lay back against her, relaxed and rather baby-like.

During the photographs he wanted to be near his mother. She wanted to pose him, but did not want to have her own picture taken. Every time she moved off he followed her, not crying and not rushing, but obviously uneasy. When we went back into the house he sat quietly near his mother, yawning occasionally. Soon he moved onto his mother's lap, and lay back drowsily. Finally he did go to sleep and she carried him off to bed. The contrast between his sturdy independence and rebellion earlier and his baby-like relaxation in her arms was quite striking.

His mother told us that she was still delighted with his response to weaning. His improvements had continued without relapse, and he was developing well. She told us of his new accomplishments. He was generous with his little aunt; he did not eat before offering her some food, not even when very hungry. He had never broken anything in the house. Whenever he heard the horn of an automobile on the road, he ran out of the house toward the road, calling *nzije* (I'm coming!).

Gesell testing

When Sembajwe was twenty-seven months old he was given the Gesell Developmental Schedules by Dr. Géber. His DQ was only 70, which is so out of line with his whole course of development that the testing could be assumed to be unreliable, even without Dr. Géber's note that he was very negativistic and did not cooperate.

PART IV

Infant Development

19

SENSORIMOTOR DEVELOPMENT

Most of the babies in this sample were clearly accelerated in their rate of sensorimotor development. The rate of their physical growth, as checked by measurements of height and weight upon visits to the clinic, was not accelerated. On the contrary, most of the babies were average in height and weight when compared with Western norms. But they sat and crawled and stood and walked much earlier than the average baby in Western societies. Although the focus of my interest was upon the development of interpersonal relations, the striking acceleration of these Ganda babies in sensorimotor development merits consideration.

Although I lacked training in infant testing, I had intended to teach myself from a test manual and to administer an infant intelligence test at regular intervals to each baby in order to have some kind of base line of developmental rate against which I could check my findings in regard to social development. Test equipment was ordered, but delays in shipping prevented it from arriving in time to be used. In order to obtain the base line which I sought, I made note of each baby's locomotor attainments and of his language development, both in terms of first words and language comprehension. I soon realized that the infants in my sample were very accelerated in regard to these aspects of development, and much regretted the lack of test equipment.

I was delighted when Dr. Marcelle Géber arrived in Kampala just before the end of my project. She was not only expert in infant testing but also wished to test a sample of Ganda infants. It was agreed that I should introduce her to the families in my sample on the occasion of my last visit and seek to gain their cooperation in her work. Then, a week or so after I had left Kampala, she was to visit each home, accompanied by Mrs. Kibuka, to administer the Gesell

DOI: 10.4324/9781003629337-23

Developmental Schedules.[1] In about half the cases this plan worked out. In a few instances we had been unable to arrange a joint visit to introduce Dr. Géber; in other instances families who had agreed to cooperate refused to do so when Dr. Géber came at the appointed time.[2] Consequently test results are available for only thirteen children.[3]

When I began my project it was not generally known that African infants are accelerated in sensorimotor development, especially throughout the first year of life. Dr. Géber's findings, not only with the Ganda but also with infants in other African societies, were the first to draw widespread attention to this significant phenomenon. Since there is some controversy about the factors responsible for this acceleration in development, and since I believe that my observations have some light to throw on the issue, I wish to present what I found, despite the fact that my observations of sensorimotor development are imprecise.

Working retrospectively I have ascertained the age level of each of the items of behavior which appear both in my records of home visits and in the Griffiths Infant Intelligence Scale[4]—the infant test with which I am now currently working—and estimated an Intelligence Quotient on the basis of the discrepancy between the age of the child when observed and the age level at which the behavioral item appears in the test norms. In all but one case there was fairly close agreement between this estimated IQ and the DQ found by Dr. Géber. This agreement lends support to the validity of the conclusions that can be drawn from my relatively imprecise observations.[5]

1 The Gesell Developmental Schedules are included in *Developmental Diagnosis* by A. Gesell and Catherine S. Amatruda (2nd ed.; New York: Harper, 1947). Dr. Géber used a revision of these schedules which had been standardized on French infants.

2 Mrs. Kibuka subsequently wrote to report the reasons for the refusal. Dr. Géber was working in cooperation with Dr. R. F. A. Dean, director of research in infant nutrition supported by the National Research Council of Great Britain. Dr. Dean's unit wished to make anthropometric measurements on the same occasion that the Gesell Tests were to be given. Being unaware of this plan, Mrs. Kibuka and I had not prepared the families for the prospects of two male visitors in addition to Dr. Géber, nor for the fact that they wished to photograph each baby when naked and to measure his physical dimensions with calipers. Some of the first babies visited cried with fear when faced with male strangers and the strange procedures, and the mothers found it incomprehensible and somehow improper that their babies were stripped naked for the photographs. Word spread through the villages, and some of the families refused to cooperate when the team came to visit them at the appointed time.

3 I am much indebted to Dr. Géber for providing me with her findings and with permission to use them here. For some cases only the Development Quotient was recorded. For other cases she sent a full report of details of the test behavior and findings for the four separate scales of the Developmental Schedules. These reports have been summarized and appear at the end of each of the summaries of case history.

4 Griffiths, Ruth, *The Abilities of Babies* (London: University of London Press, 1954).

5 The discrepancy occurred in the case of Sembajwe (see Chapter 18). His DQ of 70, which falls in the borderline-defective range, does not match the picture of healthy development which I report, and was, I believe, misleadingly low because he was so uncooperative in the testing.

Locomotor development

In the case of all infants, I inquired from the mother about the age of the infant when the locomotor milestones were achieved—sitting alone, crawling, standing alone, and walking. Although only the mother's retrospective report is available for milestones achieved before our observations began, my notes of the baby's behavior during visits provide a check on the achievement of later milestones and also provide details that could not be obtained in interview.

Sitting

Sitting alone is a very important milestone for the Ganda infant. I suspect that its importance traditionally was that the naming ceremony could not take place until the infant was able to sit. None of the mothers in our sample made any reference to the naming ceremony, which among Christians has been replaced by christening. Nevertheless, it was generally acknowledged that a baby ought to be able to sit alone by the time he was three months old. My informants of ancient customs told me that a baby was given training in sitting as he approached three months of age. A hole of suitable size was dug in the ground. Barkcloth was wrapped around the baby to give support to his trunk, and he was placed in the hole in a sitting position for about fifteen minutes a day, until he was able to sit unsupported. Sixteen babies in this sample (see Table 12) were given "training" of this sort. In only one case was a hole actually dug. More usually a basin of suitable size was used, and in some instances the only support was given by the cloths (no longer barkcloth) that were wrapped around him.

Can a baby be trained to sit? Or does he just naturally sit when maturation has proceeded to the point that his is able to? Widespread opinion in Western countries favors the maturational view, and even though the work of Piaget[6] and others leads to the inescapable conclusion that experience plays an important role in the development of intelligence and in the sensorimotor development that is the forerunner of intellectual development, there are grounds for skepticism that training of this sort imposed on an infant could substantially facilitate development. This sample can provide no support for the belief that training helps a baby to sit earlier than he might otherwise have done. But before considering the evidence, it is first necessary to consider a definition of what is meant by a baby's sitting "alone."

6 Jean Piaget, *The Origins of Intelligence in Children* (New York: International Universities Press, 1952). Further, for an excellent exposition of the role of experience in the development of intelligence see J. McV. Hunt, *Intelligence and Experience* (New York: Ronald Press, 1961).

TABLE 17 Locomotor achievements and developmental quotient

	Training in Sitting	*Sits with Slight Support*	*Sits Alone, Sustained*	*Crawls*
Griffiths' Norms		*6 mos.*	*9 mos.*	*9 mos.*
Name				
SECURE – ATTACHED				
1. Paulo	yes	6 [a]		6 [a]
2. Sembajwe	yes	3 [a]		6 [a]
3. Juko	yes	4 [a]		5 [a]
4. Senvuma				
5. Petero	yes	8		
6. Mutebe	yes	5 [a]		6 [a]
7. Nakiku	no	4½ [a]		6 [a]
8. Alima	yes	3		6
9. Aida	no		4½	
10. William	no		5	5½
11. Senkumba	yes	3	4½	4½
12. Kyimba			5½ [a]	5 [a]
13. Samwendi	no	4	4½	
14. Maryamu	no	4 [a]		9
15. Lusiya	yes	5 [a]		6 [a]
16. Nabatanzi	no	3 [a]		5½ [a]
INSECURE – ATTACHED				
17. Muhamidi	no	4½ [a]	5	4½ [a]
18. Magalita	no	3 [a]		6 [a]
19. Sulaimani	no	3 [a]		6
20. Nakalema	yes	4 [a]	5½	8
21. Kasozi	yes	4 [a]		6 [a]
22. Waswa (1)	yes	4 [a]		6 [a]
23. Nakato (1)	yes	4 [a]		5 [a]
NON – ATTACHED				
24. Nora	no	3 [a]		7½
25. Kulistina	yes	6½		7
26. Waswa (2)	yes	5½	6½	7
27. Nakato (2)	yes	5½	6½	7
28. Namitala	yes	3		

[a] Based on the mother's retrospective report.

[b] Gesell Developmental Quotient, courtesy of Dr. Marcelle Géber.

Creeps	*Stands Held*	*Stands Alone*	*Walks*	*Trots*	*DQ* [b]
11 mos.	*10 mos.*	*13 mos.*	*14 mos.*	*16 mos.*	
6½		9½	11	13	114
			8½ [a]		70
7	7				
			11		
	8				108
	7	11½			102
7½	6½		10	11	120
4½					
7½	6½		9		122
8½					
		6½ [a]	9		
	4				
9½		11½	11½	13	107
		7 [a]	8½		102
7		8½	9½	10½	
7½	7	7½			130
		8 [a]	12		104
6½	7½				
9					
		10[a]	11½		109
		15	17		
		13	14		
9	9	9½	10½		
	9	10½			
	5½				105
	5½				120

In several instances we observed the infant shortly after he was able to sit "alone." In these instances the mother placed him in a very special position to help him keep his balance. The soles of his feet were placed together in front of him, and he was tipped forward slightly so that his hands rested on the ground beyond his feet. His hands kept him from falling forward, and the spread of his legs counteracted a tendency to topple sideways. But the babies positioned thus nevertheless looked pretty wobbly and some expressed insecurity by crying. There are no norms in the infant tests for this item. The closest that one can approximate it is "sits with slight support," which Griffiths places at the end of the sixth month. Being able to sit unsupported for a short time she places in the eighth month, and being able to sit on the floor more or less indefinitely she places at the end of the ninth month. With the few Ganda babies we observed who were seen first to sit when positioned and then at the next visit to sit indefinitely unsupported, there appeared to be a gap of two to four weeks between the two achievements. In cases where we have only the mother's report to guide us it seems safest to assume that she refers to the baby's being able to sit alone when positioned.

Combining mothers' reports with our own observations, babies who were "trained" to sit achieved sitting "alone" at a mean age of 4.6 months whereas babies who were not so trained achieved sitting at a mean age of 3.9 months. These figures must be taken as very approximate, however. Mothers' retrospective reports are notoriously unreliable, and this might be suspected to be the case especially in a non-literate community where calendars are less important and written records are not kept in baby books. For those babies who were already able to sit when we began to visit and for whom we had to rely on mother's reports, the mean age of sitting alone was 4.0 months. For those babies whom we actually observed at, or close to, the achievement of sitting, the mean age was 4.8 months. I consider these figures essentially equivalent, for we could pinpoint the precise age at the time of observation whereas the mother was reporting in "months old"; moreover, in some instances our observation did not take place until the baby already could sit without support for extended periods. All things considered, the mother's reports match our own observations quite well, and a discrepancy of 0.8 months must be considered negligible. By the same token the discrepancy between those who were trained and not trained must be considered negligible. Our figures give no grounds for arguing that training slows the development of sitting. Indeed, it may well be that some babies were not trained because they sat spontaneously at the expected age and others were trained because they were considered to be slow. Nevertheless, and regardless of the difficulties discussed above, it is clear that this sample of Ganda babies was accelerated in sitting in comparison with the London babies on whom Griffiths standardized her test.

Crawling and Creeping

We followed the standard usage in distinguishing between crawling and creeping. The term "crawling" was used when the infant, placed in a prone position on the floor, moved body and limbs in such a way as to make some progress, even though he was still flat to the floor. Griffiths' norms place this behavioral item at the end of the ninth month. The term "creeping" was used for locomotion on the hands and knees or on all fours—a "bear walk." This item is placed by Griffiths at the eleventh month. In interview I was not careful to make a distinction between these two modes of locomotion, although I did so when recording observations. Therefore, I assume that when the mother reported the age at which locomotion was first achieved she meant "crawling"— the earlier form.

The findings suggest that the Ganda child achieves locomotion first at about six or six and a half months of age and is able to creep effectively about a month later. The mean age of "crawling" from the mothers' reports was 5.6 months; that from our own observations 6.6 months. The mean age of "creeping" from our own actual observations was 7.5—but this could not refer to the very onset of creeping. All we knew was that the child was able to creep on the occasion of one visit and that we had not seen him do so on an earlier visit. On the basis of our own observations crawling occurred about two and a half months earlier than the Griffiths' norms and creeping about three and a half months earlier.

Standing

Standing alone is not quite as momentous a milestone as sitting or crawling or walking, and the age at which it is achieved is sometimes not remembered. But limiting ourselves to those babies in which standing alone could be pinpointed by our own observations, the mean age of achieving this milestone was eleven months—two months in advance of the Griffiths' norms. Moreover, the intermediate stages in development of standing were observed to be well in advance of the Griffiths' norms. Standing firmly when held supported was observed to occur at about seven months (Griffiths' eleven months); being able to pull oneself to a standing position while holding onto furniture was observed at about seven or eight months (Griffiths' eleven months).

Walking

Walking is an important landmark in present-day Ganda society because it is, more often than not, the signal that a child is old enough to be weaned. Fourteen of the sample were able to walk, and with one exception (Sembajwe) we were on hand to witness the event. The mean age of achievement of walking was eleven months, Sembajwe excluded. We used as our criterion for walking the ability to take a few steps before falling. Griffiths places this item at fourteen months. For those whom we observed long enough to ascertain when they could "trot about well," we found this to occur at about twelve months whereas Griffiths places it as sixteen months. The intermediate steps toward walking were observed infrequently. Only four babies, ranging in age for seven and a half to eleven months were observed to "cruise," that is, to side step while holding onto something—an item which Griffiths places at twelve months. We did not inquire about this—and indeed the sparse furniture in the typical house would make it difficult for a baby to cruise while holding onto furniture. We saw only one child walk when led with both hands held— Juko. He was seven and a half months old; Griffiths places the time at twelve months. My impression was that, despite the significance attached to walking, few of these mothers walked the child about while holding his hands whereas this is fairly common among the "Western" mothers I have known.

Language development

Unless one deliberately sets out to observe an infant's vocalization, one tends to ignore it because it is so undifferentiated. And even when one deliberately attempts to note and record it, this is a difficult task—difficult because the untrained person cannot reproduce in writing the sounds (phonemes) the baby makes. An exhaustive examination of my field notes made me realize that it was not until the baby was capable of the repetition of four or more syllables—and I most frequently recorded "da-da-da-da" and "ma-ma-ma-ma"—that I made notes of vocalization, except crying of course. When vocalization got to the point of approximating a word, I, as an alien, found it difficult to detect—except in the case of *mama*, which is the same in Luganda and English. I had to rely, therefore, on the mother's reports of the child's acquisition of words—although having been told, I could sometimes verify the report through my own observations. Similarly, we had to rely on the mothers' reports of what the child was able to comprehend—although, again, there was some opportunity for direct observation. In regard to locomotor development my inquiries about achievements were repeated frequently and observations were easily made. In regard to language development, my specific inquiries tended to be made toward the end of the project; consequently I missed some of the milestones, and direct observations were more difficult. Thus, my records of language development are much more incomplete than those pertaining to locomotor development.

But, since I found locomotor development to be so accelerated, it is a fair question to ask whether the acceleration was limited to locomotor achievements or was more general. It is only because of this question that I turn to my scanty notes on language development.

I recorded four-syllable vocalization in the case of nine infants, but there is no reason to suppose that my record caught anything approximating a first achievement. The mean age at which I observed this type of vocalization was thirty-eight weeks; Griffiths places this item at the beginning of the ninth month. My notes suggest that the mean age at which it was reported that the child "knew his own name" was about eight and a half months; Griffiths places this at fourteen months. We inquired about all children who had begun to say words the number of words they could use appropriately. Of those who could use three or more words appropriately the mean age was ten and a half months. Griffiths places this item at the end of the twelfth month. She lists only one item pertaining to early language comprehension; thus she places appropriate response to simple requests, such as "give me the cup," at twelve months. Although the nature of our inquiries did not give us a longitudinal picture of the development of comprehension, a number of children were responding appropriately to simple commands— "come," "stop," "go away," "hush," "give it to me," and the like— by the time they were nine or ten months old.

Géber's findings

In all, Géber examined 252 infants and young children in or near Kampala. Her findings[7] not only substantiate but greatly elaborate our own. She found precocious psychomotor development to be common and particularly marked in the first year of life. She found momentary sitting to be achieved at four months and sustained sitting at five months. Standing without support was achieved at seven months and the first steps alone at nine months. Although locomotor development was most accelerated, all aspects of development were precocious—prehension and manipulation, adaptivity, language, and personal-social behavior. All of the babies under six months of age had Developmental Quotients of better than 100, and the same was true of 95 per cent of the babies between six and nine months of age. The superiority of the African group to the European norms was less marked in the second year of life, but even then, 75 per cent of the DQ's exceeded 100. From then on the rate of development slowed down even more, until after the age of three years the DQ's tended to be below the European norms.

Although Géber found that even the newborn baby was in a more advanced state of development than newborn European children,[8] she placed most emphasis upon methods of infant care as the factor responsible for the accelerated

7 Marcelle Géber, Développement psychomoteur de l'enfant africain. *Courrier*, 1956, *6*, 17–29. Marcelle Géber and R. F. A. Dean, Gesell tests on African children. *Pediatrics*, 1957, *6*, 1055–65. Marcelle Géber, Problemes posés par le développement du jeune enfant africain en fonction de son milieu social. *Le Travail Humain*, 1960, *23*, 97–111.

8 Marcelle Géber and R. F. A. Dean, The state of development of newborn African Children. *Lancet*, 1957, *1*, 1216–19.

development of African babies. She particularly emphasized the close infant-mother relationship throughout the first year of life, the breast feeding on demand, the intimate physical contact, and the mother's constant availability. She also suggested that the way that the baby is carried on his mother's back may strengthen his ability to hold his head steady by forcing him to compensate for her various movements, and that the "sitting position" on her back may help him to sit alone earlier.

Furthermore, I was very much impressed with the way that the Ganda baby is held sitting face outward on his mother's lap as she pauses to visit with family or guests; this brings him, from the beginning, into the midst of the social group and gives him much stimulation. I also noted that from an early age he is often held standing. As soon as the baby can sit alone, he spends some time on the floor rather than being held or confined, and when he can crawl he is given complete freedom to move about. I have no doubt that this absence of confinement interacts with social stimulation to account for his very precocious locomotor development, and I agree with Géber in attaching importance to postural adjustments to being held and carried during the earliest months.

Géber suggests that the decline in rate of development is attributable to abrupt and traumatic weaning and the great diminution of mother-child interaction that follows, often culminating in mother-child separation. The findings on weaning reported in Chapter 24 suggest that it is a misunderstanding to characterize Ganda weaning as abrupt, but there is no doubt that the advent of a new baby in the family very substantially reduces the amount of time that a mother has free for the toddler who has been weaned. Although William's mother managed not only to interact with him often but also to spread her attention over all the members of her large family, I felt that she was exceptional. The general impression I received was that the Ganda mother's all-absorbing preoccupation with the infant made it impossible for her to give adequate stimulation to her other young children. Additional factors contributing to too low a level of stimulation in childhood beyond the first year or so of life are the dearth of toys and other playthings, the absence of organized activities for the young child, and the traditional training in polite, submissive behavior.

Géber reported two additional sets of findings that lend further support to the view that the course of sensorimotor development of the Ganda child is much influenced by child-care practices. One group of children attended a nursery school; these children showed much less of a decline in DQ in the third and fourth years of life than the children without nursery school experience. Géber points out that their mode of life and the socioeconomic level of their families were essentially the same as those of the group as a whole. Secondly, she reports[9]

9 Marcelle Géber, L'enfant africain occidentalisé et de niveau social supérieur en Uganda, *Courrier*, 1958, *8*, 517–23.

that a group of infants from highly acculturated Ganda homes failed to show precocity of development during the first year of life. They were slower than babies in village families and approximated the European norms. They tended to be kept in their cribs much of the time and were held and carried much less than the village children. They were also fed on schedule, and breast feeding was on the whole less satisfactory. But when they could walk they had a much richer experience than did the village children—more toys, more attention, and the stimulation of parents with a relatively high degree of education, and in due course nursery school. These children did not enter into the decline in rate of development characteristic of the village children after the first year of life but rather proceeded to develop regularly at an average or somewhat above average rate.

When Géber's findings first became known in this country, some psychologists in my acquaintance received them with critical disbelief. The belief that intelligence is predetermined by genetic endowment and develops through a process of maturational unfolding is so ingrained in our society that it is difficult for many to assimilate evidence that experiential factors could either facilitate or retard its course. Géber's methods were criticized.[10] The old argument was revived that tests of infant sensorimotor development do not examine the same abilities that are measured by intelligence tests at later ages, and, moreover, they have been found to have limited predictive value. Another argument implied that Africans must be viewed as a species other than Western man; chimpanzees are accelerated in early development in comparison to humans, but this early precocity is associated with a much lower limit for potential development. The relevance of this issue to the controversial question of the intellectual potential of Negroes versus whites is all too painfully evident.

If the issue of the role of experience in the development of intelligence rested solely upon Géber's reports and upon my own observations reported here, I would have to acknowledge that confirmation from other studies was required. But there is in fact a great deal of evidence from a variety of sources other than these which makes continued belief in predetermined intelligence uninfluenced by experience untenable. J. McV. Hunt[11] has summarized and discussed this evidence; it is beyond the scope of this book to repeat it here.

10 The criticisms were as follows: Her sample was relatively small and not selected in a way to ensure that it was representative; she does not provide adequate data in regard to measures of scatter and significance of statistical differences; she counts the same children twice or more by combining retest data with cross-sectional data. These criticisms are quite justified, and certainly my own data reported here are from an even smaller sample—some are based on retrospective report and are equally open to criticism.

11 *Intelligence and Experience*.

Assuming, therefore, that the major issue—that intellectual development is influenced by individual experience—is resolved, the question then can be examined: What kinds of experience, at what periods of development, can facilitate intellectual growth? Obviously much careful and intensive research is needed before this important question can be answered. In the meantime Géber's and my studies of the Ganda suggest that during the first year of life development is facilitated by the kind of infant care the Ganda give—with much physical contact, much interaction between the infant and his mother, much social stimulation, prompt gratification of creature-comfort needs, lack of confinement, and freedom to explore the world. Just which of these features are the crucial ones in facilitating development cannot, of course, be ascertained, for they are confounded in these studies. Furthermore, Géber's findings suggest that traditional Ganda methods of child rearing in the second year of life and beyond provide less adequate stimulation to development than the Western methods characteristic of the more acculturated members of the society.

20

PATTERNS OF ATTACHMENT BEHAVIOR

The development of the baby's attachment to his mother was the center of interest in our study of infant development. As the research took shape in the field, the original focus of the study— on the infant's responses to weaning and to separation—shifted to the development of attachment. At the beginning our interest in the infant's attachment to his mother was specifically as a base line, in terms of which his response to weaning and separation could be evaluated. Thus, for example, it was expected that a baby who had formed a strong attachment to his mother would be more distressed when separated from her than would a baby whose attachment was weak or non-existent. In order to assess the strength and nature of this attachment it seemed desirable to observe the baby's relations with his mother for some months in advance of weaning and separation. From the beginning, therefore, infant-mother interaction was the chief focus of observation and had a major place in our interviews as well.

The newborn baby is not attached to his mother or to anyone else. He may be taken from her and given to a foster mother without any apparent distress or disturbance. But in the course of the first year of life he forms an attachment to his mother, and after this attachment had developed he is distressed if he is separated from her and he protests the breach of ties. How does this attachment develop? What factors facilitate this development or delay or prevent it? What are the criteria which enable us to judge that an attachment has been formed?

Since distress at being separated is an obvious criterion, I was careful to observe and to inquire about the baby's response to the separation situation in everyday life. Did the baby cry when his mother left the room? Did he follow her? Did he cling to her to try to prevent her going, or did he greet her return by clinging? In this sample, however, there were some babies who

DOI: 10.4324/9781003629337-24

seemed clearly attached to their mothers, who did not dependably cry, follow, or cling when their mothers seemed about to leave them. Were these babies less attached than the children who clung to their mothers and would not let them go? Or were they perhaps simply more secure in their relationships with their mothers?

These questions led me to re-examine in detail the notes from my field visits in an attempt to specify the behavior that had given me a clear impression that a baby was attached to his mother in the relative absence of distress in everyday separation situations. I arrived at a catalog of behavior patterns that seemed characteristic of babies who could be judged to be attached to their mothers.[1] The list of patterns of attachment behavior is as follows:

1. Differential crying
2. Differential smiling
3. Differential vocalization
4. Crying when the mother leaves
5. Following
6. Visual-motor orientation
7. Greeting through smiling, crowing, and general excitement
8. Lifting arms in greeting
9. Clapping hands in greeting
10. Scrambling over the mother
11. Burying the face in the mother's lap
12. Approach through locomotion
13. Embracing, hugging, kissing[2]
14. Exploration away from the mother as a secure base
15. Flight to the mother as a haven of safety
16. Clinging

Perhaps it would be unjustified to infer an attachment from any one of these responses. In particular, the differential responses—crying, smiling, and vocalization—may occur when the baby is still so young that it seems doubtful that he has yet formed a firm attachment to his mother, although certainly he can discriminate her from other people (and this is a necessary first step toward attachment). But further reflection led me to the hypothesis that it is through

1 The author has published two earlier accounts of these patterns of attachment behavior: The development of infant-mother interaction among the Ganda, in Foss (ed.), *Determinants of Infant Behaviour, II*, 67–112, and Patterns of attachment behavior shown by the infant in interaction with his mother, *Merrill-Palmer Quarterly*, 1964, *10*, 51–58.

2 No Ganda infant was observed to hug, kiss, or embrace. Nevertheless, this pattern is included in the list since it does occur with babies in Western societies.

these responses that the infant develops his attachment and that the responses serve to mediate his attachment once it is formed. Therefore, a longitudinal examination of these behavior patterns was undertaken in order to elucidate the development of attachment.

It is now proposed that we consider each of the behavior patterns in turn—to see how frequent it is in the sample, at what age it first appeared, and to trace its developmental course. In so doing I have had to rely upon my field notes, both the record of my observations and the interview record. It must be remembered that I was not specifically searching for the occurrence of most of these patterns and hence did not regularly inquire about them; I may well have failed to note instances of their occurrence. Both because of this and because the infants were admitted to the sample at varying ages rather than being observed from birth, it is certain that the first time I noticed a pattern was unlikely to have been a reliable indication of its first occurrence. Nevertheless, a study of the ages at which each pattern was first observed or reported yields some interesting information.

The first three patterns imply little more than discrimination of the mother from other people and differential responsiveness to her.

Differential crying

Crying was judged to be differential if the baby cried when held by someone other than the mother and stopped crying when taken by her; or when the baby cried and continued to cry when someone else attempted to comfort him, but stopped crying immediately when taken by the mother. For example:

Samwendi (nine weeks) was restless when I held him, despite my efforts to quiet him. When Mrs. Kibuka held him he was restless also, despite several shifts of position, and finally he cried violently. He stopped crying as soon as his mother took him. She did not give him the breast.

Petero (eleven weeks) protested when his mother handed him to me to hold but stopped crying immediately when she took him back. She did not give him the breast then, although she did a while later in response to a demand from him.

Alima (fifteen weeks) had been used to being held by other people. At this age, however, if crying, she would stop when picked up by her mother, but she would not stop if anyone else picked her up. Her mother said: "Now she has started noticing me; she doesn't care about other people at all."

The earliest occurrence of this pattern was noted at nine weeks. It may conceivably have occurred in younger Ganda babies, but there was only one baby we observed earlier than the age of eight weeks —Namitala—and she failed to develop any differential responses during the four months we visited.

Two other instances might be classified as differential crying. Thus, if a baby cried more when left with other people than with his mother, this seemed to indicate some discrimination, even though the baby did not yet cry at the moment of his mother's departure.

Senkumba (eight weeks) was said to cry very little when he was with his mother but usually to cry when he was left with other people while his mother gardened. Nevertheless, when I visited at this time he was alone in the front room and was crying when we arrived. He stopped crying when I picked him up.

Furthermore, if a baby cried when his mother put him down but did not protest being put down by someone else, this too could be considered differential. We have no clear record of this in the youngest babies of the sample, but it was certainly observed in some of the older babies—but long after other signs of attachment were clear-cut.

Differential smiling

Smiling was judged to be differential if the baby smiled more frequently, more readily, and more fully in response to his mother than in response to another person. This was one of the patterns of behavior that we did not set out to observe from the beginning. Indeed, smiling was noted only when it was particularly striking. In our American households the parents, loving relatives, and interested visitors alike bend over the baby as he lies in his crib, presenting him a smiling face, and waggle their heads and talk to the baby in an effort to coax a smile. This kind of face-to-face confrontation was not observed to occur in this Ganda sample. Indeed, it was rare for an adult even to hold a baby so that there could be a face-to-face confrontation, for the baby was, at least from about eight weeks on, usually held in a sitting position on the adult's lap, facing outward and leaning back. Therefore, the differential smiling that we noted occurred without exception after the baby was old enough to smile across a distance, to initiate smiling without requiring the stimulus of a face-to-face confrontation, or to manage the face-to-face confrontation himself by twisting his head or body in the direction of the adult. I mention this because in a subsequent study of American infants it is quite clear that differential smiling in response to a face-to-face confrontation emerges very early and is one of the first differential responses. In the Ganda sample the earliest instance occurred in Muhamidi.

Muhamidi (ten weeks) kept tipping his head up to smile at his mother as she held him. Once he smiled at me from across the room. All of these smiles were given on his own initiative.

Differential smiling was specifically observed in several other cases: Alima (twenty-six weeks), Aida (twenty weeks), Samwendi (nineteen weeks), and again Muhamidi (twenty-two weeks). Had we properly searched for it, it would undoubtedly have emerged more commonly.

Differential vocalization

Vocalization was judged to be differential if the baby vocalized more readily and more frequently in interaction with his mother than in interaction with other people. This is another pattern of behavior to which we were not alert during the field visits and which we noted only when it was particularly striking. What these mothers did when they were alone with their babies we do not know, of course. During our visits their attention was chiefly directed to the visitors, and we noticed no instance of the mother attempting to elicit a vocalization from the infant—until the end of the first year of life when there was sometimes an attempt to coax the child to demonstrate his knowledge of a new word. Therefore, again, differential vocalization emerged during our visits in terms of the baby's own spontaneous vocalizations. However, there is also some interview evidence:

Aida (twenty weeks) was said to make cooing noises, especially in response to her mother when she spoke to her. She squealed when excited, laughed aloud, and made "much noise."

Petero (twenty weeks) was dependent on vocal contact with his mother. He would accept being left in a room alone provided that his mother talked to him from a distance. He uttered many sounds in response. He and his mother "talked" to each other from room to room. We also noted that when picked up face-to-face with his mother he responded to her vocally.

For the most part, however, our observations of differential vocalization occurred well after other signs of attachment had clearly emerged.

The next group of patterns have in common a concern on the part of the infant for the whereabouts of his mother—a concern that implies the use of distance receptors, especially vision.

Crying when the mother leaves

The baby cries when his mother leaves his visual field and cannot be brought back into it through visual-motor adjustments. An example of this situation is when his mother leaves the room, in contrast with times when she merely moves to another part of the same room. The earliest age at which this response was observed in this sample was fifteen weeks.

Babies younger than fifteen weeks sometimes cried when put down or when left alone. When the mother left the baby alone, having just previously put him down, it was not clear whether the baby was protesting the cessation of contact, the departure of the mother from his visual field, or being left alone. Therefore, it was of particular interest to observe whether the child cried when his mother left him when he was not left alone, and whether he cried when he had not been in recent physical contact with her. The chief criterion was, however, that the crying was prompt when the mother left the room. Usually, a child at this point in development cries promptly, as soon as he sees his mother depart, although sometimes, if he is occupied with something else, he may not notice her go, and may cry only when, after some delay, he looks up, finds her gone, looks around for her, and cannot find her.

Alima (fifteen weeks) had begun to cry whenever her mother left the room, although she was never left alone in a room except when asleep.

Aida (twenty-two weeks) was likely to cry when her mother left the room and to try to follow her, especially when she was hungry. At twenty-four weeks, during our visit her mother left the room for a little while. Aida cried as she left and continued to cry until she returned, when she stopped at once. A little later in the visit her mother left again and again Aida cried. Mrs. Kibuka picked her up and tried to comfort her, but she did not stop crying until her mother returned and took her. Her mother confirmed that she now invariably cried when left with someone else, even a familiar person—although after a while she would usually stop and accept the attentions of another caretaker.

Nakalema (twenty-four weeks) was said to cry a great deal. She invariably cried when her mother left the room, regardless of with whom she was left.

Petero (twenty-four weeks) had begun to cry when his mother left the room, even when left with his brothers and sisters, although he soon stopped crying and accepted their attentions. Whereas previously (twenty weeks) he could be reassured by the sound of his mother's voice from an adjoining room, he now required her to be where he could see her.

Paulo (twenty-nine weeks) was very rarely left by his mother, but when she went out of the room, even for a moment, he invariably cried, whether left by himself or with another member of the household. During our visit at thirty weeks his mother left the room while he was being held on Mrs. Kibuka's lap. He immediately yelled and continued to do so until his mother returned.

The instances quoted above suggest invariability of crying when the mother leaves the room. Some children, however, accepted being left with a favorite person, although they cried if left alone or with someone else.

Alima (twenty-six weeks) cried promptly whenever her mother left her alone or with a child, even one familiar to her. She did not cry, however, when left with her father, who often held her and played with her, or with the senior wife in the household, who sometimes shared in her care.

Samwendi (twenty-four weeks) had begun to cry when his mother left the room, but only if he were left alone or with someone he did not know well; he accepted being left with a familiar caretaker.

Following

In this sample the babies, once they were able to crawl, not only cried when the mother left the room, but also attempted to follow her.

William (twenty-four weeks) began to crawl and to try to follow his mother whenever she left the room, letting out an immediate cry.

Muhamidi (thirty-two weeks) wanted to be with his mother all the time. Whenever he was parted from her even for a moment, he cried and tried to follow. He was said to have been doing this ever since he could crawl (twenty weeks). At thirty-four weeks I tried to photograph him by himself, but whenever his mother moved away, he cried and tried to follow her.

Some babies cried and followed the mother under certain circumstances, but not under others.

Kyimba (thirty-seven weeks) had been accustomed to being left with his grandmother and did not cry or follow his mother when left with her, although he did when left alone or with anyone else; he had been doing so ever since he had begun to crawl at five months of age. When alone with his grandmother he cried and followed whenever *she* left the room.

Mutebe (thirty-nine weeks) was used to being left with his grandparents, and did not follow his mother when left with them. But if she left him either alone or with less familiar people, he usually cried and tried to follow her.

As the babies became older some of them tended to follow without crying, perhaps because their locomotion was more efficient and they could keep up with the mother as she moved away. But if such a child were frustrated in following, either because the mother closed a door behind her or because she outdistanced him, he would usually cry.

Senkumba (thirty-seven weeks) followed his mother if she left him alone in a room, usually without crying. He often did not follow her if he had been left with familiar people.

Sulaimani (thirty-six weeks) followed his mother wherever she went, often without crying.

Lusiya (fifty-one weeks) followed her mother whenever she left the room but she did not cry. If her mother did not want her to follow, she closed the door. Even then she usually did not cry, but banged on the door.

Nakiku (twenty-eight weeks) followed her mother without crying whenever she left her alone in a room, although she was content to stay with her father or with Pantaleo. At fifty-two weeks, and after the first stage of weaning had begun, she was much the same, although she sometimes cried if she was prevented from following her mother by a closed door.

Maryamu (forty-six weeks) followed her mother whenever she left the room, hurrying to keep up, but not crying. Her mother said she had been following ever since she could crawl at forty-one weeks. At fifty weeks, after weaning, she still followed whenever her mother left her alone for a moment, but she cried only if she had difficulty keeping up with her. When left with other familiar people she usually did not follow.

Visual-motor orientation

This is another pattern of behavior through which the baby expresses his concern for the whereabouts of his mother. After the baby can sit by himself, if placed on the floor at some little distance from his mother, he tends to keep track of her whereabouts, glancing at her occasionally, and perhaps smiling if he catches her eye. On the other hand, he is likely to show interest, curiosity, and perhaps apprehension of other people present, and, since he tends to watch a stranger, one cannot consider visual fixation or even visual following as an unequivocal manifestation of attachment. Indeed, under these circumstances, the fact that the baby's glances at his mother manifest attachment becomes clear only when she gets up to leave the room and he cries or follows, or both.

Nevertheless, there is one set of circumstances in which visual-motor orientation seems clearly to manifest attachment. If the child is held on one's lap, at some distance from his mother, he may keep his eyes on his mother and be tensely oriented toward her.

William (eighteen weeks) was given to me to hold. He smiled at his mother across the room. He became increasingly restless, giving me the impression of wanting to get to his mother, with every muscle oriented toward her, although he did not cry. Once back on his mother's lap he gave me a brilliant smile.

Nakiku (twenty-eight weeks) sat for a while on the lap of a woman who was visiting. She was much quieter than she had been when on the floor. Whereas previously she had looked around at the visitors, gurgling and smiling, now she kept her eyes fixed on her mother, reserving smiles for her.

Muhamidi (thirty-one weeks) was given to me to hold at the clinic while his mother helped comfort and control another child who was being examined. Muhamidi sat on my lap without protest, but he was tense, with his whole body oriented toward his mother, whom he watched intently.

Greeting responses

Babies can express their attachment not merely by a concern for the mother's whereabouts and by protesting when she departs, but also by giving her a warm welcome when she returns. Some babies who are accustomed to being put down by their mothers and left alone to sleep, and some who are accustomed to being left with another familiar person, show their attachment more by the enthusiastic greeting they give the mother upon her return than by a protest when she departs.

These greeting responses are not stereotyped patterns, but rather seem to combine behavior that appears also in other contexts. The earliest type of greeting to appear usually combines *smiling, vocalizing, and general bodily excitement.* In my observations of American babies the earliest greetings seem to come when the mother approaches the crib to take the baby up from his nap. The baby, still too young to sit or to pull himself up, smiles, crows, and jiggles about in excitement, jerking his arms and legs. The conditions of my observations of Ganda babies did not permit me to observe this early response, although it undoubtedly occurred—and occurred earlier than the reports we obtained during the interviews. Although smiling was sometimes mentioned—as with Alima at twenty-six weeks—more usually the report was less specific: "He is very happy to see me."

Soon *lifting the arms* is reported as part of the greeting response.

Senkumba (twenty-one weeks) was said to accept being left with the senior wife in the household and not to cry when his mother left; but when his mother returned he lifted his arms and vocalized loudly in greeting.

Aida (twenty-two weeks) was said always to greet her mother after an absence by smiling and lifting her arms.

Although I have often seen American mothers attempt to evoke this response by standing in front of a child before picking him up, offering her outstretched hands to him, I did not notice Ganda women doing this. American mothers, moreover, usually pick a baby up by placing the hands on the baby's trunk under the armpits, in a way that encourages an anticipatory movement of lifting the arms. Ganda women, on the other hand, tend to pick a baby up quickly, grasping one upper arm near the shoulder. I am inclined to believe, therefore, that the lifting the arms in greeting—at least among Ganda babies— is a gesture of reaching toward a desired object rather than an imitative gesture or a mere anticipatory response.

Clapping the hands in greeting occurred frequently in this Ganda sample, although I have not observed it in my American sample. Pat-a-cake is one of the first games an American mother plays with her baby. I inquired carefully about this among Ganda mothers, and they denied either playing pat-a-cake with a baby less than a year old or trying to teach the baby to clap his hands. My best guess is that the Ganda express delight by clapping the hands, and that babies imitate this gesture of delight, presumably in delayed imitation. I did not witness a Ganda adult expressing delight in this fashion, however; their greetings were formal when we visited and their behavior tended to be too dignified and inhibited to permit such a spontaneous exprestion. In any event, however they acquired the response, Ganda babies clapped their hands in greeting.

Aida (thirty-one weeks), who earlier had smiled and raised her arms in greeting her mother, now clapped her hands in delighted greeting.

William (twenty-eight weeks) greeted his mother after an absence by clapping his hands and then putting his arms up to her.

Mutebe (forty-four weeks) always greeted his mother's return by crowing and clapping his hands.

Kasozi (forty-eight weeks) showed his delight upon his mother's return by clapping his hands.

After locomotion was achieved, *approaching* became part of the greeting pattern.

Muhamidi (thirty-three weeks) was brought into the room by a young girl and put down on the floor. He immediately crept to his mother, smiling and crowing with pleasure.

Nabatanzi (thirty-seven weeks), who had not protested when left with the visitor, greeted her mother upon her return, creeping to her quickly and crowing with delight.

Paulo (forty-one weeks) had been left with us while his mother went out for a moment. His uncle came into the room; Paulo scuttled quickly across the room to him and crowed with glee as his uncle picked him up. At forty-four weeks he gave us a similar welcome when we arrived in the car, but we suspected that it was the car rather than we who aroused his enthusiam.

Lusiya (fifty-one weeks) always greeted the return of either her mother or her father by laughing, clapping her hands, and then approaching as quickly as possible.

Nakiku (fifty-two weeks) also was said to greet both parents by laughing joyously and approaching quickly at a trot.

As may be seen from these examples, toward the end of the first year, greeting responses are given increasingly to other favorite people and not exclusively to the mother.

Thus, attachment is shown by concern for the loved person's whereabouts, by protest at her departure (or an attempt to keep her from increasing the distance), and by delight when she returns. It is also shown by several behavior patterns that occur in the mother's presence, which involve a desire for proximity to her although there is no impending threat of separation. Approach through locomotion, already mentioned in conjunction with greeting, may occur also as a flight toward the mother as a haven of safety. On many occasions, however, approach is exclusively a sign of the baby's desire to be close to her. Scrambling over the mother is another pattern of attachment behavior which implies no anxiety. Finally, burying the face in the mother's lap or in some other part of her person often implies no anxiety, although at times it may emerge in response to the presence of strangers. Let us first consider scrambling.

Scrambling

Even before the baby is able to crawl and hence to follow or to approach, he nevertheless can take the initiative in making contact with his mother when on her lap or when placed on the floor beside her. One of the ways in which he can do so is to climb up onto her and over her, exploring her person and playing with her face, her hair, or her clothes. On occasion he may behave in this way with another person, but since he much more frequently scrambles over his mother —or over another favorite person to whom he has become (or is becoming) attached—this differential response is included in our catalog. This behavior pattern differs both from an attempt to find the breast, which has a purposiveness that is unmistakable, and from an effort to maintain a close and continuous physical contact. It appears to be a pattern of exploration, as though the baby cannot be sated in his investigation of a figure—even one as familiar to him as his mother.

Muhamidi (twenty-two weeks) spent most of our visit scrambling over his mother. He frequently smiled at her, vocalized a great deal, and sometimes hid his face in her lap. He responded readily to our advances but smiled more frequently at his mother. He was able to crawl but did not leave his mother's side.

Juko (thirty weeks) scrambled over his mother cheerfully when held on her lap, before taking off to explore the room. Again at thirty-two weeks he crawled over his mother at one point, exploring her person; this occurred in sharp contrast to the times he sought her breast in a directed way.

Petero (thirty-four weeks) scrambled over his mother, vocalizing continuously, and occasionally smiled across the room at us. Later he stood on his mother's lap, buried his face in the angle between her neck and shoulder, and in this position bounced around. Still later he scrambled over me when I held him, but somehow less intimately than with his mother.

Muhamidi (thirty-two weeks), after playing with the other children for a while, moved close to his mother and began to play with her hair, standing behind her. Then he chewed her hair. At thirty-six weeks he was fussy and scrambled over his mother for the entire visit, showing no interest in anyone or anything else.

Mutebe (forty-one weeks) spent the entire visit on his mother's lap, scrambling over her part of the time.

Burying the face

The baby, whether in the course of scrambling over the mother, or having returned to her after exploring the world at some distance from her, buries his face in her lap or elsewhere in her person. This behavior was observed only in relation to the mother. Some examples have already been cited in conjunction with scrambling. Here are a few more.

Nakiku (twenty-eight weeks) sat near her mother on the floor, bouncing about, smiling, and gurgling, and then crawled to her mother and buried her face in her mother's lap.

Maryamu (fifty weeks) stood smiling, occasionally bobbing over in a squatting position. She vocalized a great deal and imitated sounds that I made. Then she burrowed her head in her mother's lap. She stood for a while again, then burrowed some more, and repeated this over and over. She approached me and accepted being held for a while; then she explored the room; finally she returned to her mother and spent the rest of the visit crawling over her.

Lusiya (fifty-one weeks) sat close to her mother for a while, her head on her mother's lap, bouncing her bottom up and down; occasionally she smiled up at her mother and babbled.

Paulo (fifty-three weeks) went exploring outside for a while, then sat beside his mother, burying his face in her lap. Later he was very active outside and when brought back, again sat beside his mother and again hid his face in her lap.

Magalita (fifty-two weeks) first sat on her mother's lap, then got down on the floor, buried her head in her mother's lap, and wiggled her bottom back and forth in the air.

Approach through locomotion

After the child is able to crawl, he characteristically terminates his greeting responses by crawling to the loved person as quickly as he is able; also, if apart from his mother when frightened, he crawls to her as quickly as possible. But approach can also occur simply to increase proximity, without any implication of anxiety.

Nakiku (twenty-eight weeks) was said always to crawl to her mother when placed on the floor apart from her, and to try to crawl up onto her lap. There was no implication of anxiety in this response.

Juko (thirty weeks) was cheerful when held on Mrs. Kibuka's lap. When he was put down, however, he crept vigorously to his mother.

Nabatanzi (fifty-one weeks) also was cheerful when held by Mrs. Kibuka. When put down she walked across the room to her mother with arms outstretched.

Other instances have been included in the examples cited to illustrate scrambling and burying the face.

Kissing and hugging

In our society affection is ordinarily expressed—both ritually and spontaneously—by a hug, a warm embrace, and perhaps a kiss. Many mothers encourage their babies to give them a hug and a kiss—or to hug and kiss the father or a brother or sister. By the end of the first year of life, babies in our society are able to return an embrace or kiss when it is given to them, perhaps clumsily, but in distinct response to the adult's affectionate advance.[3] That this is largely a culture-bound pattern of response—whether learned through reinforcement or through imitation—is suggested by the fact that Ganda babies very rarely manifest

3 Ruth Griffiths places this response at eleven months in her Infant Intelligence Scale (*The Abilities of Babies*).

any behavior pattern even closely resembling European affection, and, indeed their mothers did not try to elicit hugging or kissing in the baby, although they themselves occasionally nuzzled the baby while holding him.

Nakiku (twenty-eight weeks) was held standing by her mother. Her mother kissed her repeatedly and tenderly, on the cheek or the back of the neck, seemingly absent-mindedly. But we never observed Nakiku reciprocating.

Lusiya (about six months) was brought by her aunt to visit me. The aunt seemed very fond of Lusiya, holding her on her lap, often putting her face close to the baby's, nuzzling and giving little kisses.

Nakalema (thirty-five weeks) began to reach to feel my face after I had been holding her for a while. Twice she put her lips to my throat, and later I observed that she did the same thing when her mother held her.

We had no evidence that Nakalema had been taught to kiss; it may be that she was merely exploring with her mouth. In any event, Nakalema was the only baby observed to give anything remotely resembling a kiss, and none of the babies were observed to hug.

The fact that Ganda babies do not hug and kiss, whereas Western babies who are encouraged to hug and kiss do so, suggests that this pattern of attachment behavior is of a different order than the other patterns considered in this chapter—is much more contingent upon a specific learning process.

Use of the mother as a secure base for exploration

When most babies are able to crawl, they do not always stay close to the mother but rather make little excursions away from her, exploring other objects and interacting with other people, but returning to the mother from time to time. The mother seems to provide a secure base from which these excursions may be made without anxiety. The child who is attached to his mother, if he is secure in this attachment, does not need to maintain constant proximity or contact with her. He is content to move away, as long as he knows that she is there. He can even leave the room on his own initiative, and his aplomb in so doing is sometimes in sharp contrast to his consternation when his secure base gets up and moves off. Indeed, one could scarcely identify this as a pattern of attachment were it not for the fact that the child still is concerned about his mother's whereabouts.

Juko (thirty and thirty-two weeks) did much cheerful exploring, even out the front door of the house. Especially at thirty-two weeks, he kept returning to his mother and seeking the breast before taking off on another jaunt.

Nakiku (thirty-three weeks) crept about very actively during our visit, occasionally returning to her mother for contact.

Aida (thirty-four weeks) wanted to be close to her mother at first but then she became active, crawling about, exploring, returning to her mother occasionally.

Senkumba (thirty-seven weeks) played actively on the floor during our visit, made excursions away from his mother, but then returned to lie back against her and smile up at her. His mother said that he was quite willing to leave her to cross the room when someone else invited him to play.

Paulo (forty-two weeks) sat on his mother's lap for the first half of our visit. When his two sisters got up and left the house he scrambled down from his mother's lap and followed them as far as the doorway. He stood up, holding onto the doorjamb. Then he became more active, creeping about, playing with a little string of celluloid balls happily and noisily. Occasionally he smiled across the room at his mother. The girls returned, but twice more they left the house, and he crawled out after them, only to be retrieved by his mother, who did not like to let him out of her sight. And yet Paulo often made a big fuss if his mother left the room and he was prevented from following.

The use of the mother as a secure base from which to explore the world manifests itself under circumstances in which danger is absent and the child does indeed feel secure. When a threatening element enters the situation the child does indeed seek close proximity to his mother, but in an intense way, which may be distinguished easily from his seemingly casual use of her as a secure base. When he feels secure he leaves his mother, returning to her only occasionally, and perhaps only glancing at her from time to time. When he is frightened or insecure he flees to her as to a haven of safety and clings, protesting any attempt she makes to release him.

Flight to the haven of safety

Both Bowlby and Harlow[4] describe infants and young children —human and monkey—as fleeing to the mother, as a haven of safety, when faced with a fear-producing stimulus or when in a strange situation. The strange situations in which we observed these Ganda infants were mainly the clinic visits and, at home, being taken outside to be photographed. The chief fear-producing stimuli were ourselves as strangers.

Aida (thirty-four weeks) was put down by her mother in the middle of the room, halfway between me and the place where her mother was sitting. She immediately crept back to her mother and buried her head in her lap.

Sulaimani (twenty-eight weeks) was distressed when left alone on a mat to be photographed. When his mother moved closer he crept toward her and stopped crying as soon as she took him up.

4 John Bowlby, The nature of the child's tie to his mother, *Internal. J. Psychoanal.*, 1958, *39*, 1–34; H. F. Harlow, The development of affectional patterns in infant monkeys, in Foss (ed.), *Determinants of Infant Behaviour* (London: Methuen, 1961), pp. 75–100.

Paulo (thirteen months) was outside the house by himself when we arrived in the car. He became quite excited when he saw us and ran inside to his mother.

Kyimba (forty weeks) tolerated being held by me for a while, but he was very tense. As soon as I put him down he scuttled to his mother as quickly as he could.

When one attempts to identify the use of the mother as a haven of safety one realizes how interlocked all these attachment patterns are and how the same general behavior may mean different things in different contexts. Thus, for example, the child, when put down on the floor, may crawl to his mother in a purposive but non-anxious way. If she arrives after an absence, he may greet her enthusiastically and creep toward her. If he has been exploring, he may occasionally return to her and make contact. But all of these approaches can be distinguished from the flight to her as a haven of safety, perhaps more because of context than because of actual behavior—although there is both speed and absence of delight in the flight. Similarly, a baby may scramble over his mother and occasionally bury his face in her person, and the impression that is given in affectionate attachment. He may venture around the room, return to her, and bury his face—the impression is the same. But he may also *bury his face* and give the distinct impression that he is using his mother as a haven of safety. For example:

Juko (thirty weeks) buried his head in his mother's shoulder and would not look at me when I approached him early in the visit offering him a piece of candy.

Aida (thirty-four weeks) scuttled to her mother when I invited her to come to me and buried her face in her mother's lap.

Clinging

Studies of subhuman primates suggest that clinging is the major way in which the infant manifests his attachment to his mother.[5] The infant monkey maintains contact with his mother or with any object placed on his ventral surface but he clutches it tightly. Although subhuman infant primates hold onto the mother with arms and hands and often also with legs and feet from their earliest days, human infants are unable to cling tightly in this fashion until later in the first year of life. Nevertheless, Bowlby[6] has suggested that clinging is one of the component instinctual responses which underlie the child's attachment to his mother. It seems likely that the prototype of the clinging response in the human neonate is his postural adjustment reflex;[7] when he is picked up by an adult, with

5 Harlow (The development of affectional patterns in infant monkeys) identifies the "contact-clasp reflex" in neonatal monkeys as the basic response out of which the subsequent infant-mother affectional pattern develops.

6 The nature of the child's tie to his mother.

7 Helen Blauvelt and J. McKenna (Mother-neonate interaction: Capacity of the human newborn for orientation, in B. M. Foss [ed.], *Determinants of Infant Behaviour* [London: Methuen, 1961],

his ventral surface held against the shoulder-chest-breast area of the adult, he cuddles closely.

My observations of Ganda babies took place before much of this theoretical interest in clinging as a possible instinctual response in humans appeared in the literature. I did not have the opportunity to observe neonates—with one exception—but even with a child of two or three months of age or older I paid no special attention to his postural adjustment or to the circumstances under which he held onto his mother; I noted only conspicuous instances of clinging. Those instances in which clinging occurred so intensely that it forced itself to my attention tended not to occur until toward the last quarter of the first year of life. In some cases this intense clinging occurred in response to strangers or to a strange situation.

Mutebe (forty-one weeks) spent the entire visit on his mother's lap, either clinging to her or climbing over her. He seemed apprehensive of me, watching me warily from the shelter of his mother's arms. At forty-six weeks he again seemed very shy of the visitors and clung to his mother. Whenever I looked at him he cried and clung to her. At fifty-two weeks he was clinging to his mother as she brought him out after his nap. His mother started to hand him to me, but he cried immediately, and spent the rest of the visit clinging to her.

Magalita (fifty-two weeks) wanted to be close to her mother always. When we went out to take photographs her mother tried to put her down on a table. Magalita screamed and clung, resisting being put down.

Paulo (forty-three weeks) had accompanied his mother to the hospital when she was ill. When we visited them there, Mrs. Kibuka picked him up from his crib and held him for a while. When she tried to put him down again in his crib he caught onto her and would not let go.

In some instances clinging seemed to occur as a manifestation of insecurity in times of illness or following weaning rather than as a response to a specifically frightening situation.

Kasozi (fifty-seven weeks) responded to the dropping of his daytime breast feeding by crying a great deal and clinging to his mother.

Lusiya (fifty-nine weeks) was still disturbed by the final weaning that had taken place seven weeks before. During our visit she was close to her mother the whole time, either clinging while sitting on her lap or staying close to her on the floor and leaning back against her. Her mother left her behind when she worked in the garden, but when she returned Lusiya clung to her and would not allow her mother to move away for a moment.

pp. 3–35) describe this orientation reflex, although most of the paper describes the orientation of the head and face in response to tactual stimulation.

Nabatanzi (forty-eight weeks) had suffered a severe burn on her foot. Throughout our visit she sat on her mother's lap, fussing, and frequently clutching her mother.

Finally, there is the kind of clinging usually implied when one describes a child as "clingy"—a child who seeks constantly to maintain close physical contact and is distressed when put down, even though he may not actually clasp his mother with his arms or hold onto her.

Sulaimani (forty weeks) cried immediately when his mother put him down but stopped when she picked him up again. Again she tried to put him down; he screamed, and did not stop this time even when she took him up again. Later he permitted her to set him down on the floor but he played in a desultory way and protested whenever she moved away.

William (forty-three weeks) was ill and very subdued and "clingy." Throughout our visit he sat on his mother's lap, leaning back against her breast, sucking his thumb.

Magalita (forty-nine weeks) sat on her mother's lap, snuggled in, her head on her mother's breast, sucking her thumb and seeming very much the little baby. This was said to be quite characteristic of her, and her mother believed that it was because she was ill so much of the time.

These, then, are the patterns of behavior by means of which an infant shows his attachment. Their importance is greater, however. They are the patterns of behavior *through which attachment grows.* The baby is not attached to anyone at first. He does not somehow become attached and *then* show it by smiling at the loved person and crying when she leaves him. He gradually becomes attached through smiling and crying—and through adjusting his posture to his mother, suckling her breast, looking at her, listening to her, vocalizing when she talks to him, scrambling over her, approaching her, following her, and clinging to her. The course of development of attachment behavior will be described in Chapter 22.

21

RESPONSES TO OTHER FAMILIAR FIGURES AND TO STRANGERS

Attention has long been directed to the baby's relationship with his mother—first in theoretical accounts of personality development and much more recently in empirical research. From Freud onward, personality theorists have assumed, with convincing plausibility, that the baby's first significant relationship is with his mother, that he becomes attached to her before becoming attached to any other person, and, indeed, that the nature of his relations with her colors the nature of all subsequent interpersonal relationships. Nevertheless, the infant does have relations with other people during his first year of life, although the particular figures concerned and the nature of his relations with them depend in part upon the structure of his particular family group and upon the infant-care practices of this group. These practices are, of course, influenced by the society in which the family lives—at least to some extent. The relations of the infant to familiar figures other than his mother have been the subject of very little research, although surely no account of early social development can be complete without them.

More attention has been paid to the infant's response to strangers than to his response to familiar figures in the home environment. This is because fear of strangers emerges suddenly at about eight or nine months of age, and is a very conspicuous response. Moreover, some theorists have especially directed attention to fear of strangers as a criterion for the infant's attachment to his mother.

DOI: 10.4324/9781003629337-25

Attachment to familiar figures other than the mother

Nearly all the babies in this sample who became attached to their mothers during the period spanned by our observations became attached also to some other familiar figure—father, grandmother, or other adult in the household, or to an older sibling. In many instances these other attachments were formed to persons who shared to some extent in the routine care of the child, although in most instances it was the mother only who undertook the feeding—of supplementary solids as well as breast feeding. In other instances babies became attached to adults or older children who took no part in routine care and even sometimes to persons who were not constant members of the household.

In some families in this sample the father was either altogether absent or away so much of the time that the baby had little opportunity to know him. Nevertheless, it seemed to be especially to the father that these other attachments were formed, even in the cases of babies who saw their fathers relatively infreqently. One can only assume that there was some special quality in the father's interaction with his child—whether of tenderness or intense delight—which evoked in turn a strength of attachment disproportionate to the frequency of his interaction with the baby.

Schaffer[1] reports that some of the babies in his Glasgow sample formed attachments to other figures at the same time that they developed an attachment to the mother, or even earlier. Since Schaffer's visits were made at intervals of four weeks, however, it is quite possible that seemingly simultaneous attachments might have been successive. The present study of Ganda babies does not clear up this point. Although in most instances the infant seemed to direct his attachment behavior first to the mother, the intervals between visits were too long to enable us to ascertain the time lag, if any, between the formation of the first attachment and the formation of succeeding attachments. There was one child—Nora—who directed attachment behavior toward her father but not toward her mother. Otherwise, all babies became attached to the mother if they became attached to anyone. In any event, the findings of this study confirm Schaffer's findings to the extent that attachment behavior was directed toward other specific persons very soon after it was directed toward the mother, if not at the same time or even earlier.

Differential responses to the mother seemed to be followed fairly rapidly by differential responses to other figures.

Senkumba (twelve weeks) was said to "know" his father, who liked to hold him and play with him and who sometimes gave him his evening bath. At

1 H. R. Schaffer and Peggy E. Emerson, The development of social attachments in infancy, *Monog. Soc. Res. Child Develpmt.*, 1964, *29*, No. 94.

twenty-one weeks he could be left with the senior wife in the household without crying, but otherwise he cried whenever his mother left the room.

Samwendi (twenty-four weeks) cried when his mother left the room unless he was left with his aunt, who lived in the same household and shared in his care.

Sulaimani (twenty-five weeks) could be left with relatively little protest with a young neighbor boy, but he cried continuously when left with his grandmother, whom he did not like.

Actual attachments, as manifested by greetings and other positive responses, seemed to emerge in the third quarter of the first year. This is the same quarter in which the first really clear-cut attachments to the mother were observed.

Nakiku (twenty-eight weeks) was fond of her father. She greeted him enthusiastically when he returned from work. She did not protest when left with him—or with a young boy, Pantaleo, who lived in the household and who baby-sat. Nakiku's father had great affection for her, and in the evenings and over the weekends he enjoyed helping to care for her; he played with her a great deal.

Juko (thirty weeks) also was said to be very fond of his father and to "want to be with him."

William (thirty-two weeks) had had his father at home for a week after an absence of some months. At first he did not recognize him, but after the father had been home for a few days, William showed excitement whenever he saw him. His father was fond of him and held him a lot when he was at home. William was on good terms with his brothers and sisters, who helped keep an eye on him while his mother was in the garden, but he became attached to none of them as clearly as he was to his parents. If he cried when his mother left him, he could, however, be comforted by them. He differentiated them from other children.

Kyimba (thirty-seven weeks) was attached to his father, who came home every evening, who held him, played with him, and went for walks holding him in his arms. He was also attached to his grandmother, who lived in the household, who was fond of him, held him frequently, and shared in his care. When his mother worked in the garden, the grandmother looked after him. He became used to this arrangement and often did not cry when his mother left. When alone with his grandmother he tended to cry and follow if she left the room.

Nakalema (thirty-nine weeks) was said to be fond of her father and to accept being left with him. When her mother was absent, she followed her father if he moved off. She was also attached to her paternal uncle, who lived in the household. She did not seem attached to her siblings. She showed some liking for one sister, but she rejected the other and had little interaction with her brothers.

Mutebe (thirty-nine weeks) lived in his grandparents' home. He was attached to them and to his great-grandmother, as well as to his mother. His grandmother shared her bed with him; she also helped to feed him and looked after him while his mother worked in the garden. He was obviously attached to his mother but did not protest her departure if he was left with any of these familiar figures. He even got to know his father, who visited very rarely.

Nabatanzi (thirty weeks) was attached to her grandmother and great-aunt, who lived in the same household, and who were affectionate with her and sang to her. She was also strongly attached to her mother. Sometimes she protested her mother's departure when she was left with one or the other of the older ladies; sometimes she did not.

The specificity of attachments and the sharpness of preferences among familiar people was very striking in some instances.

Magalita (forty-three weeks) was attached to her mother, her father, a twelve-year-old half-sister and an adult half-brother. Her father was said to give her much attention and was good at soothing her when she was fussy. Although her half-sister was usually at school, Magalita was said to prefer her to anyone else; we witnessed the joyous greeting Magalita gave her. We also witnessed her excited greeting of her half-brother. She played with her three-year-old sister, although she often hit her. She was not especially interested in her brothers or half-brothers except for the one favorite. She rejected her grandmother, seeming to be afraid of her.

Paulo (forty-one weeks) was attached to his maternal uncle, who lived in the household. He gave him a big greeting when he entered, scuttled to him, and was picked up. He later protested being put down by him. His mother said that he was very fond of his uncle but would not let anyone else pick him up. The uncle took no part in Paulo's routine care; he merely held him and played with him. Paulo also seemed to be attached to one of his sisters, whom he followed, but not to the other.

Some babies seemed to be even more closely attached to their fathers than to their mothers.

Nakiku was one of these. She was said to prefer her father to her mother whenever he was at home, despite the fact that she seemed to have a very good relationship with her mother. Her mother said that this preference for the father was first expressed when she learned to crawl at six months of age. The preference held even if she was tired or ill. After final weaning at fifty-three weeks, Nakiku's preference for her father had in no way altered.

Sulaimani (thirty-six weeks) was said to prefer his father to his mother, even when he was tired or ill, and to obey him better. He did not try to follow his mother when left with his father, unless he was hungry.

Nora (fifty weeks) had showed no signs of attachment to her mother. A half-sister and her father were said to be her favorite people. When her father was at home Nora woke at night calling *taata*; during the day she was exceptionally active, going to him, going away, and coming back, laughing.

And yet the general trend was for the child with several attachments to make it clear that it was the attachment to the mother which was the focal one. Under conditions of hunger, fatigue, or illness the child usually turned to the mother. For example:

Magalita (forty-three weeks) was one with several attachments. But when she was ill she returned to her earlier overwhelming preference for her mother and wanted to be held by her all the time.

William (forty-two weeks) was ill and less willing to be left in the care of his brothers and sisters than previously; he wanted his mother.

In instances where there was an intense and fairly prolonged disturbance after final weaning, babies who had previously seemed to show no striking preference for the mother over other figures to whom they were attached were "clingy" and insecure and wanted to be with the mother all the time.

Lusiya (fourteen months) at two months after final weaning was still disturbed. Although previously she had seemed quite attached to her father, she now cried whenever her mother left her, even when she was left with her father. Previously, she had been content to be left with Nighty, who had always been her nursemaid, or with her aunt, but this was no longer the case.

Nabatanzi (fifty-eight weeks) had been weaned two weeks earlier. She wanted to be with her mother all the time and cried and followed whenever she left. Her attachment to the two substitute mothers who had always looked after her while her mother gardened did not compensate for the disturbance weaning caused in her relationship with her mother.

Indeed, there is some evidence that an insecure type of relationship with the mother tends to prevent the child from developing attachment to other figures.

Muhamidi (thirty-two weeks) had been living for a few weeks in his maternal grandfather's household, having moved away from home with his mother and sister. He had been friendly with his father before they moved but had not become really friendly with anyone else since. In this big new household it was his mother who did everything for him. He was responsive to other people as long as his mother was present, but if left by his mother, he was inconsolable. His mother was very anxious during this period, and whatever the causal chain, this seemed to make Muhamidi anxious and clingy.

Kasozi (fifty-six weeks) had been left every day with a neighbor for six months but had not become enough attached to her to want to stay with her. He always protested his mother's departure and finally one day ran away and found his way home. His mother, who had left him for long periods in order to establish a new garden, now had to take him along to the garden with her. She had been abandoned by her husband, but in this case it seemed to be not so much her anxiety that caused Kasozi to be anxious as the rejection of him implied by her long daily absences.

Regardless of the mother's own feelings toward the child, attempts to put him at a distance may be interpreted by the child as rejection and give rise to insecurity. This, I believe, is what happened to Kasozi. And I believe that children disturbed by weaning, such as Nabatanzi and Lusiya, interpreted weaning as a rejection.

Whatever the interpretation of these facts may be, it is clear that the infant during the first year of life may establish several attachments and a complex set of interpersonal relations. Our stereotype of the infant as developing an attachment to the mother and to the mother alone during the first year is not borne out by these observations, despite evidence that when the chips are down the attachment to the mother usually seems to be the focal one.

Response to strangers

Response to strangers has come to have special significance for the student of infant-mother attachment. When a baby displays a fear of strangers it is certain that he has developed to the point of being able to discriminate between familiar and unfamiliar people. Some theorists have suggested that fear of strangers can be used as *the* criterion that an attachment for the mother has been formed; the assumption is that before the child displays fear of strangers he has not sufficiently differentiated his mother from other people to be attached to her. The findings of this study suggest that there are two phenomena here, each of which has its own course of development, even though they are not entirely unrelated to each other: infant-mother attachment on one hand and response to strangers on the other.[2] Nevertheless, it is of interest to attempt to understand the relationships between the growth of infant-mother attachment and the child's responses to strangers.

Mrs. Kibuka and I were the strangers in these visits to Ganda homes. Occasionally there were other strangers who visited when we did, and we inquired of the mother about the child's responses to strangers, but much of our evidence came from observing the babies' responses to us. It was of particular interest to observe differential behavior in the child's reactions to Mrs. Kibuka and to me. Mrs. Kibuka was a stranger, but she is Ganda, whereas I have a white skin and, at least prior to the child's visits to the clinic or to the hospital, was very likely the only European the child had encountered. In other words, I was both especially discriminable and particularly strange. On the other hand, with each repeated visit we became less strange. Given a child old enough to make

2 I seem to have arrived at this opinion more or less simultaneously with several others: Mary D. Ainsworth, The development of infant-mother interaction among the Ganda, in B. M. Foss (ed.), *Determinants of Infant Behaviour*, *II* (London: Methuen, 1963), 67–121; J. D. Benjamin, Further comments on some developmental aspects of anxiety, in H. S. Gaskill (ed.), *Counterpoint* (New York: International Universities Press, 1963), pp. 121–53; H. R. Schaffer and Peggy E. Emerson, The development of social attachments in infancy, *Monog. Soc. Res. Child Develpmt.*, 1964, *29*, No. 94; Katherine H. Tennes and E. Esther Lampl, Stranger and separation anxiety, *J. Nerv. Went. Dis.*, 1964, *139*, 247–54.

discriminations, even biweekly visits served to make us increasingly familiar figures.

I have often mentioned that when visitors come to a Ganda household it is customary to give the baby to a visitor to hold. This provided an excellent occasion for observing the baby's response to a stranger, although it was also interesting to observe his response to the stranger at a distance.

There are several variables of interest here: (1) the age of the child at the time of the visit; (2) the number of times we had visited previously; (3) the differential response to Mrs. Kibuka and myself; and finally (4) the stage in the development of attachment to the mother that the child had reached.

During the first quarter of the first year most babies accepted us even though we were strangers, and, indeed, accepted being held by anyone.

Senkumba (eight weeks) was alone and crying when we arrived; he stopped crying when I picked him up.

Muhamidi (ten weeks) accepted being held by Mrs. Kibuka for most of the visit and once gave her a spontaneous smile. In general we were impressed with how friendly and responsive he was to us.

Alima (ten weeks) did not protest when I handled her to test her motor development; she was said to accept being held by anyone.

Nevertheless, three babies showed a differential response suggesting a preference for the mother, even though it did not necessarily indicate a fear of strangers.

Samwendi (nine weeks) was restless when Mrs. Kibuka held him and later when I held him, despite several shifts of position intended to make him more comfortable; finally he cried hard but stopped as soon as his mother took him.

Petero (eleven weeks) actually protested when his mother handed him to me but he stopped crying when she took him back again.

Aida (nine weeks) was crying and did not permit herself to be comforted by the visitors who picked her up and tried to soothe her; it may be that she was simply hungry, for her mother gave her the breast as soon as she returned and Aida stopped crying and suckled.

These responses indicate differentiation of the mother from other people—and at a much earlier age than that at which stranger anxiety has usually been reported as most conspicuous (eight or nine months). Thus, the emergence of differentiation of the mother seemed in some instances to inhibit responsiveness to strangers, although in general these babies accepted being held by anyone and accepted care from people other than the mother.

Soon after these first differential responses appeared the babies began to respond to the arrival of strangers by staring. The first part of the visit characteristically found the baby quiet and inactive, wholly preoccupied with staring at the stranger. This intense visual exploration did not seem to be apprehensive, for the same babies who stared were likely to accept being held by a stranger.

Aida (twenty weeks) at first stared very intently at Mrs. Kibuka and at me—for a long time. Later she interacted actively with me, accepted being held, and, indeed, scrambled over me exploring my person. She repeated this activity when held by Mrs. Kibuka.

Samwendi (nineteen weeks) spent the first part of the visit on his mother's lap, sucking his thumb and staring at us intently. Later he was quite content to be held both by Mrs. Kibuka and by me.

Sulaimani (twenty-five weeks) sat on the floor staring at us at first. When Mrs. Kibuka held out her arms to invite him to come to her he smiled and went readily. He accepted being held by her and indeed cried when she put him down.

At the same time, babies of this age seemed quite ready to exchange smiles over a distance and even to initiate the exchange. Sometimes I got the impression that the readiness to smile and the brilliance of the smile when it came was in direct proportion to the proximity of the child to his mother. Even at this early age the baby seemed to be able to use the mother as a secure base from which to be friendly with strangers.

Muhamidi (twenty-two weeks) had such an animated expression as he bounced about on his mother's lap that it invited an exchange of smiling and vocalization. He responded readily to Mrs. Kibuka and to me, although he smiled most often at his mother.

Petero (twenty weeks) sat on his mother's lap, leaning back against her, and smiled across the room at us from time to time. When he was given to Mrs. Kibuka to hold, he grew restless and made increasingly unhappy noises until he was given back to his mother.

As implied in the example of Petero's behavior, the baby could be friendly across a distance, and yet, when held by a stranger, he would be tensely oriented toward his mother and obviously relieved when given back to her. Other examples of this have been cited earlier on page 310.

The next development came with the onset of locomotion; although still accepting the stranger, the baby, given a choice, chose to keep his distance. He did not seem to be dismayed by the presence of strangers, but, although he moved about exploring, it happened that his exploring rarely brought him to the stranger. He still tended to stare at the stranger, and could be friendly across a distance. He might even accept being held. But he did not initiate close interaction.

Nakiku (twenty-eight weeks) sat near her mother, bouncing about, gurgling, and smiling at us. Later she crawled about, exploring. Once she crawled toward me, seemingly attracted by my sandaled feet. Her mother thought that she was intrigued with the white skin of my feet. At thirty-three weeks she crawled about but did not approach the visitors. Her mother said, however, that she still accepted being held by anyone.

Juko (thirty weeks) was cheerful when held by Mrs. Kibuka, but when put down he crawled vigorously to his mother. His mother said he was friendly with stangers as long as she was present.

The first fear of strangers came in the third quarter of the first year, or just immediately before. It seemed perhaps earlier and more intense in the case of children whom we were just beginning to visit than in children to whom we were not totally strange.

Nakalema (twenty-six weeks) accepted a toy from me and manipulated it, but when I approached her she cried. She resisted when I tried to pick her up. Her fear of me seemed to stem from the fact that I was European for she accepted being picked up by Mrs. Kibuka immediately afterward.

Juko (thirty-two weeks) would not come when I held out a piece of candy to him, inviting him to come to me. I crossed the room to offer him the candy again, but he buried his head in his mother's breast and would not look at me. His mother thought that he was shy of Europeans because he was usually easy with strangers. At the end of the visit I picked him up to see what he would do. He did not protest and seemed mildly interested as well as slightly tense and apprehensive. Later he sat on Mrs. Kibuka's lap without protest.

Kyimba (thirty-eight weeks) was approached by a complete stranger as soon as we arrived. (The stranger was a Ganda woman who was substituting for Mrs. Kibuka.) When she picked him up he shrieked so loudly that she returned him to his mother.

Mutebe (forty-one weeks) clung to his mother throughout our visit. He seemed apprehensive of me, watching me warily from the shelter of his mother's arms. His mother thought he must be afraid of me because I was European, for he was usually very active. At forty-six weeks he seemed even more shy of me. Whenever I looked at him he cried and clung to his mother. I had to observe him out of the corner of my eye, not seeming to watch him. Yet at forty-eight weeks, at the end of the visit he did not protest when I picked him up and held him. He accepted being carried the long distance to the car by a Ganda woman who was a complete stranger to him, his mother accompanying us. At fifty weeks he was more friendly and smiled at me when I offered a piece of candy. Nevertheless, he whimpered when Mrs. Kibuka picked him up. When I made a move to pull him toward me, he struggled away, moving closer to his mother. From this safe vantage point he smiled at me. At fifty-two weeks his mother began to hand him to me when he was first brought out after a nap. He cried immediately and spent the rest of the visit clinging to her.

We were not complete strangers to the babies after we had been visiting for some months. Nevertheless, at about the age of eight or nine months some of these children began to shy away from us. For example:

Aida (thirty-four weeks) would not come to me when I invited her, even when I offered her candy. This was the first time she had seemed shy of me. The mother thought that this was because I was European, for she was usually friendly with strangers. The mother carried her to the middle of the room, halfway between my seat and hers. Aida scuttled back to her mother and buried her face in her lap. When I crossed the room to her and held out the candy, she took it, but with hesitation.

William (forty-two weeks) was sitting on his mother's lap when we arrived. Mrs. Kibuka approached him and he cringed away.

Nabatanzi (forty-four weeks) was quiet, seemingly subdued because of the presence of a white stranger—I had not been able to visit for two months. I touched her foot gently and she responded with a whimper. She sat quietly on her mother's lap and fixed me with an intent stare. Everyone agreed that Nabatanzi usually was not shy of strangers but that she was shy of me. At forty-six weeks she was again somewhat shy of me. She cried briefly several times, seemingly in response to my presence and to the unfamiliar situation of being photographed. By forty-nine weeks it was clear to her mother that Nabatanzi did not like strangers; her previous friendliness had given way to distrust of strangers, whether men or women, Africans or Europeans.

One puzzling thing was the inconsistency we found in some of these children in regard to their response to strangers. One of these instances has already been cited. Mutebe, who had seemed extremely afraid of me, once permitted me to pick him up and hold him and he accepted being carried some distance by a complete stranger. Other examples follow:

Paulo (forty-one weeks) protested vigorously when his mother tried to hand him to me to hold, and she did not force the issue. At forty-two weeks he explored actively, but did not approach Mrs. Kibuka or me. He accepted being held by Mrs. Kibuka, however, and when she carried him out to the car, pretending to take him away, he did not protest. At forty-six weeks his mother tried to give him to Mrs. Kibuka to hold. Seeming to anticipate her intention he began to struggle and scream, hitting at his mother. Resisting his protest, his mother placed him on Mrs. Kibuka's lap and he continued to scream until he was put down. At forty-seven weeks Paulo came to Mrs. Kibuka directly; he was content when she picked him up and held him. Another visitor came for a while and took him on her lap. He did not cry but soon squirmed off and went to his mother. At fifty-three weeks he crept out to the car while we were all in the house. I went out to get him and he did not protest when I picked him up and brought him back to his mother. Later when we were leaving his mother handed him to me through the car window, suggesting that I take him with me. He did not protest but he was quiet and subdued and did not take his previous active interest in the interior of the car. I started the car and began to turn it around. He tolerated this for a few moments and then made a slight movement of protest.

Nabatanzi (fifty-six weeks) accepted being held by Mrs. Kibuka, although she had been distrustful of strangers for several months previously. Throughout the rest of the visit she was active and happy and did not seem apprehensive. She approached me on her own initiative once, demonstrating how she had learned to give a Ganda greeting by placing her hand in mine. Yet two weeks later she barely tolerated being held by me, and her mother confirmed that she did not like strangers. A puzzling episode occurred at the very end of that visit. Nabatanzi and her mother accompanied us up the path toward the car. When the mother announced that she would turn back, Mrs. Kibuka took Nabatanzi in her arms and began to carry her up the path away from her mother. Nabatanzi did not protest, although she looked back. Mrs. Kibuka turned her so that she could no longer see her mother, but there was still no sign of distress.

Some of the inconsistencies can be explained perhaps. It seems reasonable that a baby would shrink from a stranger's advance at the beginning of a visit and become more friendly after an hour or so. It also seems reasonable that a baby might approach a stranger on his own initiative, yet reject an approach made by the stranger, particularly if it were abrupt. It is puzzling, however, that some of these babies accepted being taken away by a stranger when outside of the house, while having seemed apprehensive of the stranger in the more secure and familiar environment of the interior of the house and in the mother's presence. It is also puzzling that at times a baby would vigorously protest being held by a stranger and at other times accept it. The answer to these inconsistencies probably lies in the subtle differences in the baby's own perceptions of various situations—perceptions that these observations do not permit us to infer.

In summary, the response to strangers changes in the course of the first year of life and seems to go through the following phases. (1) The baby does not seem to discriminate between strangers and familiar people. (2) The baby is differentially responsive to his mother and to strangers but nevertheless accepts strangers fairly readily. (3) The baby stares at strangers, seemingly struck by their strangeness, but does not seem apprehensive. (4) The baby is reserved with strangers; he can initiate interaction across a distance but does not spontaneously approach a stranger; nevertheless, he tolerates being held by a stranger and, although he may be tense and somewhat uneasy, he does not seem to be clearly afraid. (5) The baby is anxious with strangers, the anxiety ranging in intensity from slight apprehension to panic. In the next chapter it will be shown how these phases of response relate to the development of attachment.

22

THE DEVELOPMENT OF ATTACHMENTS

Let us now examine the developmental sequence in which emerge the patterns of attachment behavior described in Chapter 20. Let us note how these behavior patterns are manifested to the mother in comparison with other familiar figures. Let us also examine the baby's responses to strangers in the context of his attachment behavior. It is proposed to undertake this recapitulation in two ways. First, let us consider each quarter of the first year separately and summarize the findings descriptively. Secondly, let us attempt to divide the infancy period into phases of development of interpersonal behavior—phases which transcend mere description and throw light on the developmental processes themselves. In this chapter we will consider only those infants who did in fact develop clear-cut attachment to the mother; the five infants who did not do so will be omitted from this account.

A summary of the development of attachments

First Quarter: Birth to Thirteen Weeks

Six of the twenty-three attached infants were observed in this quarter—none of them before seven weeks of age. Although at first they seemed to be undiscriminating in their responsiveness to people, all six showed some signs of budding discrimination of the mother from other people by eleven weeks of age. Samwendi and Aida manifested some discrimination on our very first visit, at eight and nine weeks respectively, and might conceivably have done so when younger, had we been there to observe.

DOI: 10.4324/9781003629337-26

The chief criterion of differentiation of the mother from other people was crying—either differential crying or the similar response of crying more when left with other people than when with the mother (see Table 13). One child, Alima, who cried very little under any circumstances, made her mother feel that she recognized her—"by smell" the mother thought. In this sample of babies, all of whom were breast-fed, it was impossible to determine how much of this prototypical differentiation was of the mother as a whole person and how much was directed toward the breast, although some of the examples of differential crying given on pages 305–306 suggest that the baby stopped crying when picked up by the mother even though she did not give the breast.

By the end of the first quarter these mothers felt that their babies "knew" them—that is, responded to them with some special recognition—although the basis for this "knowing" could not be verbalized. One baby, Senkumba, was even reported to know his father—at the age of twelve weeks. Differential smiling may have been one of the cues for the judgment of "knowing"—a cue which we ourselves were not set to observe especially. Indeed, we noted differential smiling in only one child during this quarter—Muhamidi at ten weeks.

My impression is that cross-cultural differences in infant care make for differences in the earliest differential responses. It was typical of these Ganda mothers both to hold the baby more than American mothers do and to be prompter and more consistent in picking the baby up if he cried. Differential crying was certainly more conspicuous in this Ganda sample than in an American sample which I am currently observing. The American babies, on the other hand, seemed to manifest their first discriminations more clearly through differential smiling—and American adults much more than Ganda adults attempted to interact with a baby through smile-evoking behavior.

It is interesting to note that three of the six babies made some kind of protest when held by a stranger. It seems very unlikely that this protest implied discrimination of the stranger from familiar figures—except for the mother, of course. Thus, the protest upon being held by a stranger seems to reflect mere differentiation of the mother from other people, not stranger anxiety. In general these babies were friendly with other people, even though they showed a preference for the mother. Only two of the babies were looked after exclusively by the mother; the four who had other caretakers tolerated their care at least some of the time, even though they were more likely to cry with them than with the mother.

Second Quarter: Fourteen to Twenty-six Weeks

Ten of the twenty-three attached infants were observed at some time between the ages of fourteen and twenty-six weeks. Early in this quarter differential responsiveness to the mother was the chief attachment behavior manifested,

TABLE 13

ATTACHMENT BEHAVOIR: FIRST QUARTER

Name	*Age at Beginning of Study (Weeks)*	*Differ-ential Crying*	*Cries More When Left with Others*	*Other Differential Responses to Mother*	*Discrimination of Other Familiar Persons*	*Response to Strangers*
Petero	9	11	—	—	none	protested being handed to S (11)
Alima	7	—	—	"knows M by smell" (10)	none	accepts being held by S (8)
Aida	9	9	—	—	none	cries when held by S (9)
Senkumba	8	—	9	scrambling (10)	"knows" F (12)	accepts being held by S (10)
Samwendi	8	9	—	—	none	restless when held by S (9)
Muhamidi	9	—	10	smiling (10)	none	accepts being held by S (10)

TABLE 14 Attachment behavior: second quarter

Name	*Age at Beginning of Study (Weeks)*	*Differential Responses*	*Cries When Mother Leaves*	*Follows When Mother Leaves*
Juko	18	—	22	22
Petero	9	crying (11)	24	—
Alima	8	crying (15) smiling (26)	15	no
Aida	9	crying (9) vocalization & smiling (20)	22	22
William	14	—	24	24
Senkumba	8	—	no	22
Samwendi	8	crying (9) smiling (19)	24	—
Muhamidi	9	smiling (10) vocalization (22)	—	20
Sulaimani	24	—	25	—
Nakalema	24	—	24	—

but it was much more clear-cut than it had been in the first quarter; differential smiling and differential vocalization were noted as well as differential crying. As other attachment behavior began to emerge, however, we paid less attention to mere differential responses, and these were probably more frequent than our tabulation would indicate.

The most conspicuous pattern of attachment behavior in this quarter was crying when the mother left the room. The youngest child for which this was reported was Alima, age fifteen weeks. Otherwise it was not reported until twenty-two to twenty-five weeks of age. The consistency of this response and its duration differed from child to child. Nakalema, who cried a great deal anyhow, invariably cried when her mother left, regardless of circumstance, and tended to continue crying while her mother was gone. Others—for example, Aida, Alima,

Greeting Responses	*Other Attachment Behavior*	*Attachment to Other Familiar Persons*	*Response to Strangers*
—	—	—	responsive (20, 24); stares (24)
—	visual-motor orientation (20)	none	restless when held (20)
smiling (26)	—	greets and accepts M's leaving when with F and OW (26)	accepts being held (18)
smiles & lifts arms (22)	—	none	stares but is responsive (20)
—	visual-motor orientation (18)	none	restless when held (18)
vocalizes & lifts arms (21)	—	accepts M's leaving when with OW (21)	responsive, accepts being held (21)
—	—	accepts M's leaving when with MA (24)	stares, accepts (19); cries when S approaches (24)
—	—	friendly with F	responsive (22)
—	cries when M puts him down	none	stares, accepts being held (25)
—	cries when M puts her down	none	—

William, and Petero—were fairly consistent in crying when the mother left, but after a while they would settle down and accept the attentions of others. Toward the end of the quarter, some of the children—specifically Alima and Samwendi—were consistent in not crying when left with a specific familiar figure to whom they had developed some attachment, but otherwise they cried when the mother left. With those who were not entirely consistent in this response, state seemed to make a difference. Thus, for example, Aida was likely to cry especially when hungry.

Toward the end of the quarter the response of following emerged —usually as soon as the child began to crawl or very soon afterward. Muhamidi was the youngest child to begin following—at twenty weeks. It seems entirely likely that he cried as well as followed when his mother left the room, but we neglected to ascertain this point. Three babies were still unable to crawl at twenty-six weeks, so of course they did not follow. Alima was the only child who could crawl who did not follow, and she was just beginning to crawl.

Also toward the end of the second quarter, greeting responses began to emerge. Those that were reported included smiling, vocalizing, and lifting of the arms. It seems entirely likely that general excitement also characterized these greetings and that greetings were more common than our tabulation would indicate, because we had few occasions to observe them and did not inquire about them systematically.

In a sense the second quarter is the crucial quarter for the evaluation of the criteria of attachment. It is toward the end of this quarter that one might first begin to describe the child as attached rather than merely as differentially responsive. What then are the criteria which lead to that conclusion? First, crying when the mother leaves the room—which was not only conspicuous but which also is commonly accepted as *the* criterion of attachment by those who equate attachment with separation anxiety. What then of the two children who did not cry when the mother left the room? In the case of Muhamidi we were, of course, uncertain whether he did or not. But he did follow when his mother left the room, and also his differential responsiveness to his mother was unmistakable. If Muhamidi was not attached to his mother as early as or earlier than any other child, we would be forced to re-examine all our notions of the conditions of infant care which foster the growth of attachment, for Muhamidi was cared for exclusively by his mother, who took him with her wherever she went, and even worked in the garden with him in a sling on her back. Senkumba is the other child in question. He did not characteristically cry when his mother left the room, although he did (by twenty-two weeks of age) consistently follow her. Furthermore, he was one of the three children reported to greet his mother upon her return after an absence—vocalizing and lifting his arms—and this response predated following.

Further to this argument, let us contrast Nakalema and William. Nakalema was an insecure child who cried whenever her mother left, regardless of circumstance; she cried whenever her mother put her down and although she was reared in a large family, she did not accept being left with any member of the household. William, on the other hand, was reared in an even larger family of children but accepted being left by his mother with his brothers or sisters. He cried when his mother left the room and also followed, and this was invariable; but he settled down and accepted the attention of others. Even as early as eighteen weeks of age he showed by an intense orientation toward his mother his preference for her in comparison with the stranger who held him—and this bit of attachment behavior predated crying and following when his mother left the room. I do not believe that one could identify Nakalema as being more attached to her mother at twenty-four weeks of age than William was to his, but she certainly was less secure.

Three of the ten babies seemed to have developed a secondary attachment to other familiar figures by the end of the second quarter of the first year. In the case of Alima this was clearly preceded by an attachment to the mother. As early as fifteen weeks of age Alima was described as not caring about other people at all. But by twenty-six weeks of age she showed attachment both to her father and to the senior wife in the household. When either of these two figures or her mother entered after an absence, she acknowledged their arrival with a greeting; she accepted her mother's leaving the room if she had been left with either one of these two whereas when she was left alone or with anyone else in this large, extended household, she cried at her mother's departure. Senkumba also seemed to have developed an attachment for the senior wife in the household, with whom he was frequently left and who shared in his care. He showed his attachment for his mother by following her when she left, even though he did not cry, and by greeting her enthusiastically upon her return. But he did not protest when he was left with the senior wife—moreover, he was also the child who in the first quarter was precocious in " knowing his father." Samwendi was reared in the household headed by his maternal uncle; he became attached to the uncle's wife and did not cry when his mother left him with her, although he otherwise protested her departure.

These three cases lead me to hypothesize that if an infant is reared in a household in which he has the opportunity to attach himself to an adult other than the mother, he will do so before the end of the second quarter, provided that his relationship with his mother is a secure one. Petero, Aida, and William did not have this opportunity, for there were no other adult women in the household and the fathers were home infrequently. Juko probably formed an attachment to his father before six months of age, but we neglected to inquire about it and hence must leave him out of consideration. Muhamidi, Sulaimani, and Nakalema did have the opportunity to attach themselves to other adults, but their relationship to the mother was so insecure and "clingy" that it tended to obscure other attachments during the second quarter, if, indeed, they were formed.

On the whole, babies in the second quarter continued to be responsive to strangers and to accept being held by them. Nevertheless, toward the end of the quarter, beginning as early as twenty weeks in the case of Aida, the baby's prolonged staring at the stranger made it clear that a differentiation was being made between the stranger and other familiar figures. Two children were restless when held by a stranger—Petero and William—and maintained an intense visual-motor orientation toward the mother. But only one child—Samwendi, at twenty-four weeks—was said to cry when approached by a stranger, and even then he cried at some and not at others. In short, there is no clear evidence of stranger anxiety in the second quarter, although there is clear evidence of separation anxiety and attachment—not just attachment to the mother, but in some cases to other figures as well.

Third Quarter: Twenty-seven to Thirty-nine Weeks

Fifteen of the twenty-three attached children were observed in the third quarter, although one of them—Maryamu—was not seen to show attachment behavior in this quarter. For the fourteen who did show attachment, the most conspicuous response was following the mother, or attempting to do so, when she left the room or moved off (see Table 15). Eleven babies showed this response clearly, six of them usually crying as well. One child, Petero, could not yet crawl and hence could not follow, but he had been crying when his mother left the room since the age of twenty-four weeks. (Maryamu could not yet crawl either, but she did not consistently cry when her mother left the room.) The other two children —Paulo and Lusiya—probably did follow during this quarter, but we neither witnessed this behavior nor inquired about it. Paulo invariably cried when his mother left the room, regardless of circumstance, and Lusiya was obviously close to her mother—she wanted her mother especially at night and no one else would do.

Following had occurred with some children late in the second quarter. It not only occurred with more children in the third quarter but it occurred more consistently, as though the attachment to the mother were becoming consolidated. Five children in the third quarter characteristically followed without crying. The impression they gave was that they were confident of their ability to catch up with the mother and hence were not distressed when she moved off. Two children—Mutebe and Senkumba—sometimes did not attempt to follow the mother if she left them with familiar people, but the rest tended to follow, regardless of whom they had been left with.

The overwhelming impression of attachment behavior in this quarter is the extent to which the child himself takes initiative. When his mother leaves he follows her and does not merely cry. When his mother comes back he takes the initiative in greeting her and perhaps in approaching her. At the same time he shows initiative in leaving her in order to explore his world.

Greeting responses were specifically recorded in the case of six of the fourteen children and probably occurred more frequently than the tabulation indicates. The greetings themselves seemed to become more active—lifting arms, clapping hands, and approaching, not merely smiling and vocalizing. Approach behavior appeared in this quarter for the first time, either in greeting or merely as a means of increasing proximity to the mother when put down at a short distance from her. Even when the child was in contact with his mother he sometimes took active initiative in interacting with her. Sometimes he leaned back against her passively, but other times he scrambled over her or buried his face in her person. This behavior was not observed in every case; in some instances perhaps it was inhibited by an emerging shyness of strangers, especially in the case of babies like Kyimba, Lusiya, and Mutebe whom we did not visit until they were nearly nine months old.

Finally, a highly significant form of behavior that made its appearance in the third quarter was the use of the mother as a secure base from which to explore the world. The youngest child in which this was noted was twenty-nine weeks old. Since the criterion of exploration which we used was locomotion, the emergence of this behavior obviously depended on the development of locomotion. Two babies—Petero and Maryamu—were unable to crawl; of the remaining thirteen, nine demonstrated that they could use the mother as a secure base of exploration. Of the four who did not, three—Kyimba, Lusiya, and Mutebe—seemed to be anchored near the mother because of stranger anxiety (on the occasion of our first visit), and the fourth —Nakalema—did not move about even though she was said to be capable of creeping on her hands and knees.

Of the fourteen babies who were attached to their mothers, ten were described as having clear-cut attachments to other familiar members of the household—father, grandparent, aunt, uncle, sibling, or nursemaid, and an eleventh child—Petero—at least "liked" his father, who was home on weekends only. Only three children seemed to have formed an exclusive attachment to the mother. Paulo was looked after exclusively by his mother; his father was absent and his sisters were too young to help take care of him. It is not clear when his uncle came to live with them, but in any event he did not develop an attachment to the uncle until the fourth quarter. The other two—Muhamidi and Senkumba—had moved with their mothers from home to live in the large extended household of the maternal grandfather. Muhamidi, especially, was looked after exclusively by his mother, and perhaps neither had had time to develop other attachments in the new environment. On the whole, however, it appears that Ganda babies who have the opportunity to develop an attachment to another adult in the household will do so in the third quarter, if not earlier, and very soon after a clear-cut attachment to the mother has been formed. Attachment to young siblings seems to develop more slowly, but both William and Aida appeared to be somewhat attached to siblings in this quarter.

Uneasiness with strangers was much more conspicuous in the third quarter than it had been in the second. Only two babies showed no uneasiness: Maryamu accepted being held by a stranger, although she was very quiet; William was

TABLE 15 Attachment behavior: third quarter

Name	*Age at Beginning of Study (Weeks)*	*Follows When Mother Leaves*	*Approach and Greeting Responses*	*Use of Mother as a Secure Base*
Paulo	29	? but cries	—	29
Juko	18	30	approaches (30)	30
Petero	9	cannot crawl but cries	greets (34)	—
Mutebe	39	and cries (39)	—	—
Nakiku	28	38	approaches & greets (28)	33
Aida	9	22	approaches (34); smiles & lifts arms (22); claps hands (31)	34
William	14	and cries (24)	claps hands, lifts arms (28)	32
Senkumba	8	22	—	37
Kyimba	37	and cries (22)	—	—
Maryamu	33	cannot crawl	—	—
Lusiya	38	? and cries	—	—
Nabatanzi	30	and cries (24)	approaches (37); greets with approach, smiles, & vocalizes (37)	30
Muhamidi	9	and cries (20)	approaches (37); greets with approach, smiles, & vocalizes (33)	32
Sulaimani	24	36	approaches (28)	35
Nakalema	24	and cries (35)	—	—

Other Attachment Behavior	*Attachment to Other Familiar Persons*	*Response to Strangers*
visual-motor orientation; cried when M L/R (29)	none	restless when held (29); accepted being held till M left room (30)
scrambling & burying face (30)	"wants to be with F" (30)	accepts being held (30); will not approach; tense when held (32)
scrambling, differential vocalization, burying face, differential smiling (34)	"likes F" (34)	stares (32); accepts being held (34)
—	MGF; MGF; MGGM	—
visual-motor orientation (29); burying face (28)	prefers F (28)	accepts, approaches (28); will not approach (33)
burying face (34)	accepts M L/R when left with sister (34)	will not approach; later accepts being held (34)
differential smiling (32)	accepts M L/R when left with siblings (32)	accepts women, not men (32)
—	none	slight protest when held (37)
dinging (39)	accepts M L/R when left with PGM (37); follows PGM	screams when picked up by S (37)
—	—	quiet, accepts being held (38)
—	accepts M L/R when left with F, or "nursemaid" (38)	stared, was solemn and constrained (38)
scrambling (31)	greets and accepts M L/ R when with MGM or MGA (30)	responsive (30); stares (31); subdued when left alone with S (37)
visual-motor orientation (31); scrambling (32)	none	tense, oriented toward M (31); unresponsive (36)
clinging (28)	accepts M L/R when left with F (36)	cries when taken (28); cries when held (35); accepts male S (36)
—	follows F (39); fond of PU	resists being picked up by me, but not by Mrs. K (35)

neither held nor approached closely by a stranger in this quarter. Maryamu, it will be recalled, did not yet seem to be attached to her mother. William had demonstrated uneasiness earlier—as young as eighteen weeks—and probably would have done so again had we held him. Of those who showed uneasiness there was a range of intensity from mere staring at the stranger to a panic-stricken screaming. Of greatest interest were the babies whom we had been visiting for some time, who had previously accepted us, but who now stared, failed to approach when invited to do so, or were tense when held. On the other hand, babies who had not been visited until near the end of this quarter showed the most striking anxiety.

Fourth Quarter and beyond: Forty to Sixty Weeks

Eleven attached babies were observed during the fourth quarter, and all of these were very clearly attached to their mothers. On the whole, the attachment patterns that had been conspicuous in the third quarter still seemed to be significant in mediating the infant's attachment to his mother (see Table 16). All of them followed their mothers, except for William, who had previously followed but who in the last quarter was too ill to creep about. The trend which had begun in the third quarter was now clearer, namely, for the child to follow, creeping or walking, so efficiently and with such confidence that he did not cry while following. Five babies showed this companionable kind of following and cried only when frustrated in following, either because the mother moved away too quickly or because she closed the door behind her. Lusiya did not cry even under these circumstances; instead she banged on the closed door. On the other hand five babies still characteristically cried while following. Three of these seemed generally to be insecure babies—Magalita, Sulaimani, and Kasozi. One, Kyimba, was going through a postweaning disturbance, and, indeed, after weaning Lusiya and Nabantanzi also cried when following whereas they had seemed quite secure in their following before weaning.

The other active attachment patterns characteristic of the third quarter were more frequent and clear-cut in the fourth quarter. Six children expressed attachment through approach responses. Only two did not seem to do so—William, who was too ill to crawl, and Sulaimani, whom we stopped visiting when he was forty weeks old and barely into the fourth quarter. Greeting responses were conspicuous, and only in the cases of Kyimba and Sulaimani did we fail to inquire about greeting. Maryamu was said merely to give a "happy welcome" to her favorites, but in every other case we had evidence of a more active greeting—approaching or the clapping of hands, or both.

The use of the mother as a secure base was very conspicuous in the case of six children. With these there seemed to be even less need than previously to return to make contact with the mother, and expeditions away from the mother were longer and farther, even out of sight in some instances. There seemed to be special reasons why five children failed to use the mother as a secure base for exploration during our visits in the fourth quarter. Kasozi and Mutebe seemed much too apprehensive of us as strangers to venture away from their mothers; William and Sulaimani were ill and disinclined to creep about exploring, and Magalita was both ill and apprehensive of strangers.

The active kind of attachment behavior that took place when in contact with the mother—scrambling and burying the face—continued to be conspicuous, although it did not occur in all cases.

The pattern that seemed characteristic of the fourth quarter in comparison with the third was clinging. True clinging—clasping with the arms and holding on tightly—tended to be associated with fear of strangers or of strange situations, and was not noted earlier than forty-one weeks of age. Six children were observed to cling in this fashion. "Clingy" behavior, in which the child wants to be in constant contact with the mother but may not actually hold onto her tightly, seemed less specifically a fear response and more generally an anxiety response, occurring with illness or after weaning, or as part of a generally insecure relationship with the mother. The youngest child to be clingy was twenty-eight weeks old—and this was Sulaimani, whose relationship with his mother was very insecure and ambivalent.

All eleven babies were by the fourth quarter attached to one or more familiar figures besides the mother. Two of these were said to prefer the father to the mother—Nakiku, despite the excellent relationship she had with her mother, and Sulaimani, perhaps because his relationship with his mother was ambivalent and insecure. The other nine babies seemed to be focally attached to their mother but to have other attachments as well. In some cases—for example, Paulo, Kasozi, and Magalita—there was attachment to a favorite person who held the child and played and interacted with him but who did not have any responsibility for his care. In other cases, such as Nabatanzi, Nakiku, Kyimba, Mutebe, and Lusiya, the secondary attachments were to adults and older children who did in fact have caretaking responsibilities.

A negative response to strangers emerged more consistently and more intensely in the fourth quarter than it did in the third. Over repeated visits there was considerable variability in response to strangers. There was perhaps no child who was consistently apprehensive or unfriendly. It was more usual for an ordinarily friendly child to show episodes of stranger anxiety or for a child ordinarily anxious with strangers to manifest inexplicable episodes of acceptance. Nevertheless, only Maryamu was consistently friendly and free of shyness of strangers; all of the others manifested at least one striking flash of stranger anxiety. Frantic clinging in fright occurred in only six of the eleven

TABLE 16 Attachment behavior: fourth quarter and beyond

Name	*Age at Beginning of Study (weeks)*	*Follows When Mother Leaves*	*Approaches Mother or Other Favorite*	*Greets Mother or Other Favorite* [c]	*Uses Mother Secure Base*
Paulo	29	42	41	A, S, V (41)	29
Mutebe	39	41 [a]	44	S, V, CH (44)	no [d]
Nakiku	28	28	28	A, S, V (28)	33
William	14	24 [b]	–	CH, LA (28)	no [e]
Kyimba	37	40 [a]	—	—	40
Maryamu	33	41	—	yes (50)	50
Lusiya	38	51	51	A, S, V, CH (51)	51
Nabatanzi	30	24	37	A, S, V (37)	30
Magalita	42	42 [a]	52	A, S, V (52)	no [d, e]
Sulaimani	24	40 [a]	—	—	no [e]
Kasozi	48	48 [a]	—	S, V, CH (48)	no [d]

[a] Characteristically cries while following.

[b] Previously followed M but now is ill and does not follow.

[c] The abbreviations in this column are as follows: *A*—approaches; S—smiles; V—vocalizes; *LA*—lifts arms; *CH*—claps hands.

[d] Fear of strangers seems to inhibit exploration during our visits.

[e] These children previously used the mother as a secure base from which to explore but now are ill and do not explore.

[f] This is a "clingy" response—an insecure insistence on being close to the mother—rather than an actual clinging. It may be noted that Mutebe (41), Magalita (49), and Kasozi (51), were clingy too, although at other times they actually clung.

Clings to Mother	*Other Attachment Behavior*	*Attachment to Other Familiar Persons*	*Response to Strangers*
43	burying face (53)	greets MU (41)	protests hand-over and clings (41)
41	scrambling (41)	accepts M's L/R when left with MGM, MGP, or MGGM (39)	stares, is apprehensive; clings to M (41, 46)
—	—	greets and accepts M's L/R when left with F or "nursemaid" (28)	stares (44); accepts being held, approaches (47); tense when held (52); shy (56)
43 [f]	—	greets F (28)	cringes (42)
39 [f]	scrambling (41)	accepts M's L/R when left with PGM and follows PGM (37)	tense when held (40)
—	burying face (50)	greets, follows, accepts M's L/R with F, sister, "nursemaid" (50)	friendly (50)
59	burying face (51)	accepts M's L/R with F or "nursemaid" (38); greets F (51)	stares, is solemn (51); shrinks away (60)
48	scrambling (31) burying face (58)	accepts M L/R with MGM, MGA (30); greets MGM (51)	whimpers when touched (44); cries (46); is distrustful (49)
52	burying face (52)	greets F, sister, brother (50)	stays close to M (42)
28 [f]	—	prefers F (36)	tense when held (40)
57	—	fond of MU	stares (51); cries (59)

children; it tended to occur chiefly with children whom we had begun to visit in the fourth quarter, and it tended to be more intense in response to me, the white person, than to other strangers.

Finally, events of the last quarter of the first year and of the first quarter of the second year made it clear that the development of attachment does not follow an even course, uninfluenced by changes in the environment and in methods of infant care. Perhaps the most upsetting event was weaning—in the case of babies who had been fed on demand and especially in cases where the mother attempted to consolidate weaning by withdrawing from the child. In such cases, the more insecure manifestations of attachment became acute—crying and following when the mother left, clinging to her under circumstances constituting the slightest threat, generally wanting to be with her all the time, and protesting the slightest increase of distance. Such children seemed to lose interest in other people to whom they had been attached previously and to have an exaggerated fear of strangers.

Phases of development of attachment

Although the four quarters of the first year may be distinguished one from the other in regard to attachment behavior, nevertheless, the quarterly divisions to some extent cut across functional divisions. Let us turn now to a distinction between phases of attachment, where less emphasis is placed on chronological age.

Phase I: The Undiscriminating Phase

The first phase is characterized by the lack of discrimination between people. Even here one could distinguish two periods, although perhaps not in this particular Ganda sample. Nevertheless, both from my more intensive work with an American sample and from an examination of the findings of other investigations I would propose that this undiscriminating phase has a first, neonatal period in which the baby is unresponsive to social advances, except that he makes a general postural adjustment when held and a specific reflex adjustment to the feeding situation. The second period in the undiscriminating phase is characterized by undiscriminating social responsiveness. The baby smiles when presented with adequate stimulation, especially when presented with the human face in a face-to-face confrontation, and most especially if this is accompanied with head-wagging and vocalization. But at this time it does not matter whose face it is; the baby responds to a stranger just as readily as to his mother, given the same close confrontation.

In this study of Ganda babies, observations began at the very end of the undiscriminating phase; hence, there is nothing that our observations can add to what is already known.

Phase II: The Phase of Differential Responsiveness

The baby begins to discriminate between his mother and other people and to behave differentially. The chief ways in which he can express this differentiation are differential crying, differential smiling, differential vocalization, and a differential postural adjustment. In this sample the only response that was systematically explored was differential crying. The baby cried when held by someone else but stopped when taken by the mother. When crying the baby could be comforted more readily by the mother than by anyone else. Perhaps another manifestation of differential crying was that the baby cried when put down by the mother, but did not protest being put down by someone else—although this was not explored in the present sample. In this sample the earliest instance of differential crying was observed at nine weeks and the latest at eleven weeks—but the cases were so few that no generalization can be validly made.

As I have mentioned before, we did not set out to observe any other kind of differential response. Nevertheless, I am sure that discrimination may be shown by differential smiling—by smiling more frequently, more readily, and more fully to the mother than to anyone else—and that in some societies differential smiling might well precede differential crying. In all societies differential vocalization is likely to be later than either differential crying or differential smiling, if only because non-crying vocalization is sparse at the beginning. Nevertheless, future studies of the development of attachment should attend to this differential response, especially because studies of maternal deprivation have shown that the amount of vocalization differentiates significantly between deprived and non-deprived babies.

After having completed a study, researchers sometimes suffer from regrets regarding the significant behavior that they did not adequately observe, behavior that was relevant to their problem and which should have been observed. I feel this way about postural adjustment. I now believe that the baby's postural adjustment when held is the first response that becomes differential, perhaps excepting sucking and rooting and the whole complex of responses associated with feeding. It is now known that babies who are bottle-fed by more than one parent figure learn very early to adjust differentially if they are held in different feeding positions by different figures. Discrimination between different modes of being held was shown by three of the six Ganda babies observed in the first quarter; they indicated their appreciation of the difference by protesting being held by a stranger and quieting when taken by their mothers. These protests began to be noticed in the range of from nine to eleven weeks.

In this Ganda sample the second phase of discriminating behavior seems to last from nine weeks of age at the earliest to twenty-five weeks at the latest.

Phase III: The Phase of Differential Responsiveness at a Distance[1]

In this phase discrimination is manifested through distance receptors and perhaps especially through vision. This is shown when the child cries when his mother leaves the room—as early as fifteen weeks of age in one child but more characteristically between twenty and twenty-four weeks. At about the same time, babies began to greet their mothers across a distance. And they began to indicate recognition of the strangeness of strangers at some distance by staring at the newcomers.

Phase IV: The Phase of Active Initiative

The fourth phase is characterized by active initiative in making, sustaining, and renewing contact and interaction. Following the mother when she leaves the room is a criterion of active initiative and so is approaching. Although both of these behavior patterns depend upon the emergence of locomotion, active greeting by lifting the arms or clapping the hands does not. Scrambling and burying the face are other active patterns, and so, of course, is clinging. One child—Petero—clearly manifested these active patterns before the onset of locomotion, but in this sample they were, in general, observed at the same time as, or after, the onset of following and locomotion. The earliest age at which active initiative was manifested in this sample was twenty weeks, and in several babies it seemed to succeed Phase III very rapidly. The last child to reach this phase was Maryamu— sometime between thirty-eight and forty-one weeks.

The active initiative manifests itself also in behavior which is directed away from the mother. At the same time that babies show themselves so active in seeking contact, they also begin to use the mother as a secure base from which to explore the world, leaving her and returning to her or at least checking on her whereabouts. Furthermore, active initiative in seeking interaction with other familiar figures also emerges, and it is not merely a response to familiarity because there is a high degree of specificity shown by some babies in their preferences. Finally, during this phase of development the typical response to strangers is one of some reserve—reluctance to approach strangers and constraint or tension when held by a stranger, but with no marked stranger anxiety and usually with some willingness to warm up to a stranger after the period of reserve.

1 In my earlier accounts of the phases of development of attachment behavior I did not distinguish Phase III from Phase II.

Phase V: The Phase of Stranger Anxiety

The chief developments in this phase are stranger anxiety on the one hand and marked clinging to the mother (or other object of attachment) on the other. Babies to whom we were not total strangers tended to show a more marked constraint or avoidance than they had in Phase IV, and babies to whom we were quite new manifested intense anxiety. It was the intense anxiety in response to strangers which seemed to evoke the clear-cut clinging response—clasping tightly and actively resisting any dimunition of contact, not merely the fussy clinging of the baby who is insecure, hungry, tired, or ill. In our sample it was the mother to whom the child clung in most instances, but another person to whom the child was attached could serve as a haven of safety if the mother was absent. In this sample the earliest panic to strangers was observed at thirty-seven weeks, but generally Phase V seemed to coincide fairly well with the last quarter of the first year of life.

In what phase of development can the baby first be described as attached? If the criterion is separation anxiety, then it is Phase III, when the baby cries at seeing his mother leave the room, although previously he had been content to be at some distance from her. If the criterion is stranger anxiety, then it is Phase V. But if we apply Piaget's stringent criterion of object permanence[2] to attachment, requiring that the child demonstrate that he conceives of his mother as having an identity and a permanence independent of his own subjective experience, then attachment probably is not fully consolidated until the middle of the second year of life. My own inclination is to believe that attachment begins to be consolidated in Phase IV, after the first indications of separation anxiety and before full-blown stranger anxiety, and this inclination has been reflected throughout Chapters 20 to 22. But it is obviously a question of which objectively observable patterns of behavior can be taken as criteria for attachment because attachment itself must consist of some inner representation or structuring that cannot be observed directly and that can only be inferred from behavior.

Even though this study of Ganda babies does not enable us to answer some of the most crucial questions about attachment, it has highlighted several very significant points: attachment develops in an orderly way; a number of patterns of behavior have been identified as attachment behavior and emerge in orderly sequence over time; separation anxiety and stranger anxiety also undergo a developmental sequence, and although interlocked with the development of attachment, neither seems to be an adequate sole criterion for attachment; attachment to familiar figures other than the mother can emerge very soon

2 J. Piaget, *The construction of reality in the child* (New York: Basic Books, 1954).

after attachment to the mother (if not simultaneously), and this is perhaps particularly noteworthy in a society in which there is an especially close and intimate infant-mother relationship. Furthermore, it is believed that infant-care practices influence the development of attachment, facilitating it or delaying it and shaping the quality of the attachment relationship. This is implicit in some of the discussion in this chapter which contrasts Ganda practices with American practices. But even among the babies in this Ganda sample, differences emerge which are related to infant-care practices. This is the concern of the next chapter.

23

VARIABLES INFLUENCING THE DEVELOPMENT OF ATTACHMENT

The title of this chapter reflects the belief that attachment does not develop willy-nilly according to some inner, genetic, regulating mechanism, but rather is influenced by conditions in the baby's environment. This does not imply that inner, genetic regulators are negligible. On the contrary, the orderly sequence in the emergence of attachment patterns—as well as the fact that there seem to be striking similarities between this sequence among the Ganda and the sequence observable in our society—suggests that the development of attachment is correlated with other processes of development and that all these processes are in part determined by genetic factors characteristic of the human species. Furthermore, as an article of faith, we must concede that there are genetically based individual differences between babies, as well as differences stemming from prenatal development, circumstances surrounding the birth process, and from environmental influences in the neonatal period. In the present study it is quite impossible to differentiate genetic, prenatal, and perinatal influences from environmental influences since only one baby was observed from birth onward, and even in this case observations were too widely spaced to be helpful. Nevertheless, the fact that some environmental variables can be demonstrated to have a significant influence on the development of attachment among the babies of this sample demonstrates that genetic factors are not overwhelmingly important and that infant-care practices can make a difference.

The assertions in the paragraph above may seem obvious to many readers. Nevertheless, there are some scientific students of infant behavior who attach almost exclusive importance to constitutional determinants of development, who view development as a maturational process of unfolding of genetic potential, who believe that a child can only learn a specific behavior pattern when his

DOI: 10.4324/9781003629337-27

maturational level makes him ready, and who do not believe that methods of infant care and child rearing have any significant effect in accelerating or retarding development. There are other psychologists, chiefly concerned with animal learning, who believe that a person's responses can be controlled largely, if not entirely, by environmental contingencies, and who equate development with learning, thereby implying that developmental level is of little significance as long as the environmental contingencies are right. Because these two divergent views are widely held, it seems necessary to assume a stance and to assert that my position rests on a thorough-going belief that development is an interactional process—an interaction between the constitutional elements and environmental circumstances.

But here we are concerned with environmental influences. Let us begin with the end result insofar as it is known in the babies of this sample.

Classification of infants according to strength and security of attachment

The sample may be divided into three groups according to the strength and security of the baby's attachment to his mother: (1) a secure-attached group consisting of sixteen children, subjects #1 to #16; (2) an insecure-attached group of seven children, subjects #17 to #23; and (3) a "non-attached" group of five children, subjects #24 to #28. In all of the tables interspersed throughout the book, the order in which the babies are listed corresponds to these divisions.

The babies in the two attached groups were those who manifested the patterns of attachment behavior found to be typical of their age—at least as judged by the norms of this sample. The third, "non-attached" group did not show any of the patterns of attachment behavior (directed toward the mother) throughout the entire period of observation. Let us consider this third group first, since they have not been dealt with in previous chapters.

The "Non-Attached" Group

First, let it be said that "non-attached" has been placed in quotation marks because the implication is not that these babies are not attached and never will be, but rather that they are not yet attached, and, although they are delayed in the development of attachment, it is entirely likely that they will become attached. Nevertheless, the fact that this small group is behind the rest of the sample in regard to the development of attachment makes it deserving of notice.

The "non-attached" (or "not-yet-attached") group consists of Nora, Kulistina, the younger set of twins—Waswa and Nakato—and Namitala. We shall immediately exclude Namitala from consideration. Although she did not develop any signs of discrimination of her mother from other people during the fifteen weeks she was observed, it could easily be said that she was somewhat delayed in discrimination, and that one cannot expect attachment to have developed by fifteen weeks of age. The other four children were, however, observed long enough to ascertain that they were deviant from their age peers in the development of attachment. In no case do I consider that conditions were such as to prevent the development of any attachment; but, certainly, attachment was delayed in these cases.

Nora, even when one year old, did not show any discrimination between her own mother and Kulistina's mother, who was a familiar caretaker and a member of the household. She did not cry when her mother left the room nor did she attempt to follow. We did not observe any greeting responses, and none were reported to us. Nora liked to explore her world after locomotion developed, but there is no evidence that she used her mother as a secure base for this exploration. Indeed, one might describe her tentatively as precociously independent. The only sign of attachment was to her father. On the weekends when he was at home, Nora was exceptionally active, approaching him, laughing, then retreating, only to approach him again. And at night she called out to him—*taata.* She also showed some preference for one of her half-sisters—one who was home only for occasional visits. Nora was not at all apprehensive of strangers. During our visits she sometimes responded to our advances, sometimes smiled spontaneously, but mostly she wanted to explore without interference from her mother or anyone else.

Kulistina had the unenviable distinction of being the baby in the sample whose start in life had been worst. Her mother did not, or could not, breast feed her, and she did not flourish on artificial feeding, not, at least, until pediatric advice was obtained and put into practice. Kulistina was a friendly baby and smiled a great deal. Her smiling seemed to be quite undiscriminating, even at forty-seven weeks of age. She accepted the attentions of the other wife in the household as readily as she accepted the attentions of her own mother. At thirty-three weeks of age we noted that she was more active and "scrambled" with her mother more than with other people—but aside from this observation, there seemed to be very little differentiation in her mode of responding to different people. At forty weeks Kulistina was said to "know" her mother, and also to "know" her father when he came home—but other babies could make these discriminations in the first quarter of the first year. In short, she seemed to be just beginning to make differential responses in the last quarter of the first year, whereas by this time most of the other babies in the sample were making their attachments clear by active, preferential behavior which showed initiative.

The Younger Twins—Waswa and *Nakato.* The twins manifested very little attachment behavior during the period of investigation At twenty-three weeks they were described as lifting their heads up and vocalizing (as though they wanted to sit) in response to the approach of a person, but the response seemed quite non-differential. Nakato at thirty-two weeks was characterized as likely to cry when strangers were present, but Waswa "liked people." Neither baby cried when the mother left the room and both were described as behaving toward the mother no differently than they behaved toward others. The only hint of differential response came from Nakato, who was described as being less likely to cry when with her mother or father than when left with the young girls who were her "nursemaids." Waswa seemed to show no discrimination whatsoever.

One could perhaps argue that these babies were not wholly "non-attached." Nakato showed a few differential responses; Nora seemed especially excited by her father. But, on the whole, there seems little doubt that these four, including Nakato and Nora, were lagging markedly behind their age peers in regard to the development of discrimination and differential response—let alone the development of clear-cut attachment.[1]

The Secure-Attached Group

This is the largest of the three groups, consisting of sixteen children. These children were designated as "attached" according to the criterion of manifesting age-appropriate attachment behavior. Fourteen of the sixteen had reached at least Phase IV in the development of attachment behavior—showing following, approaching, active greeting, and the like. The other two—Alima (twenty-six weeks) and Samwendi (twenty-four weeks)—displayed Phase III behavior, which was appropriate for their age at the end of our period of observations. These sixteen children were judged to be secure in their attachment to their mothers according to the criterion of infrequent crying, as discussed in Chapter 10. To be sure, they might cry if parted from their mothers, or if particularly hungry, or they might be fussy during a period of illness or after weaning, but on the whole they cried very little, and when they were with their mothers they seemed especially content.

Frequent reference has been made to the attachment behavior of fourteen of the babies in Chapters 20, 21, and 22. Two babies, classified as secure-attached, were not mentioned there.

Sembajwe was older than any of the other babies at the beginning of our visits to him—over 19 months old—and hence his behavior was not pertinent to an examination of the development of attachment during the first year of life. Nevertheless, as the case notes in Chapter 18 make clear, Sembajwe was clearly

1 If one can judge from brothers and sisters, I could predict that these four babies, and also the fifth—Namitala—would eventually develop attachment to the mother. On the other hand, it seems likely that the attachment developed after the delay might be different in quality from the attachment of other babies who had less of a setback at the beginning.

attached to his mother before weaning, and, indeed, after weaning as well, but with a difference in behavior.

Senvuma was observed to be very clearly attached to his mother during the period of informal observations I made during my month in the village before the actual beginning of the project, although after weaning and separation, as described in Chapter 16, he was disturbed.

The Insecure-Attached Group

This group consists of seven babies. All of them had reached at least Phase IV in the development of attachment behavior and thus were classified as attached. They were designated as insecure according to the criterion of frequent crying. They were fussy babies who cried not just when parted from their mothers but even when with their mothers. As pointed out in Chapter 10, they cried to be picked up and cried when their mothers put them down and they sought to be in almost continuous physical contact with their mothers. Although seeking for proximity shows attachment, these seven children differed from the secure-attached group both in their relative inability to tolerate a little distance and in the fact that even when in proximity to the mother they continued to be fussy.

This was obviously a mixed group. Although they were all insecure, they were apparently insecure for different reasons. Two were chronically hungry and malnourished:

Waswa and *Nakato*, the older twins, were still breast-fed, although the mother obviously had insufficient milk to nourish two babies of their age. They were over thirteen months old when we began to visit and twenty-one months old at the end of the study—and still unweaned. The mother, having been deserted by the father, did not have any money with which to buy milk or any of the protein foods the twins so sorely needed to supplement their diet. As may be seen from the case summary in Chapter 13 the twins characteristically fussed during our visits, competed in their attempts to be picked up by the mother, and when picked up, persistently sought the breast and could not be soothed. Although after we provided dried milk supplement for them they began to gain and were somewhat less fussy, they still cried more frequently than the secure-attached babies.

One was chronically ill and fussy—*Magalita.* Although some of the secure-attached babies had periods of illness during which they were fussy, Magalita was ill and fussy throughout most of the first year of life. *Nakalema*, too, was ill a lot, although perhaps not more than some of the secure-attached babies. The mothers of four of the babies—*Muhamidi*, *Kasozi*, and the older twins—were themselves highly anxious, having been separated from or deserted by their husbands and finding it difficult to establish satisfactory mode of life apart from them. *Sulaimani's* mother must have been preoccupied with marital difficulties and with her conflict with the other wife in the household, and, indeed, Sulaimani seemed more secure after the other wife left the household.

There was some evidence that Nakalema was rejected by her mother, and this was perhaps the chief reason for her insecurity. Nevertheless, there may well have been an element of rejection in the other cases as well. Even Muhamidi's mother, who seemed so devoted and over protective, was so anxious and depressed that she could not give Muhamidi delighted attention even though she gave him the physical contact that he so constantly demanded. The mother of twins was at her wits' end; she constantly frustrated the babies by withholding the breast that they sought, and their persistent demands obviously contributed to her anxiety. In all of these cases there seemed to be a vicious spiral in which the baby's fussy demands exasperated the mother, who then overtly or covertly rejected the baby, who in turn responded to the rejection by anxiety and by increasing his demands. The mother's and the baby's anxiety seemed to be in spiraling interaction.

Furthermore, the infant-care practices used by the mothers of the insecure-attached babies may have contributed to the babies' insecurity. Kasozi's mother, for example, had to work most of the day in a desperate effort to establish a new garden in order to provide food for her family and she left Kasozi with a neighbor. The father's desertion thus affected Kasozi both through the mother's anxiety and by making it necessary for her to give him less care and attention than most of these Ganda mothers gave their babies. The same was true of the mother of twins, and, moreover, the lack of money for supplementary milk resulted not only in the twin's hunger and malnutrition but also in a frustrating practice of scheduled feedings, for this harassed mother could not possibly accede to the twins' demands for the breast.

Maternal-care variables related to the strength and security of attachment

On the basis of all that we know about the effects on subsequent development of deprivation of maternal care in infancy and early childhood, it is an essential condition of subsequent satisfactory interpersonal relations for a child to have formed an attachment to someone—his mother or a substitute for her. On the basis of all of our clinical knowledge of the relationship between early parent-child relations and later intimacies, it seems desirable for a baby to have a secure attachment to his mother rather than an insecure one. How then can infant-care practices foster the development of a secure attachment?

This question can be answered only tentatively on the basis of a sample as small as this one and observations as discontinuous and incomplete as ours of necessity were. Nevertheless, a search was made for variables in terms of which the three groups of babies could be differentiated, on the assumption that such variables might help us to understand how it came about that some babies became attached during the first year while others did not, and that the attachment of some was secure while that of others was insecure.

With respect to some of the variables we examined, even this small sample is heterogeneous enough that hypotheses of cause and effect relationships between infant care and "outcome" can be formulated; with respect to other variables the sample is too homogeneous for statistically significant relationships to be found, however significant such relationships may be in another population of cases. Moreover, our search for cause and effect relationships is a retrospective search. Therefore, it has the strength of exploiting to the utmost the relationship between an antecedent condition which appears to be a cause and a consequent outcome which appears to be the effect. It also has the weakness of the *post hoc ergo propter hoc* fallacy in reasoning, because not all antecedent conditions are in a cause and effect relationship to events that follow them.

In full realization of these dangers and limitations let us ask the question: "In terms of what variables can these groups be distinguished from one another?" Both a priori considerations and an examination of the case summaries suggest a number of possibilities. The variables that seem possibly significant may be classified roughly into two groups: those which are related to the feeding situation and those which are not. Let us first consider those which are not directly associated with feeding.

Warmth of mother

On a priori grounds it might be assumed that the warmth and affection expressed by the mother in interaction with her baby would have much to do with how secure and attached he became. All but two of these mothers, however, seemed warm and affectionate with their children. The exceptions were the mother of the non-attached twins, Wawsa and Nakato, and the mother of the insecure child, Nakalema, who struck me as rejecting. The others all seemed warm with their babies, holding them easily, seeming to enjoy the contact and treating them with apparent affection. In this sample, therefore, the warmth of the mother and her observed affectionate contact behavior do not explain the differences between groups, although there is no reason to suppose that warmth would not emerge as a significant variable in another sample with wider range.

Multiple caretakers

The deleterious effects on infants and young children of prolonged periods in institutions and hospitals have been attributed at least in part to the fact that in the typical institutional setting a child is given care by a large number of people, who do different things for him at different times and who come and go with shifts of assignments and changes of job so that the child has no opportunity to establish an attachment with any one of them. Moreover, under these circumstances a caretaker who is responsible for several children is unable to be sensitive to the signals of all and consequently does not time her caretaking interventions in synchrony with the individual child's needs and rhythms.[2] In the context of discussing maternal deprivation, Bowlby[3] said that "what is believed to be essential for mental health is that the infant and young child should experience a warm, intimate, and continuous relationship with his mother (or permanent mother-substitute) in which both find satisfaction and enjoyment."

Margaret Mead,[4] on the other hand, disputed the view that care by a single, continuous mother figure was a necessary condition for the development of healthy interpersonal relations. On the contrary, her experience in non-literate societies led her to believe that it was not necessary for a child to attach himself to any one person. Indeed, multiple mother-figures serve as catastrophe insurance. The loss of his mother is less disastrous for a child who has been used to other caretakers than for one who has had an exclusive relationship with his mother.

These two points of view are tangential to each other because care by multiple figures in an institutional setting is obviously a different case than care by several figures who spell each other off but who each have the opportunity to give individualized and sensitive attention. Nevertheless, the controversy directs attention to the possible effect of multiple caretakers on the development of attachment.

Although the mothers of the non-attached children in this study all shared their mothering duties with other people, most of the mothers of the other two groups of children did likewise, so that this variable fails to distinguish between the groups at a statistically significant level. Therefore, there is no evidence that care by several people necessarily interferes with the development of healthy attachment. And yet if the sharing of mothering duties unduly reduces the amount of care the mother (or any other one person, presumably) gives the baby, this does seem to have an adverse effect on the development of attachment, as may be seen in the next section.

Amount of care given by the mother

Each mother was rated in regard to the amount of care she gave her baby. The rating scale is given in Chapter 10, pp. 92–94, and the ratings are listed in Table 9. Ratings of 1 or 2 occur only in the non-attached group. The mothers of the

2 Myriam David and Genevieve Appell testify to this point: A study of nursing care and nurse-infant interaction, in B. M. Foss (ed.), *Determinants of Infant Behaviour* (London: Methuen, 1961).

3 John Bowlby, *Maternal care and mental health* (Geneva: World Health Organization, 1951), p. 11.

4 A cultural anthropologist's approach to maternal deprivation, in *Deprivation of maternal care, Public Health Papers, No. 14* (Geneva: World Health Organization, 1962), pp. 45–62.

non-attached infants regularly left their babies for long periods and shared their mothering duties with others even when they themselves were available to give the babies care. Three of the four ratings of 7 occurred in the secure-attached group. These mothers gave their babies much motherly care, and, indeed, took them along wherever they went. This variable does significantly differentiate between the three groups.[5]

Total amount of care

According to Margaret Mead's position, it might be expected that the total amount of care received from all caretakers combined might be the most crucial variable. A case such as Nabatanzi fits in with this position. Although her mother regularly left her for long periods, she had three other caretakers who gave her much care; she was alone and uncared for only when asleep. And she was clearly secure and attached until the time of weaning; her disturbance at weaning was, however, especially intense and prolonged.

Each child was rated in regard to the total amount of care he received. The rating scale is given on pp. 93–94, and the ratings are listed in Table 9. It may be seen from the table that nineteen babies received ratings of 7 or 6, implying much total care, and that this was true for five of the seven insecure-attached babies as well as for thirteen of the sixteen secure-attached babies. It is probably because of this very skewed distribution that this variable fails to differentiate significantly between the groups. The condition that is not adequately represented in this sample is a high amount of total care and a relatively small amount of care given by the mother, i.e., more infants like Nabatanzi, or with an even greater discrepancy between the ratings. Under these circumstances, and depending on the size of the discrepancy and the extent to which the supplementary care was given by one rather than by several people, one might expect either that the child would become more attached to another caretaker than to his mother or that he might become insecure because he had enough interaction with his mother to become attached to her but not enough to prevent him from feeling rejected, as, indeed, Nabatanzi seemed to feel after weaning.

In any event, the infants in the non-attached group all received low ratings in both total amount of care and in amount of care given by the mother. Nora and Kulistina were both left in cribs for much of the day, each in her own separate room, quite isolated. The younger twins were together, but spent much of the day by themselves either in a gocart outside the house or in an empty house.

5 A median test shows a $p < 0.05$; d.f. 2. The N used in the test was 27. Namitala was excluded from this and subsequent statistical tests on the grounds that she was so young that she may merely have been slightly delayed in the development of attachment behavior.

The term "motherly care" is too unspecific. The connotation is one of routine care, of tending to the baby's physical needs. Two more specific variables, which have emerged as highly significant in my subsequent study of American babies during the first year of life, are: (1) the sensitivity of the mother in responding to the baby's signals and (2) the amount and nature of the interaction between mother and baby. Sensitivity of response to signals implies that signals are perceived and correctly interpreted and that the response is prompt and appropriate. The signals may be of need and distress or they may be social signals. Sensitivity to signals tends to ensure that the care the mother gives the baby, including her playful interaction with him, is attuned to the baby's state and mood—at the baby's own timing, not at the mother's timing. Routine care may be undertaken with little interaction, It is interaction that seems to be most important, not mere care, and particularly conspicuous in mother-child pairs who have achieved good interaction is the quality of mutual delight which characterizes their exchanges.

These more subtle and complex variables are subsumed in the present ratings scales of amount of maternal and total care, but they are also obscured by being included together with notions of routine care, amount of time the mother is available, and the like. Unfortunately, a much more intensive and prolonged type of observation is necessary for assessing the subtleties of interaction than was undertaken in this study, and hence more subtle assessments cannot be made even retrospectively. Nevertheless, it is believed that the reason that the amount of care given by the mother emerges as a variable significantly related to the development of attachment is that interaction and sensitivity to signals have as a necessary condition that the mother is available to the child. If the mother is elsewhere, she obviously cannot respond to and interact with the baby, although her mere presence is no guarantee of sensitivity or interaction.

Mother's excellence as an informant

This variable first suggested itself as worthy of exploration when it was realized that the information that had been collected about the non-attached babies was more meager than that accumulated about other children to whom we had paid fewer visits. The rating scale devised for this variable is given in Chapter 5, pages 41–42, and the ratings are listed in Table 3.

Of course, more than mere excellence of information is implied by this scale. Implicit in a high rating is that the mother is sufficiently interested in the baby, that she is free enough of preoccupations and anxieties of her own, that she is sensitively perceptive of his idiosyncratic ways of behaving and of the ways in which he expresses his needs, wishes, and preferences, and that she takes enough interest and pleasure in him to want to talk about him, volunteering information about him rather than talking about other things. Implicit in a low rating is that the mother has not been attentive to her baby, so that she really does not know very much about his special ways of behaving—either because she is with him infrequently or because she is pre-occupied with other thoughts or activities when they are together. Also implicit in a low rating is that the mother, when interviewed about her baby, is more interested in other topics of conversation than she is in her baby.

The mothers of the non-attached infants were below the median in excellence as informants, while a higher proportion of the mothers of the secure-attached babies had really high ratings than did the mothers of the insecure-attached babies. This variable significantly differentiates between the three groups and hence seems related to the development of attachment.[6] Of course, in future research it would be better to rate directly the mother's perceptiveness of the baby and her pleasure and interest in him than to infer it from her excellence as an informant. Moreover, it is conceivable that a mother might be uncommunicative in interview for reasons totally unrelated to her attitude toward the baby—although this did not seem to happen in this sample. Next let us consider the variables related to the feeding situation.

Scheduled versus self-demand feeding

It will be recalled that eight babies were fed according to a schedule, and that of those fed " on demand," some were fed when the mothers judged them to be hungry and some also for comfort, even though they were obviously not hungry. An examination of Table 5 shows that the schedule-fed babies are found in each of the three groups, as are those fed on demand. There is a tendency for the mothers of the secure-attached babies to give the breast for comfort whereas none[7] of the mothers of the non-attached babies did so; this tendency, however, was below the level of statistical significance.

Repeated investigations of the effects of scheduled versus demand feedings have yielded similar inconclusive results.[8] If one believes, as I do, that the mother's sensitivity to the baby's signals significantly influences their interaction and his development, it is difficult to accept these findings. One reason for inconclusive findings is that the mothers interviewed defined self-demand feeding in so many different ways. It is common for women in this country to say that they feed on demand—when the baby is hungry—but to believe that he cannot possibly be hungry until four hours after the previous feeding, and in such cases a distinction between demand and scheduled feedings is negligible.

6 The median test yields $p < 0.05$; d.f. 2.

7 Except Namitala's mother, who has been excluded from these comparisons.

8 An excellent review of these investigations is given by Bettye M. Caldwell, The effects of infant care, in M. L. Hoffman and Lois W. Hoffman (eds.), *Review of child development research* (New York: Russell Sage Foundation, 1964).

In the Ganda investigation an effort was made to obtain a statement from the mother of how she defined demand feeding, and, moreover, we could observe how hunger signals and feeding were managed during our visits. In this case, it seems likely that the distinctions broke down by reason of the unavailability of the mothers who left their babies behind when gardening. Kasozi's mother fed him for comfort when they were together, for example, but she was absent for at least seven hours a day. It is hoped that future research will overcome difficulties such as these and settle the matter of whether or not demand feeding is better than scheduled feeding.

Mother's milk supply

Some of the mothers claimed to have considerable difficulty in maintaining an adequate supply of milk (see pp. 50–54 and Table 5). If the difficulty is a real one, it could make for insecurity as well as hunger in the baby—as indeed it did in the case of the older twins—both directly and indirectly, because it makes the mother anxious. If the difficulty is imagined, it could nevertheless affect the baby through the mother's anxiety. There were eleven mothers who reported no difficulty in milk supply; nine of them were mothers of secure-attached babies. The statistical test shows that the tendency in this sample is below the level of significance,[9] but since the sample is such a small one, the influence of milk supply on the nature of the infant-mother relationship with breast-fed babies cannot be dismissed as negligible.

Mother's attitude toward breast feeding

Fourteen mothers stated without qualification that they enjoyed breast feeding—thirteen when Namitala's mother is excluded (see Table 5). Twelve of these were mothers of secure-attached infants, one a mother of an insecure-attached infant; none were mothers of non-attached babies. It is thus obvious that this variable significantly differentiates the groups.[10]

The relationship between a mother and a breast-fed baby is undoubtedly a complex one in which the feelings of the mother and the response of the infant can interact in vicious or virtuous spirals. Suffice it to say that twelve of the sixteen secure-attached babies not only enjoyed their interaction with their mothers but had mothers who enjoyed at least the feeding interaction with them.

9 Chi square yielded a $p < 0.20$; d.f. 2.
10 Chi square yielded a $p < 0.01$; d.f. 2.

Summary

In summary, then, there were three variables which were found to be related significantly to the development of security and attachment: the mother's attitude to breast feeding, the amount of care she gave to the baby, and her excellence as an informant. A fourth variable—mother's milk supply—was only slightly below the level of statistical significance. All of these variables could be described as mere rough approximations of underlying variables which are more crucial in determining the development of infant-mother attachment.

These rough approximations served the useful purpose of directing attention toward a much more elaborate set of refined variables, which can be assessed only in a more intensive study. Some of these, which are believed to be significant in this Ganda sample and which are emerging as significant in my present study of American infants, are: the sensitivity of the mother in responding to the baby's signals of need and distress and to his social signals, and the promptness and appropriateness of her response; the amount of interaction she has with him and the amount of pleasure both derive from it; the extent to which her interventions and responses come at the baby's timing rather than her own; the extent to which she is free from preoccupation with other activities, thoughts, anxieties, and griefs so that she can attend to the baby and respond fully to him; and finally and obviously, the extent to which she can satisfy his needs, including his nutritional needs.

24

WEANING

To wean is "to teach (a child) to feed otherwise than from the breast." In Western societies where bottle feeding has supplanted breast feeding for all or part of the suckling period for many babies, the term "weaning" has become ambiguous. It can refer to the cessation of breast feeding, or it can refer to cessation of nutritional sucking. Thus, a child can be weaned from the breast to the bottle, and then finally from the bottle. In Buganda traditionally, of course, cessation of breast feeding meant also cessation of suckling as a means of gaining nourishment. Despite the fact that bottle feeding is becoming more common in Buganda, in this chapter we will concern ourselves only with weaning as the simultaneous cessation of breast feeding and nutritional sucking.

To clarify this issue does not clear up all difficulties, however. Should the term "weaning" refer to the whole process of introducing sources of nutrition other than mother's milk, or should it be reserved for the final "going away from the breast?"[1] It is our belief that *weaning* properly refers to the extended process of instituting feeding "other than from the breast"—otherwise what is the significance of the qualifiers "abrupt" or "gradual" or "final" weaning? Surely "final" weaning refers to the point at which the breast is no longer proffered to the child. It seems reasonable to reserve the terms "sudden" or "abrupt" for weaning which constitutes a change from a state in which the child is entirely or almost entirely breast-fed to one in which he is not fed by breast at all. On the other hand, "gradual" weaning refers to the processes of either gradually

1 The Luganda term for *weaning* is *okuva ku mabeere*, which may literally be translated "to go away from the breast."

DOI: 10.4324/9781003629337-28

dropping out breast feedings or gradually introducing foods or types of feeding that substitute for mother's milk and for breast feeding, or both. "Traumatic" weaning should, strictly speaking, be a term reserved for weaning under circumstances that produce unusual distress for the child. Thus, the term has idiosyncratic implications, for that which is traumatic for one baby may not be traumatic for another. Loosely speaking, however, traumatic weaning usually implies a method of weaning that introduces psychological stresses, such as rejection of the child, over and above mere cessation of breast feeding.

To anticipate the fuller presentation of our findings, weaning among the Ganda nowadays is gradual in both senses—foods other than mother's milk are gradually introduced to the child for some months before final weaning takes place, and the number of breast feedings during the day is gradually reduced, although perhaps not according to deliberate plan until a few weeks before final weaning. Whether weaning is traumatic or not in present-day Buganda is an individual matter—how the particular mother in question handles the transition with the particular child. Some mothers make every effort to avoid trauma by attempting to compensate the child for the loss of the breast by giving much loving attention and close physical contact. Others, from whatever motivation, make the occasion more traumatic by adding rejection to denial of the breast.

In the old days breast feeding was prolonged for as long as three years among the Ganda. Mair[2] observed that suckling continued until the child was three years old, although solid foods were begun as supplements to his diet when he was only a few months old. My three informants of ancient customs differed in their notions of the customary age of weaning. Mariamu, the oldest informant, said that it usually took place when the child was three or three and a half years old. The other old woman thought it was two or two and a half. The male informant, who was the youngest of the three, said that weaning took place at about one and a half, provided that the mother had not become pregnant in the meantime. The difference of their opinions seems nicely graded to the gradient of their ages, and probably reflects the way in which the age of weaning has in fact changed among the Ganda. All of the informants agreed that the most usual reason for weaning was a new pregnancy.

It seems likely that pregnancies have tended to follow one another in increasingly rapid succession in the years since the earliest European influence until the present day. The reason most commonly given by the Ganda for decreasing intervals between pregnancies is the influence of Christianity and the consequent decline in the incidence of polygynous marriages. Mariamu, my oldest informant, insisted, however, that the waning influence of old customs is a more important cause of increased rate of pregnancy and consequently of early

2 *An African People*, p. 56.

weaning than the decline of polygyny, for she points out that since polygyny was the privilege of the rich, it was not common even in ancient times.

All three informants of old customs agreed that it was wrong for a woman to continue to suckle her child after she became pregnant again, and hence weaning was obligatory as soon as a new pregnancy was discovered, regardless of the age of the child. The two younger informants expressed the belief that the mother's milk turns sour when she becomes pregnant, and the child would become ill if he suckled.[3]

It was agreed by my informants that weaning in the old days was abrupt in the sense that the breast, which had previously been available on demand, was suddenly and completely denied to the child. It was not necessarily abrupt in the sense of a sudden transition from unsupplemented breast feeding to solid foods, for these were customarily given at least by the time a child could walk. The abruptness of withdrawal of the breast was reinforced by putting chili powder (*kaamulali*) on the nipple so that if the child tried to suck he would find it unpleasant. In this regard the old Ganda custom resembles that of the Zulu[4] who use bitter aloes for the same purpose. Although with the Zulu the custom of making the nipple unpleasant to the child was observable at least in rural districts as late as 1956 or thereabout, one of our informants (who must have been about sixty years old) said she had only witnessed the procedure once in Buganda. On the other hand, our oldest informant, Mariamu, claimed to be quite familiar with the practice. She said that some babies persisted in suckling and managed to suck off the hot-tasting substance. If this happened, the mother smeared an even more evil-tasting substance on the nipple and told the child that it was feces and would make him sick if he sucked it (At three years of age, presumably, a child could understand this statement.) The other old woman who informed us about Ganda customs volunteered that most mothers gave the child both food and cuddling at the time of weaning to compensate for withdrawal of the breast.

3 These informants used the term *obwosi* for the illness that resulted from breast feeding during pregnancy. My Luganda dictionary defines the term as used in the phrase *akaana kalina obwosi*, which is translated: "the child suffers from lack of mother's care because she is expectant or has a new baby." Welbourn informs me (personal communication) that *obwosi* is sometimes used as a translation of kwashiorkor. Although kwashiorkor is known to be a protein-deficiency disease, it is known also to be affected by psychological factors. Thus, for example, Géber and Dean report a high incidence of mother-child separation after weaning in a sample of children with kwashiorkor; they found also that the mother's care during treatment was a significant factor in determining outcome. (M. Géber and R. F. A. Dean, The pyschological changes accompanying kwashiorkor, *Courrier*, 1956, *6*, 1—14.)

4 Ronald C. Albino and V. J. Thompson, The effects of sudden weaning on Zulu children, *Brit. J. med. Psychol.*, 1956, *29*, 183.

Today, if one inquires when a baby is to be weaned, there are two standard replies: "when he can walk," or "when he is a year old."[5] Since it is usual for a Ganda baby to be able to walk at about a year, these replies amount to the same thing, and some informants included both in their reply.

Eleven babies in our sample were weaned from the breast before the termination of the research. Excluding Kulistina, who was not put to the breast after the third day of life, the range of age at weaning varied from seven and a half to twenty-two months, with the median at twelve and a half months.[6]

We inquired of the mothers in our sample when their other older children had been weaned. Excluding one child, who was weaned at the age of three months because "something went wrong with the breast," the range was from six to eighteen months, with a median of twelve months. Gone are the days when a baby was suckled at the breast for two or three years—gone, at least, among the semi-acculturated families near Kampala. Sembajwe, who was not weaned until the age of twenty-two months, is an exception and is therefore of particular interest.

Although the norm for weaning in this semi-acculturated population is about one year of age, some mothers planned in advance to wean their babies earlier. In every instance these mothers—the mothers of Nora, William, and Nakiku—were guided by European customs, and so was Kulistina's mother when she determined the weaning date of two older children.[7] As it turned out, of these babies only Nora was weaned before she was a year old. Kyimba and Maryamu were in fact weaned earlier—at thirty-four and thirty-seven weeks respectively—Maryamu because her mother became pregnant, and Kyimba possibly for the same reason.

In the absence of a new pregnancy, failure of the mother's milk was not in itself considered sufficient cause for weaning. Both Aida and Magalita were suckled for months after their mother's milk supply had dwindled to an insignificant amount. On the other hand, Lusiya's mother weaned an older child abruptly when a year old because she had been bitten by a snake and feared the venom in her system would poison the milk.

5 Welbourn states in *Baganda Childhood* that weaning marks a period of intensive promotion from infantile dependence. Although this "promotion" used to take place at about three years of age, now, when weaning occurs at about one year of age, the infant is obviously less well equipped to manage an independent and self-sufficient role. The belief that a child should be able to walk before being weaned is, perhaps, a significant residual of an implicit belief that weaning marked the end of dependent, indulged infancy and the beginning of self-sufficiency.

6 This median agrees closely with the figure of 12.7 months given as the age of weaning for Ganda babies from uneducated or slightly educated families. Welbourn, Bottle Feeding: A Problem of Modern Civilization, p. 159.

7 Welbourn (*ibid.*) reports that the mean age of weaning of babies from highly educated families in Buganda is 8.9 months.

Some babies in our sample were not weaned as early as their mothers had originally planned. William was one of these; he had a prolonged attack of diarrhea about the time that his mother intended to wean him; thus weaning seemed unwise. Similarly, Kasozi had even been started on the weaning process when he became ill, and weaning was stopped and postponed till a later date. On the other hand, some children, like Nabatanzi and Lusiya, were weaned according to plan, despite being ill at the time.

The ability to ingest other foods was a factor taken into consideration. Nora's weaning was delayed a month or two because of her refusal to take milk other than mother's milk. The mother of the younger twins said that the date of weaning would depend not merely upon the ability to walk, but also upon the ability to tolerate solid foods and upon her own milk supply. Sometimes walking does not occur at the anticipated time, and so weaning is delayed—as with Mutebe, Magalita, and Paulo's retarded older sister. Moreover, mere ability to take a few steps is not considered the criterion; walking should be well established before weaning.

Availability of milk substitutes was another consideration for the mothers in our sample.[8] The mother of the older twins weaned two of her three older children before they were a year of age, and explained that their father had then been available to buy milk for them. Similarly, Muhamidi's mother thought she might wean him earlier than fifteen months (her chosen date) if her estranged husband could be persuaded to provide money for milk. The older twins themselves were unweaned at twenty-one months, partly because there was no money available for milk, but perhaps chiefly because the mother believed that custom demanded that the father give permission for twins to be weaned, and he was many miles away and out of touch. As for Sembajwe—who was not weaned until twenty-two months—his mother made her own rules; she apparently believed in long breast feeding, even though this was out of fashion among her contemporaries.

It is commonly believed that present-day weaning among the Ganda is abrupt, as it was in the old days. The reason for this is that when one asks when the baby was weaned, the mother always mentions a specific day, and does not imply in any way that the process of weaning occupied an extended period. From the beginning of our inquiries we were interested to ascertain whether weaning was an abrupt transition from ad libitum access to the breast to none, or whether it was a more gradual transition. From the beginning it became clear that contemporary weaning, at least in the semi-acculturated group, is gradual rather than abrupt. Not only are solid foods, as well as juices and milk, introduced into the diet

8 Richards (personal communication) states that it is very uncommon elsewhere in Buganda to have milk available for babies. The implication is that in the area close to Kampala, from which our sample is drawn, the influence of child welfare clinics and other health educators has radiated out and modified practices even in families which did not previously attend the clinic.

when the child is but a few months of age, but also the number of breast feedings a day is gradually reduced until finally breast feeding is stopped altogether.

There are two main phases of deliberate weaning. In the first the breast is denied to the baby in the daytime, although he is allowed his accustomed access to the breast at night. The second phase is the final weaning, in which the breast is denied also at night.

To us this seems an inverted kind of procedure, for our usual practice is to gradually reduce the number of nighttime feedings, and when these have been dropped, to cut down on the feedings during the day. The Ganda system makes more sense after consideration than it does at first glance. First of all, weaning, in all but exceptional cases, is a shift from breast feeding to adult modes of eating,[9] and not from breast to bottle and then from bottle to adult modes of eating. It is only the abnormally early weanings among the Ganda—weanings necessitated by some disastrous interference with the mother's milk supply—that are from breast to bottle. Secondly, Ganda babies are fed, for the most part, on demand and often for comfort. Therefore, it is not as simple to be systematic about dropping a specific feeding as it is when feedings are scheduled. Finally, there is the fact that supplementary foods are introduced at an early age and (at least in our sample) in variety and quantity almost as rapidly as the baby can tolerate the change.

Since the baby approaching final weaning is already receiving much nourishment through supplementary feedings of milk, juices, and/or solids throughout the day, he tends to demand the breast far less for the reason of hunger. Especially if he is a schedule-fed baby who has never been able to gain access to the breast by simple demand, it is an easy matter to drop daytime breast feedings. Even the baby fed on demand may well have become accustomed to long periods during the day without the breast while his mother is away working in the garden. Thus it is that Ganda mothers tend to view the dropping of daytime feedings as an easy first step in weaning.

At night, even the schedule-fed babies tend to be released from their schedules and are fed when they awaken and cry. There did not seem to be any tendency for the babies in our sample to wake less frequently as they grew older. Somehow it is the nighttime feedings that seem most special—perhaps both to mother and to child—and it is these that are left until the last. (Since only one of the mothers voiced objection to nighttime feedings, and a fairly high proportion of the

9 Traditionally, the Ganda ate with their fingers, and even among families who now use spoons, it is considered appropriate for babies to eat with their fingers. All of the babies in our sample who were weaned were given milk to drink from a cup, in addition to solid foods that could be eaten with the fingers. In a preliminary draft, I used the phrase "weaned to the cup," but was informed by both Welbourn and Richards that in most of Buganda, people, including babies, drink only tea from a cup. See Hebe F. Welbourn, Weaning among the Baganda, *J. trop. Pediat.*, 1963, *9*, 14–24.

mothers made an unqualified statement that they enjoyed breast feeding, it may well be that there is special enjoyment in the relaxed intimacy of a nighttime feeding.) And in the case of babies fed on demand, the final phase of weaning is an all-or-none affair. No one dreams of trying to train a baby who has been fed three times a night to wake only once to be fed before finally training him to sleep through. All the nighttime feedings are dropped at once. Nowadays, few babies sleep in their mothers' beds until weaning; most of them have been in their own beds for some time. One can imagine how senseless and depriving final weaning must seem to a baby who sleeps with his mother; little wonder that in the old days babies had a ritual separation of two days at the time of weaning.

Although any extended inquiry about the weaning process will elicit the information that it is gradual, the Luganda phrase for weaning, translated as "going away from the breast," focuses upon the final withdrawal of the breast, which occurs with the cessation of nighttime feedings. This focus constituted a great difficulty in our research. We made a practice of inquiring about weaning plans in the case of any baby who was old enough to be facing weaning in the foreseeable future. In every case but one, the mothers explained in detail a gradual weaning procedure. We then explained our special interest in the child's response to weaning and exacted a promise that we would be informed in advance of the weaning process so that we could plan to visit immediately after the first step was taken and frequently until the weaning was completed. The mothers agreed, but in every case they nevertheless began weaning—i.e., dropping the daytime feedings—without informing us. Despite all the gradual preliminaries, weaning to them meant "final weaning"—the final dropping of nighttime feedings. The most cooperative mothers were as much at fault in this regard as those who were less willing to cooperate.[10]

All but one of the mothers planned a gradual weaning. Muhamidi's mother, however, did not approve of it. She believed that a child could not understand that he was to be denied the breast during the day if he still received it at night. Thus, in order to avoid frustration and misunderstanding, she planned to wean Muhamidi abruptly, as she had with older siblings. The only abrupt weaning that actually took place in our sample, however, was in the case of Senvuma. Senvuma's mother, who was unmarried, had an opportunity to marry a man, not Senvuma's father, who did not welcome the baby. Consequently Senvuma

10 Although the semantic difficulty was clear enough, I am inclined to believe that the same trouble could occur in the absence of any language barrier. In the course of a similar research project in the United States, I have noted that mothers can express their allegiance to one plan or practice and they suddenly shift to quite another, prompted by the exigencies of the moment. I cannot imagine that they would either refrain from the shift because of what they had previously told me or postpone it until they had informed me. Infant care is much more than the application of preplanned procedures; it involves personal interaction between baby and mother, and the interaction can modify the plan, as can other events and influences in the life of mother and child.

was weaned, sent to relatives, and the mother was married—all within a day or so. The only other departure from the norm of the sample in regard to mode of weaning came with William's mother—in respect to her practices with her other children —for William himself was not weaned. William's mother adhered to the practice of scheduled feeding; like Europeans she first cut down nighttime feedings, and then gradually she cut down on the daytime feedings until there was only one left; weaning was complete when this final feeding was eliminated.

That weaning was expected to be traumatic was demonstrated by the number of mothers who asked our advice about methods of weaning that might reduce its distressing effects. We have some information about how the mothers intended to respond to their babies' distress at weaning and further information of how older siblings had been treated. We also have information of how nine of the ten[11] weaned babies in our sample were treated.

Some of the mothers, in one way or another, adhered to the customary belief that a complete break was the best way to handle weaning. Petero's mother had sent her four other babies away to live with relatives at the time of final weaning. In our sample this was done with Senvuma, as stated above. Muhamidi's mother also believed in abrupt weaning but not in concomitant separation. She kept the baby with her, even sleeping with him, but bound her breasts so that baby could not reach them. Lusiya's mother believed that it facilitated weaning to stay away from the baby as much as possible. When Lusiya cried at night she did not pick her up but directed the father to do so. Moreover, she left Lusiya in the care of the nine-year-old girl who lived with them more often than she had before weaning. The purpose of this practice was to make Lusiya more independent of her mother now that she no longer needed to be fed by her.

Most of the mothers in our sample did not share these traditional beliefs. They believed that a baby at the time of weaning must be reassured of his mother's love for him and must not be allowed to interpret withdrawal of the breast as a rejection. Consequently, they believed in picking up the baby when he cried and in soothing him, although in doing so the mother tried to comfort him in such a way that he was not frustrated by an available breast that was denied to him. Thus she held him with his head to the right side away from the dress opening, or bounced him about on her back. The mothers of six of our weaned babies carried out these beliefs in practice while Nabatanzi's mother, who always had given much physical contact anyhow, merely continued to behave as she did before, giving no more and no less. Sembajwe's mother added verbal explanations of weaning to her cuddling, and Sembajwe was old enough to understand.

11 We are excluding Kulistina from the total of ten since she was bottle-fed throughout the study. The tenth child, about whom we have no information, was Magalita, who was weaned just as our field visits came to an end.

Even some of those who recognized that the baby might react badly to the rejection implicit in weaning nevertheless thought that offering milk—dried skim milk prepared with tea or water or fresh cow's milk—might lessen the disturbance when a child cried at night wanting his mother's breast. In the cases of Nakiku and Lusiya the father was detailed for this duty, but Nabatanzi and Kasozi, who had been deserted by their fathers, received the milk from their mothers.

Despite their awareness of the significance of weaning for a baby as marking a change in his relationship with his mother and its possible significance as an occasion for hunger, few of these mothers gave thought to its significance as a loss of sucking satisfaction. A very young baby might be bottle-fed if breast feeding were impossible, as in the case of Kulistina, who was bottle-fed from the third day of life, and also with Mutebe's older brother, who was weaned to the bottle at three months of age when his mother developed "trouble with her breast." There were only two reports of babies being weaned from the breast to the bottle after reaching the age of being able to ingest any significant proportion of solid food; these were older siblings of Kulistina and Maryamu. Maryamu's sister was weaned to the bottle at six months of age when her mother became pregnant again and was fed according to a four-hour schedule as she had been when breast-fed. Kulistina's mother weaned two of her babies at the age of eight months, first to the bottle, and then, two months later, to a cup. For a month after that they were given milk to drink during the night; only then were they considered old enough to get through the night without being hungry. Throughout these accounts the emphasis was upon relief of hunger and providing proper nutrition; there was no recognition of a baby's need for sucking as such.

We have information about the response to weaning in only eight[12] cases.

Three of these babies had been schedule-fed—Maryamu, Nakiku, and Nora—and five had been fed on demand—Sembajwe, Nabatanzi, Kasozi, Kyimba, and Lusiya. Although eight babies are too few to generalize about, it is of interest to note that the weaning disturbance was much less marked in the schedule-fed babies than in the babies who had been fed on demand.

Nakiku and Nora showed little disturbance when the daytime feedings were discontinued. They cried very little, although they did try to get at the breast, despite the fact that they had shown no initiative in reaching for the breast before weaning began. Maryamu showed somewhat more disturbance and cried a lot for the first few days. A week later when she was thirty-seven weeks old, Maryamu's nighttime feedings were eliminated. She cried a lot the first night but showed no further disturbance, and her general behavior seemed unchanged.

12 Senvuma is not included, since his weaning was both abrupt and complicated by separation from his mother.

Nakiku, finally weaned at fifty-two weeks, was only slightly disturbed. She cried a lot the first night and again on the third, but after this she slept through without waking. She had shown a very strong attachment to her mother before weaning, following her mother everywhere she went. After final weaning she followed her mother less, and seemed much more independent of her. Nora, finally weaned at forty-nine weeks, cried the first night and was fussy for two days, but the fussiness may have been due partly to a cold. Neither Maryamu nor Nora followed their mothers before they were weaned; Maryamu had not yet learned to crawl, and Nora was one of the few babies who seemed not to have developed any significant degree of attachment to her mother.

The five babies who had been fed on demand showed considerably more disturbance either in the first phase of weaning or in the second, or in both. Three of them were considerably disturbed at the cessation of daytime feedings. Sembajwe, the oldest, was very fussy for three weeks before the nighttime feedings were discontinued also. He wanted to be near his mother all the time and was constantly hanging onto her skirts. He kept trying to get at his mother's breast; he lost his appetite; he refused to drink milk; and he wet the bed more than usual. When he was finally weaned at twenty-two months of age, he cried the first night and then the disturbance was over. His general behavior changed markedly. He became much more independent—no longer a baby but a sturdy little boy. Moreover, he spontaneously assumed responsibility for his own elimination control; he stopped wetting the bed and went outside the house when he wanted to pass water.

With the other four demand-fed babies the story was different, perhaps because they were considerably younger. All of them showed disturbance which continued for some weeks, and, indeed, until the end of our field visits. Nabatanzi was forty-nine weeks old and scarcely recovered from an illness when her daytime feedings were discontinued. Then, for three weeks or more, and again for some weeks following final weaning at fifty-six weeks, she was much fussier than usual and wanted to be close to her mother all the time, protesting the slightest separation. Her appetite diminished. The most marked change in her behavior was the emergence of sharp displays of temper in which she would hit her mother. Her mother interpreted her anger as directed at the breast, which she was said "not to care for" and yet sometimes tried to reach.

Kasozi's daytime feedings were dropped when he was fifty-seven weeks old, although a week earlier his mother had tried to drop them but had reinstated them when he became ill. For two weeks he clung to his mother more than before and stayed close to her. He could no longer be left with a neighbor while his mother worked in the garden but had to be taken along with her. When he was fifty-nine weeks old the nighttime feedings were dropped. He cried a lot during the first three days, and four out of the five first nights were very disturbed. For a week his appetite was poor, and for a month he continued to cling to his mother and protest the slightest separation. Shortly after final weaning he began to cover up his mother's breast if he saw it. "He doesn't like it; he doesn't want to see it."

Lusiya's weaning began when she was fifty weeks old. She was said to show little disturbance. At fifty-two weeks the nighttime feedings were also dropped. For the first five nights she cried a great deal, and if her mother came near her, Lusiya hit her breast. She cried whenever her mother was not in sight, however, and during the day she followed her mother much more than she had before and more frequently demanded to be picked up and held. For some time she continued to wake twice every night and cry, and her clinging behavior continued unabated for eleven weeks, when our study came to an end.

Kyimba was only thirty-two weeks old when his mother dropped his daytime feedings, and we do not have information about his response to this. He was thirty-four weeks old when he was finally weaned. For five weeks afterward he protested when his mother left him for a moment and he tried to follow her. He fussed to be picked up and continued to fuss even when his mother held him. He cried almost continuously the first night and hit his mother for withholding the breast. For five weeks he continued to cry so much at night that he was given phenobarbitone at the clinic. Until the end of the study, when he was forty-three weeks old, he continued to be fussy and to demand frequently to be picked up, although he no longer showed quite so much separation anxiety.

These findings, although stemming from only eight cases, suggest that weaning from the breast means different things to babies fed according to a schedule than to babies fed on demand, and especially (as in the case of four of our five demand-fed babies) if the breast is given at least on occasion merely for comfort. To the schedule-fed babies, weaning seems to cause little or no change in the baby's relationship with his mother. To the demand-fed babies, weaning seems to imply rejection by and separation from the mother. The baby tends to respond with separation anxiety, and also with increased ambivalence, as indicated by hitting the breast or other behavior that the mother interprets as disliking the breast. The disturbance cannot be attributed to traumatic weaning procedures, for only Lusiya's mother withheld the baby from herself as well as her breast, and Sembajwe's, Kasozi's, and Kyimba's mothers tried to give their babies special comfort and soothing to make up for withholding the breast.

My own explanation of the difference stems from my view of the way in which a baby's attachment to his mother develops. The hypothesis that I believe best fits the facts is that a baby's attachment to his mother is founded on and grows out of his own behavior towards her, strengthened (or weakened) by the kind of response his mother makes to his behavior. One of these behavior patterns is the whole constellation of responses related to feeding—first the innate responses of sucking and "rooting" or searching for the nipple. If, whenever the baby emits this kind of behavior, he is pretty consistently given the breast, he in a true sense is permitted to take the initiative and to gain control over feeding. If breast feeding continues long enough, the initiative is more conspicuous to the observer, as in the case of these Ganda babies who could reach for the breast, fumble in their mother's clothing, and succeed eventually in managing the breast by themselves; and once locomotion was acquired, these babies could crawl across the room to the mother and scramble up onto her lap, no longer needing to be picked up. Under these circumstances, it would seem, feeding behavior becomes an integral part of the whole organization of attachment behavior. Thus, when the time for weaning comes, frustration of the baby's demand and search for the breast disturbs the whole organization of his attachment to the mother.

In contrast, the baby who is fed according to schedule is not allowed to take initiative in the feeding relationship and never gains control over feeding. Under these circumstances it would appear that his feeding responses do not get built into the organization of his attachment behavior; consequently, weaning does not affect his attachment to his mother. He is forced to be passive in regard to feeding, and it appears that to passively receive satisfaction from his mother does not contribute to his relationship to her as a loved person. The argument here is that attachment does not grow through receiving but through actively reaching out and attaching oneself. The schedule-fed baby may attach himself to his mother through other attachment behavior but not through feeding behavior—which remains more or less independent of his relationship to his mother as a person.

This study of Ganda babies does not throw any light on responses to weaning from the bottle, which is what *weaning* now means to many Western babies. My guess would be that there is little disruption of the mother-infant relationship as a result of the weaning of bottle-fed babies. Furthermore, this study does not give evidence of the effects of weaning from the breast in cases where the weaning occurs early in the first year of life, say, at four months of age. Since this early weaning takes place before the infant has become attached to his mother, it seems inconceivable that it could disrupt the infant-mother relationship. If a mother, having weaned her baby, entered into much less interaction then than before weaning, the establishment of a secure attachment might be delayed or distorted, but an attachment cannot be disrupted before it has been formed.

25

MOTHER-CHILD SEPARATION

In 1951, John Bowlby,[1] commissioned by the World Health Organization, published a review of research and practices pertinent to the care of young children separated from their families. He concluded that two sets of circumstances could have adverse effects upon development—effects that sometimes were lasting and resistant to reversal. First, infants and young children were adversely affected by the severe deprivation they experienced in institutions and hospitals where both understaffing and the organization of nursing duties precluded adequate substitute mothering, especially when the children's exposure to such deprivation was prolonged. Secondly, a young child old enough to have formed an attachment to his mother, but not yet old enough to be able to maintain a relationship with her throughout a period of absence, was disturbed by the breach of ties when he was separated from his mother. This disturbance could have adverse long-term effects, particularly if the separation ushered in a period of deprivation or if the experience of separation was repeated. Most of the research evidence available to Bowlby made it impossible to disentangle the effects of separation from those of deprivation, because both had occurred.

Bowlby's monograph attracted more widespread attention than had the research reports upon which it was based and it stirred up a storm of controversy.[2] In part, the controversy hinged upon the question of whether an infant or young

1 *Maternal care and mental health* (Geneva: World Health Organization, 1951).

2 A discussion of the controversial issues and subsequent research pertinent to them is reported by the present author in a paper entitled The effects of maternal deprivation: A review of findings and controversy in the context of research strategy, in *Deprivation of maternal care: a reassessment of its effects, Public Health Papers No. 14* (Geneva: World Health Organization, 1962), pp. 97–165.

DOI: 10.4324/9781003629337-29

child could experience any adverse effects as a result of mere separation from his mother, and whether these could not all be attributable either to an unstimulating institutional environment or to the trauma of illness or family disruption that necessitated the separation in the first place.

In 1954 there was no incontrovertible evidence that the sheer breach of mother-child ties could lead to adverse consequences in the absence of other pathogenic circumstances. Therefore, a study of mother-child separation as it occurred among the Ganda seemed to offer the critical case of "pure" separation. Since separation had traditional sanction, it did not necessarily imply either that the child was being rejected by his mother or that the family was disorganized. The child, when separated, was not sent to an institutional environment but to live with a substitute mother who was, often enough, eager to have him and to give him loving care. If, under these circumstances, the child experienced distress upon leaving his mother and a setback in his development, this would provide the crucial proof that "pure" separation could have adverse effects.[3] This issue made an examination of mother-child separation among the Ganda of particular interest, and I inquired very carefully about it.

My informants of traditional customs had much light to throw on the matter. They made it clear that there were two traditional forms of separation. The first was a ritual separation at the time of weaning and was obligatory by custom. The second occurred later and was optional and variable. Let us consider the ritual separation first. At the time of final weaning, when the child was no longer to be given the breast, not even at night, he was taken to either the maternal or paternal grandmother, kept by her for two days, and then returned to the mother. It was believed that this separation enabled the child to "forget the breast." In some cases the child then remained at home, in other cases he was sent back to the grandmother. But it was believed that unless he was returned to his mother for at least one night—the third night after weaning—he would become ill and might even die.

After the child had been returned to his mother, it was common, but by no means invariable, for him to be separated from her for a second time. The reasons for this second separation varied from one case to another and, in general, were ostensibly in the interests of the child's welfare. The period intervening between the first brief ritual separation and a second, long-term separation was variable.

My oldest informant, Mariamu, stated that it was usually the grandmother, either maternal or paternal, who was chosen by the parents as the child's foster mother. The choice was made, however, according to who was known to love

3 In the meantime, other evidence has accumulated to answer this question' For example, Leon J. Yarrow (Research in dimensions of early maternal care, *Merrill-Palmer Quarterly*, 1963, *9*, 101–14) found clear-cut separation disturbance in 86 per cent of children aged six months when separated from a foster mother (who had reared them from birth) and placed in an adoptive home.

the child and to want to have him. If neither grandmother wanted the child, another female relative might be selected as the foster mother, preferably either the father's sister or the mother's sister. If no one seemed really to want the child, and the parents were nevertheless set on the separation, they might take him surreptitiously to the home of the grandmother and leave him without seeking her consent. Under these circumstances the grandmother was obliged to accept the child.

Mariamu said that in the "old days" it was desirable to send a child to live with the maternal grandmother or another of the mother's relatives. She explained that it was customary for the *Kabaka* to recruit young children to be brought up in his court. Although this was an honor and had certain advantages, including the possibility of advancement through favoritism, the danger was always great. Mariamu said that in the old days the *Kabaka* was cruel and often had members of his household thrown to the crocodiles if they incurred his wrath—or sometimes at a mere whim. Children were recruited for the court by the heads of the clans, each recruiting only within his own clan. If the child was absent from his own home when the recruiting officer came, he could escape recruitment; if he lived with his mother's relatives, who were not of his own clan, he was safe when the recruiting officer arrived—for he belonged to another clan. This informant offered no other explanation of the common practice of separation.

The other female informant, who had no firsthand experience of the period during which evasion of the *Kabaka*'s recruiting officers was a cogent reason for separation, offered as a reason the birth of a new baby in the family. The mother sent the older child away so that she would have her full attention to devote to the new baby. The separation might occur at or just before the birth of the new baby, or it might occur earlier in the period of pregnancy. She agreed that a grandmother was the customary foster mother but stated that if there was no grandmother living, the child would not be sent away.

The above was the sum total of what I could find out about traditional customs of mother-child separation. As I talked to informants about present-day customs, however, the picture became more complicated. The consensus was that the chief reason for separation was the birth of a new baby and the mother's need to be relieved of the demands of the toddler in order to devote her full attention to the baby. In a society in which each woman was tied to her garden, the grandmother could not come to visit and help out; she could help with the older children in the family only if they were sent to visit her.

Although children were no longer taken from their families to be reared at court, nor sent away to avoid being taken, the present-day equivalent was to send a child away in the interests of his education. Among the relatively well-to-do, school-age children were sent to boarding schools. Among the less well-to-do, a school-age child might be sent to stay with relatives who lived close to a school that the child might attend as a day pupil. Furthermore, a child might be sent to live with relatives who, either because of wealth or education, or both, might give him more advantages than his own family could offer him. Paulo's parents repeatedly suggested, for example, that I take Paulo back to America with me because I could give him so much that they were unable to provide for him.

Finally, the instability of marriages and other more informal unions resulted in mother-child separation. The child belonged to the father and the father's clan. If the parents separated, the father might permit the baby or very young child to go with his mother, but he had the right to keep the child or to claim him at any future time.

How frequent is mother-child separation among the Ganda at the present time? In 1954 Dr. Hebe Welbourn[4] informed me that 16 per cent of the children between one and three years of age attending child welfare clinics were living with a grandmother or an aunt and were apart from their mothers. She suggested, however, that this sample was probably not representative of the village populations in regard to separation because the clinic mothers had been taught that separation was dangerous for young children.

At the outset of my study it had been my intention to focus on the effects of separation. I was under the misapprehension that separation commonly took place at the time of weaning, that is, at about a year of age. I expected that from one-third to one-half of the sample might be separated at that time, and that it would be interesting to follow both separated and non-separated children for a period of weeks after weaning in order to compare the groups. As it turned out, only one child in the sample was separated. This was not only because —as I later discovered—separation tended to take place not at weaning but later when or just before a new baby was born, but also because the mothers in my sample felt that the research was bringing so many benefits to the children in the sample that it would be disadvantageous for the child to be sent away from home.

But inquiry about separations of older siblings suggested that the practice of mother-child separation was quite common. In our sample twelve mothers practiced mother-child separation. Nine mothers are excluded from consideration, eight because the child was an "only" child and still unweaned, and one because of inadequate information about the older children. This leaves only five who had not sent any of the older children away from home—the mothers of William, Maryamu, Nora, and Kulistina (all of whom were relatively acculturated) and the mother of the older twins.

Seven mothers had sent older children away to be reared elsewhere. Namitala's mother regularly sent away one child as soon as the next was born, and thus had four children being reared elsewhere. Muhamidi's mother did likewise, although she did not always permit the separation to continue indefinitely; indeed, in

4 Annual Report for Child Welfare Unit, 1954–55.

her case I got the impression that the older children had multiple separation experiences, being brought home then sent away again several times, which could be expected to be more disrupting than a single shift. Aida's mother had sent her two older children away to be reared by relatives and four others had died during the first two years of life. I had the impression that she was afraid that the other two would die also if they were brought back home. Lusiya's mother had sent a two-year-old child away when she discovered she was pregnant with Lusiya and had not brought her back. Mutebe's mother had done the same with a ten-month-old baby when she became pregnant with Mutebe, although she subsequently brought him home again. The mother of the younger set of twins had left behind a young child of a previous marriage when she married again. Finally, Nakiku's mother had left behind a daughter born out of wedlock when she became married, although the child was ten years old and thus was outside the age range of greatest vulnerability to separation.

Four of the mothers in the sample practiced short-term separation. Petero's mother had sent each of her four older children away for several months at the time of weaning. Paulo's mother had sent a toddler away when she discovered she was pregnant with Paulo but had brought her back again after Paulo was born. Magalita's mother usually separated her babies for a few months at the time of weaning. Kasozi's sister was two years old when he was born; she was sent to stay with her aunt, but it was a relatively brief separation, lasting only a few weeks.

During the period of the project only one of the children in the sample was separated—Senvuma. But of the thirteen children who were tested by Dr. Géber, only six were available for all retests. Kasozi's family had moved and Sembajwe's mother refused, but five were unavailable because they had been separated. Lusiya was sent away to live with an aunt when she was two years old, Muhamidi was sent to a grandmother at the age of four, and Magalita was sent to a grandmother when she was five. Mutebe was sent to his grandmother when two, and at three his mother left home and he was claimed by his father, with whom he had never lived. Nakiku's mother also went away and left her with her father when she was four.

The overwhelming impression is therefore that mother-child separation was frequent in this sample of Ganda families. The circumstances of our observations make it impossible, however, to assess the effects of separation on the development of the children in all but a few cases.

Senvuma

Senvuma's story has been told in more detail in Chapter 16 and will merely be reviewed here. He was born out of wedlock. At ten months of age his very close, intimate relationship with his mother was abruptly terminated when

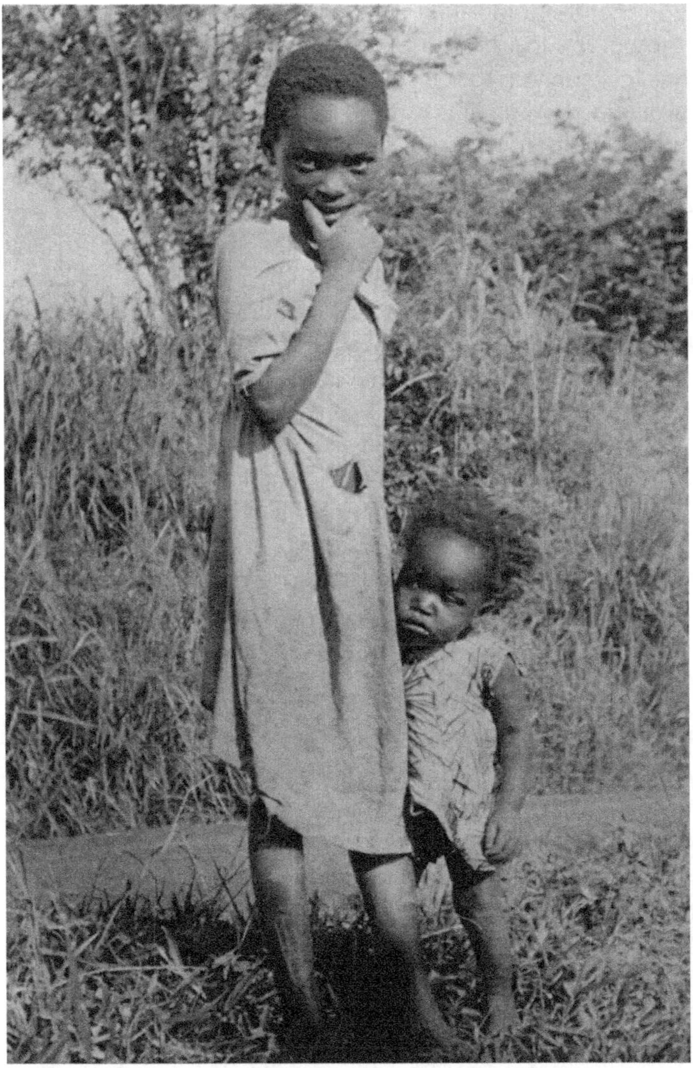

FIGURE 35 Senvuma at thirteen months with his nursemaid. Since his weaning and separation from his mother he has been unkempt and unresponsive.

she decided to marry a man, not his father, who did not wish to rear him. He was weaned suddenly and sent to live with relatives. Before weaning he had been an active, responsive baby, robustly healthy and accelerated in his development. After weaning and separation we found him unresponsive, passive, expressionless, and seemingly neglected and unkempt. He was perhaps not a fair test of the proposition that pure separation can have adverse effects in the absence of adequate substitute mothering, for it was apparent that he was cared for by a variety of young girls and adults, who together did not give him the kind or amount of care that his mother had given him before separation. His foster mother was found at home only once. Although Senvuma manifested some attachment to her, his behavior otherwise was in striking contrast to the other babies in our sample of the same age. He was less friendly to us as visitors, but, more important, he was quite impassive at the clinic when his young nursemaid left him totally alone for a protracted period in the midst of strangers. Whereas most children of his age would have expressed acute distress upon being abandoned by a familiar person in a strange situation, he did not protest; on the contrary, he accepted attention from me—a stranger—neither welcoming it nor rejecting it. He was said not to have recognized his mother when she visited him. But, even more important was the fact that he was so listless, unresponsive, and unsmiling, and that he accepted being taken by a stranger away from his home without any protest of any kind. Despite the fact that he was described as attached to his foster mother, he seemed quite withdrawn and indifferent to who held him—indeed, to who was present or absent.

Kitala

This is the story of Namitala's brother. The mother believed in separating her young children from her when a new baby was imminent so that she could have time for both the new baby and for her absorbing preoccupation in her garden work. There were at least four other children in the family, and all had been separated—most of them being sent to live with the maternal grandmother in the same village and thus having the possibility of some continued although intermittent contact with the mother.

When we first visited the family to see Alima, Kitala's half-sister, Kitala was very much in evidence. He was cheerful, active, and friendly. He trotted about, constantly intruding into the situation—into the conversation, into the foreground of photographs. He was fifteen months old. Although he had the charm of a happy and active child, despite his persistent intrusiveness, he was capable of bitter protest. His mother, who was pregnant, seemed to be trying to force an even greater distance between herself and Kitala than a recent weaning had imposed. When she got up to leave the room she went quickly and without any acknowledgment of his concern. Kitala always let out an immediate howl and scrambled after her. Sometimes she left him behind, and he yelled inconsolably; sometimes she heeded his protest and returned to pick him up and take him with her. But as long as she was present he was a delightfully vigorous child, dancing about, banging his playthings or interacting with people.

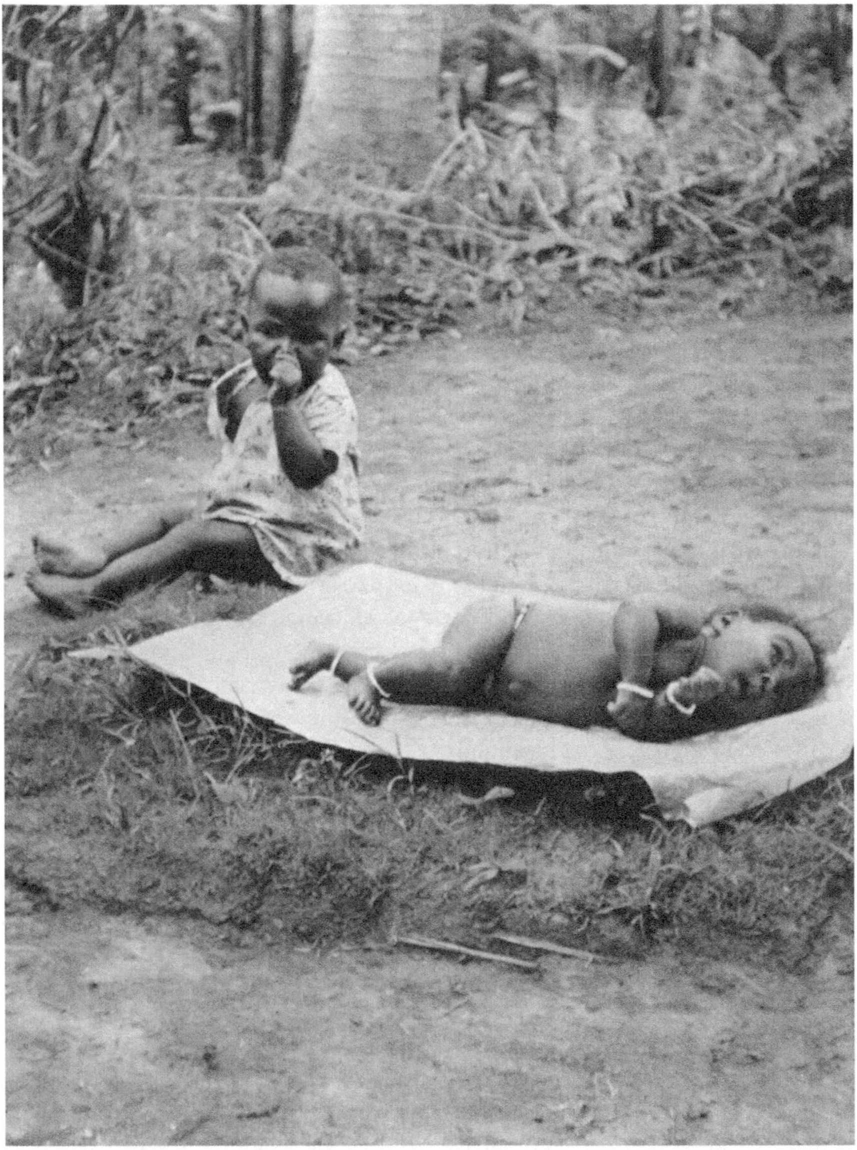

FIGURE 36 Kitala at eighteen months. He has been unhappy since he was separated from his mother. In the foreground is Namitala, eight weeks old—the cause of it all.

When Namitala was born, the mother visited the maternal grandmother for a while. She kept Kitala with her during the day but sent him home at night. Kitala was miserable, lonely, and jealous with the birth of the new baby. His father appreciated this and took him with him, riding him on the handle bars of his bicycle. When the mother returned home she left Kitala behind with his grandmother. The father did not approve of this action, appreciating the child's attachment to his mother and his distress at separation. But his intervention was useless.

The mother visited Kitala regularly—twice a week—and, of course, at the same time visited the other children and the maternal grandmother. Sometimes Kitala was at home for a visit for a day or so. The maternal grandmother complained that after a visit from or to his mother Kitala cried the rest of the day and all night afterward and became very difficult to manage.

These difficulties persisted. When he was at home during one of our visits, two months after separation, his behavior was in striking contrast to his preseparation behavior. Before, he had been active and cheerful. Now he was quiet and unresponsive. Before, he had thrust himself forward, intruding into conversations and photographs. Now he sat with his back to the visitors throughout the visit and responded not at all. Gone was his previous sturdy adventurousness. He cried at the slightest provocation and did not explore at all. If a visitor held him, he accepted this impassively. Previously he had been gentle and affectionate with Alima, his half-sister; now he was rough and rejecting. For most of our visit he sucked his thumb.

We observed Kitala from time to time for three months after his separation, and for all of this time he continued to be passive and withdrawn. He became a little more friendly to visitors but never regained his previous charming vigor and joyousness. He seemed to have reconciled himself to his separation from his mother, in that he no longer protesed parting from her at the end of a visit. But he was a changed child.

Ruthie

This little girl, the younger twins' half-sister, was four and a half when we first visited. When she was two years old, her mother, who had been living with William's family, left her and married. Ruthie was reported to have shown no disturbance, but, on the other hand, she had already become attached to William's mother, who was responsible for much of her care. She seemed to have become so assimilated into her foster family that she perceived no great difference when her mother left. She still saw her mother from time to time, for they lived in the same village. It was felt that somehow she knew that she was her mother's daughter, but no one could quite say how. She never said anything pertinent to this issue, and when her mother visited there was nothing special between them.

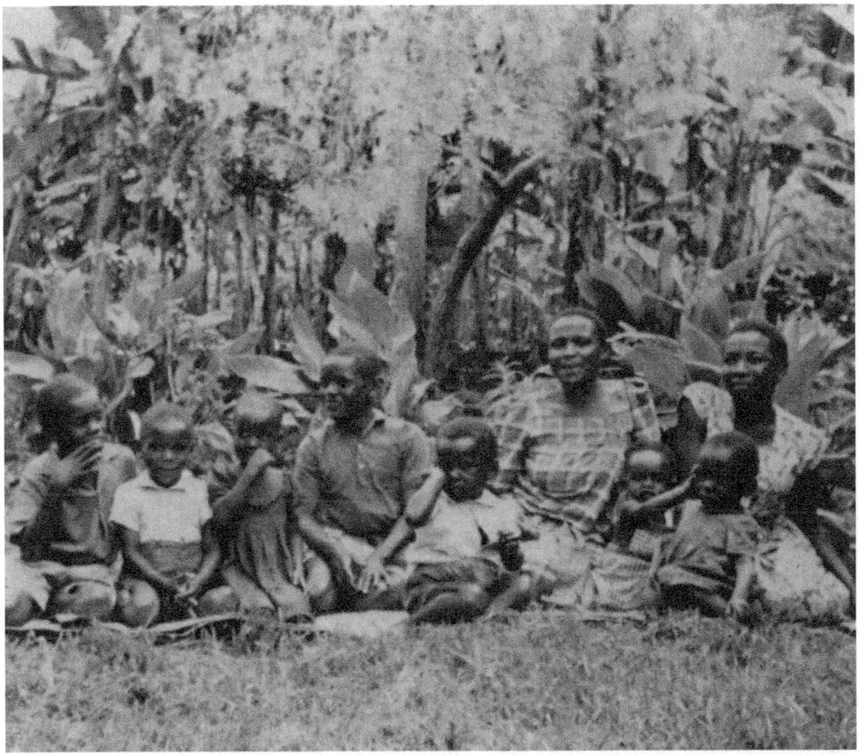

FIGURE 37 Ruthie, third from the left, is one of the family. Her foster home is with William's family.

Once her father came to claim her, but William's mother staved him off, insisting that she was too young to be wrenched away from her foster family to whom she was so obviously attached.

Three cases are too few to offer any critical evidence, of course. I did not, however, observe anything in the course of my visits to Ganda homes that was incompatible with the view that the disruption of ties between a young child and his mother can be disturbing and can set back development. The three cases are of interest in that they represent three degrees of disturbance. Although we did not witness Ruthie's initial responses to separation, it seems likely that, under the circumstances, her foster mother's report of absence of disturbance was accurate. But even in Uganda it is a very exceptional case in which the child before separation has been able to build up close ties with his foster mother. And after her own mother left, Ruthie had the care of an unusually good foster mother who treated her as she did her own children. If Ruthie suffered any setback in development, the effects of it are not apparent now.

Senvuma, on the other hand, had an especially traumatic kind of separation coincident with weaning. Moreover, it seems clear that his response to separation was confounded with his response to the insufficient maternal care that he received in his foster family. He was looked after by several people, including two young girls, but none of them seemed to be deeply committed to his welfare, and in aggregate he received less motherly attention than the other babies in our sample after weaning. Although he was reported to show some signs of attachment to his foster mother, his interpersonal relations as we observed them showed a striking degree of detachment.

Kitala is the middle case. As far as I could judge, his grandmother, who also looked after two of Kitala's siblings, was glad to have him and gave him a reasonable amount of interaction. Moreover, he had been weaned some time before being separated, and he still saw his parents at regular intervals. Yet the change in his behavior at the time of separation demonstrates that he was profoundly disturbed, and in his case it seems clear that it was the separation itself that was the major cause of the disturbance.

Welbourn[5] contrasted a group of ninety children from fifteen "good" families who had faithfully attended child welfare clinics with a group of thirty-six children from nine families who had first attended the clinic with a child suffering from malnutrition. Only seven of the children from "good" families were separated during the period of the study; all the "malnutrition" children had been sent away to realtives at some time, and three were living with grandparents while they were observed. Three of the "malnutrition" babies had suffered separation during the first few months of life. Welbourn acknowledged that some toddler-age children seemed to benefit from separation. Some who became ill with malnutrition after the birth of a new baby and with the consequent withdrawal of the mother's attention recovered and regained good spirits when sent to live with a grandmother. But, more frequently, the separation from the mother made matters worse rather than better. Too often a child was moved to a household where he belonged to no one in particular, like Senvuma, and where he was left very much on his own and was valued only as he grew older and could help with chores.

Géber and Dean[6] found a history of mother-child separation in thirteen of twenty-five consecutive hospital admissions with the diagnosis of kwashiorkor. Although kwashiorkor is a protein deficiency disease, Géber and Dean suggest that against an unsatisfactory dietary background and a history of slow growth something happens to turn the child's progress downhill. This event may be an infection or anything that further decreases his protein intake, or, they believe,

5 *Baganda Childhood.*
6 The psychological changes accompanying kwashiorkor, pp. 3–15,

it may be a psychological trauma such as mother-child separation. Furthermore, although all their patients were treated with a high-protein diet based on milk protein, Géber and Dean considered that the admission of the mother to hospital with the child was a vital part of the treatment and that the kind of relationship the mother could sustain or re-establish with her child had much to do with the course of recovery. If the relationship was good, the recovery was rapid. If the relationship was bad, the psychological symptoms of the disease—apathy, and withdrawal, with intense resentment at any intervention—tended to persist even though the physical state might be much improved.

The suggestion of linkage of malnutrition and deficiency disease with early mother-child separation therefore leaves us no grounds for complacency that "pure" separation, without the adverse influence of an unstimulating institution, has no consequences of significance. To be sure, there is evidence that young Ganda children may suffer from insufficient mother-child interaction after weaning, and especially after displacement by a new baby in the family, and that sometimes they may do better with a foster mother than when rejected and neglected by their own mother. Nevertheless, the weight of evidence —both in Uganda itself and extrapolated from other societies—is that the young child experiences distress upon being separated from his mother, and that even when this has been preceded by relative rejection and neglect, the distress can set in train processes which make it difficult for him to establish trusting relationships with a substitute figure. If, as all too frequently happens, the child is thrown as Senvuma was into a large household in which no one is deeply committed to him, this action will interact with his own feelings of misery and abandonment and will make it difficult for him to pick up the threads of closeness and intimacy.

26

IMPRESSIONS AND CONJECTURES

In Swahili, the lingua franca of East Africa, any journey is called a safari.[1] Whenever I left Kampala to spend an afternoon with a village family I made a safari. These many small safaris were, however, only the beginning of a much longer safari—one that has lasted eleven years—a journey in understanding. My report of this safari would be incomplete without an attempt to tell what emerged at the journey's end. What has emerged is a new way of viewing the origins and early growth of first love—the attachment of a baby to his mother.

This new point of view stems directly from my observations of Ganda babies and their mothers, but owes so much to a study of the viewpoints and findings of other scientists that only a limited originality can be claimed for it. It comprises a network of scientifically oriented conjectures, but it goes so far beyond the slim body of observations of a few infant-mother pairs in one society that it cannot be described as the incontrovertible conclusion of a scientific study. It marks the end of one safari, but it is hoped that it is the fruitful beginning of other ventures which will do much to test and to expand its component premises.

We are here concerned with nothing less than the nature of love and its origins in the attachment of a baby to his mother. According to this viewpoint, attachment originates in a few specific patterns of behavior, some of which are manifest at birth and some of which develop shortly afterward. Attachment is not present at birth, however; it emerges gradually through a course of development, and it is perhaps a matter of more or less arbitrary definition to identify the point at which it could be said to have finally emerged. Attachment is manifested through these

1 The Luganda word is *ssaffaali*.

DOI: 10.4324/9781003629337-30

patterns of behavior but the patterns do not themselves constitute the attachment. Attachment is internal. We can conceive of attachment as somehow being built into the nervous system, in the course of and as a result of the infant's experience of his transactions with his mother and with other people. This internalized something that we call attachment has aspects of feelings, memories, wishes, expectancies, and intentions, all of which constitute an inner program[2] acquired through experience and somehow built into a flexible yet retentive inner mechanism (which we identify with central nervous system functions) which serves as a kind of filter for the reception and interpretation of interpersonal experience and as a kind of template shaping the nature of outwardly observable response.

Patterns of attachment behavior are viewed as being analogous to Piaget's concept of the schema.[3] According to Piaget, the infant is born with a number of simple schemata—sucking, grasping, listening, looking, vocalizing, and moving the limbs. Each of these behavior patterns is the part of the schema that is objectively observable, but the schema includes also the inner representation of the behavior which is not itself directly observable. These original schemata constitute the infant's sole equipment for dealing with the world. It is through them that he processes the information he receives from the world; it is through them that he has effect on the world, both upon the physical objects and upon the people which surround him; and it is through them that he learns what the effect of his actions has been. Through an interactional process of acting and observing the consequence of his actions his simple sensorimotor schemata become modified. The inner structure of their representations is changed through experience, and at the same time the outward behavioral manifestation is modified as the child becomes more competent in producing the effects he wishes. Human intelligence originates in these simple sensorimotor schemata. Through a long course of transactions with his environment, which Piaget describes in exquisite detail,[4] the person gradually builds up a whole set of "operations" or strategies for coping with more and more complex and difficult tasks, and it is these strategies which constitute intelligence.

Piaget was not concerned with the development of attachment, but it appears to me that his developmental theory is applicable in broad terms to the development of attachment. The prototypical patterns of attachment behavior

2 Like a computer program. As many others do, I find the computer model a useful one. See *Plans and the structure of behavior*, by G. A. Miller, E. Galanter, and K. H. Pribram (New York: Holt, Rinehart and Winston, 1960).

3 J. Piaget, *The origins of intelligence in children* (New York: International Universities Press, 1952).

4 The reference to Piaget earlier cited deals only with the sensorimotor period of development. References to the later periods of development are too numerous to cite here. J. H. Flavell provides a comprehensive bibliography and a good introduction to Piaget's work in his book *The developmental psychology of Jean Piaget* (Princeton: Van Nostrand, 1963).

overlap and to a large extent are identical with Piaget's sensorimotor schemata. Development appears to take place through transactions with the environment, but the transactions are with people rather than with the physical objects Piaget emphasized in cognitive development. Furthermore, in the development of attachment as well as in the development of intelligence it is appropriate to emphasize the infant's own actions and his experience of the consequences thereof.

In my opinion, the most significant yield of my study of Ganda infants is the identification of patterns of attachment behavior presented in Chapter 20. It is in these patterns of behavior that attachment originates. They also serve to mediate the manifestations of a baby's attachment to his mother, and may be used as criteria thereof, even though the attachment itself must eventually become largely internalized. This list of behavior patterns should be useful in subsequent investigations of infant-mother interaction by directing attention to specific behavior upon which observation can focus. This list is acknowledged to be incomplete; it is weak especially in its omission of descriptions of the prototypical behaviors of the first two months of life. To the list should be added the neonate's postural adjustment when held and the whole complex of reflex-like feeding patterns, including sucking and rooting.

If Piaget's developmental views have been an important influence on my viewpoint, so has a broader and less specific application of biological evolutionary theory. The science of ethology has stemmed from Darwinian evolutionary theory. It concerns itself with the study of animal behavior, emphasizing those patterns of behavior which are just as specific to a species as bodily structure, conformation, and external distinguishing features. These species-specific patterns of behavior are viewed as having evolved because by and large they facilitate the survival of the species. They are viewed as having evolved in a specific "environment of adaptation" and as facilitating species-survival within the context of that particular environmental niche. Some species, among which primates and especially the human species are outstanding, have been able to survive within a great range of environmental variations through having developed the capacity for great modifiability of behavior. This capacity for modifiability is correlated with both a very complex central nervous system and a long and relatively helpless period of infancy during which the immature creature learns much from and through his parents and throughout which he must be protected and nurtured. The patterns of behavior, both infantile and parental, which favor the maintenance of physical proximity, protection, and nurturance are therefore of particular interest to ethologists.

Although Darwin's work drew attention to the important function of instinctive behavior, the concept of instinct soon became discredited in the study of human behavior. Instinct was usually conceived by the psychologist as an innate, automatic, and unmodifiable pattern of behavior, which might be typical of bees and spiders and migrating birds, but which was scarcely characteristic of human beings. The new ethological view of instinct,[5] which we do apply to human behavior, does not exclude the notion of modifiability. According to this view a baby's smile may be viewed as an example of instinctive behavior. It is a behavior pattern, characteristic of the human species, which emerges without a specific individual learning experience and which can most readily be evoked by an identifiable stimulus configuration—the human face, full face, or a model thereof, especially when the face is in movement—although it may fail sometimes to be elicited by this stimulus and may sometimes be given in its absence. The smile serves the biological function of inviting or sustaining tender attention from an adult and thus is part of the reciprocal set of behavior patterns which provide for the care of the young. In these respects the smile meets the criteria defining instinctive behavior, despite the fact that as the child grows older his smiling and not smiling is influenced by cultural patterns of socially desirable behavior and despite the fact that the life experience of some children is such that they smile rarely and perhaps not at all.[6]

Among students of child development it was Bowlby[7] who first drew attention to the relevance of the concepts and methods of the ethologists for the study of human development. He suggested[8] that the human infant, like the infants of other species, has at least a few instinctive patterns of behavior which serve the important biological function of binding child to mother and mother to child. He specified five such patterns: crying and smiling, which serve to evoke maternal behavior, and sucking, following, and clinging, through which the infant is active on his own account in seeking and sustaining contact or proximity.

The five patterns of behavior, identified by Bowlby as "component instinctual responses" forming the basis of the child's tie to his mother, have an obvious social function that may readily be viewed as significant for species survival. But the list of patterns of attachment behavior detailed in Chapter 20 includes some which are not exclusively social. The baby may manifest his budding attachment to his mother by his visual orientation to her, but he watches things as well as people, especially when they move. He orients himself to sounds of all sorts, although the sound of familiar voices may be especially significant to him. He reaches out to grasp things as well as to lift his arms to his mother when

5 A recent and definitive account of this view, but avoiding the terms "instinct" and "instinctive," is given by Robert Hinde in *Animal behavior: a synthesis of ethology and comparative psychology* (New York: McGraw-Hill, 1966).

6 For example, young children reared from early infancy in depriving institutions or subjected to a series of separations from mother figures may come to smile very rarely.

7 John Bowlby. Critical phases in the development of social responses in man, in *New Biology, No. 14* (London: Penguin, 1953), pp. 25–32.

8 John Bowlby, The nature of the child's tie to his mother, *Internat. Jour. Psychoanal.*, 1958, *39*, 1–34.

she approaches. He creeps and later walks to fulfill a variety of purposes and not merely to follow his mother as she moves about or to rush to her as a haven of safety when he feels threatened. Most of the behavioral components that mediate attachment in the human infant have multiple functions, and attachment must be viewed as having great overlap both in origins and development with the sensorimotor processes which underlie intelligent behavior.

Bowlby points out that the component instinctual responses that bind a child to his mother are not necessarily specific to her from the beginning but become, through experience, organized with the mother as the object. This implies that no one behavior pattern is crucial for attachment but rather that the particular organization of behavior patterns which the individual child has established through experience constitutes the basis for his attachment to a particular person. One component instinctual response may, because of individual experience, fail to become built into the attachment configuration, either disappearing from the child's repertoire or becoming part of his habitual transactions with some other person or object. Thus, although biological perspective identifies sucking as one of the behavior patterns which most characteristically bind the infant mammal to his mother, a bottle-fed baby may be attached to his bottle through his sucking behavior and attached to his mother through an organization of other behavior which altogether omits sucking. (And even a breast-fed baby can become attached to a pacifier!) Similarly, although clinging is likely to be an instinctive attachment pattern,[9] some babies, having been discouraged from clinging to their mothers as much as they would like to, may become attached to the blankets or cuddly toys to which they cling, and attached to their mothers through a behavioral organization in which clinging is not a central feature.

The human infant is equipped with the potential for a number of patterns of attachment behavior, in which it is likely that no one is essential and crucial. If the environment in which the baby is reared differs strikingly from the original environment of adaptation of the human species—in that some biologically appropriate behavior is discouraged in present-day society—attachment can still be mediated by other patterns which are neither stifled nor deflected to other

9 Clinging is an important instinctive behavior pattern throughout primate species, although human clinging appears later than subhuman clinging and seems more environmentally labile. The infant monkey, for example, attaches himself to his mother through very strong, innate clinging—although he too will cling to something else if he has no mother to cling to, whether another monkey, an inanimate model, or even the cloth on the floor of his living cage. Clinging behavior in infant monkeys reared in captivity is described by a number of authors. See H. F. Harlow, The development of affectional patterns in infant monkeys, in B. M. Foss (ed.) *Determinants of Infant Behaviour* (London: Methuen, 1961), pp. 51–74. See also Thelma Rowell, The social development of some rhesus monkeys, in B. M. Foss (ed.), *Determinants of Infant Behaviour, II* (London: Methuen, 1963), 35–52. A convenient introductory reference to primate field studies is I. DeVore (ed.), *Primate Behavior* (New York: Holt, Rinehart and Winston, 1965).

objects. Nevertheless, it is possible to rear an infant under circumstances which are so inappropriate biologically that attachment fails to develop—as we know from the now extensive literature on the effects of maternal deprivation.[10]

Although most of the ethological studies of animal behavior have been undertaken in the field—in the animal's natural environment—experimental interventions have proved to be highly instructive. They demonstrate that although in the "natural" environment instinctive patterns are most likely to be evoked by biologically appropriate stimulus configurations and to serve species-survival functions, they can be deflected from "natural" objects and modified to greater or lesser extents. Thus, for example, a chick, duckling, or gosling soon after hatching will follow the first moving object that it encounters, and through this following is "imprinted" on the object and subsequently follows only it.[11] Although in the average expectable environment into which the little bird hatches the first moving object is the mother bird, and he therefore follows her, in the laboratory or in other unnatural circumstances he may become attached to a biologically inappropriate object—a human being, a wooden model, or a red ball. It is, of course, evident that the human infant does not become attached to his mother as quickly as does the chick, and that following, although a human pattern also, is by no means the first attachment behavior to emerge. A cardinal rule of ethology is that one cannot impute the behavioral characteristics of one species to another. Only research can demonstrate the extent to which behavior patterns are shared by two or more species.

Nevertheless, laboratory studies of infant-mother interaction in mammalian species, such as rats, cats, and monkeys,[12] yield broad principles which seem to hold across species. One principle is that infant behavior and maternal behavior interact with each other, the behavior of the infant serving as stimulus to the mother, and vice versa, in a continuing sequence of interactions. Another principle is that the development of the infant and of his behavior changes the character of

10 See reviews of the literature by Bowlby, Yarrow, and Ainsworth which have been cited earlier, and for a more popular treatment see Bowlby's *Child care and the growth of love* (2nd ed.; London: Penguin, 1964), to which the present author contributed two chapters.

11 The phenomenon of imprinting was first drawn to widespread attention by K. Lorenz. See Companionship in bird life, in Claire H. Schiller (ed.), *Instinctive behavior* (New York: International Universities Press, 1957), pp. 83–116. For a review of subsequent research on imprinting, see W. Sluckin, *Imprinting and early learning* (London: Methuen, 1964).

12 In the volumes edited by B. M. Foss may be found reports of some relevant laboratory studies: in *Determinants of Infant Behaviour* (London: Methuen, 1961) there is a paper by J. S. Rosenblatt, G. Turkewitz, and T. C. Schneirla on Early socialization in the domestic cat as based on feeding and other relationships between female and young (pp. 51–74), and one by H. F. Harlow which was cited earlier; Harlow in the second volume (1963) follows up his theme in The maternal affectional system (pp. 3–34); and in the third volume (1965) J. S. Rosenblatt writes of The basis of synchrony in the behavioral interaction between the mother and her offspring in the laboratory rat (pp. 3–46).

his transactions with his mother so that the nature of their interaction is specific not only to the species but also to the developmental stage of the infant.

There have been three major influences that have shaped the viewpoint I present here. I have acknowledged my debts to Piaget's investigations of the development of intelligence in infancy and to the biological viewpoint currently advanced by ethologists. The third debt I owe to psychoanalytic theory. The way in which my approach has been shaped by psychoanalytic theory is so pervasive that I should like to believe that the findings and views reported here could be assimilated into the main body of contemporary psychoanalysis. Nevertheless, there are not only differences in terminology but also differences in approach and in concepts, which may make it difficult for the reader to perceive the compatibilities that are present. Furthermore, in a few respects my viewpoint seems to depart sharply from classical Freudian theory.

Let me first acknowledge the obvious and most general debts. Freud was the first to draw attention to the significance of infancy as a time when processes are set up, which, although modified by later experiences, nonetheless are potent in influencing the later course of development. He was thoroughgoing in his insistence that psychological processes are firmly anchored in bodily processes and drew heavily upon the biological science of his day in formulating his views. He was the first to assert the significance of the interaction between mother and child in the earliest years of life, holding that the mother-infant relationship was the prototype of all later interpersonal relationships. In a very real sense the whole study of mother-infant interaction was inspired by the Freudian emphasis.

Freud stressed the importance of inner experience, however, and psychoanalysts since Freud have attended more to what goes on inside, and especially in fantasy, than to externally observable behavior. For many years the psychoanalytic view of infancy was arrived at by a process of reconstruction, a piecing together from the adult's—or older child's—recollections and fantasies, with an admixture of shrewd inference, of what the inner life of an infant may perhaps be like. The psychoanalyst also had to become a keen observer of behavior, although he is mainly concerned with the behavior of a patient while in the interview situation in his office (and not in the patient's everyday life setting), and his observations supported his inferences about the patient's early experiences. We shall never know what the inner life of an infant truly is, for the infant cannot tell us about it and the person later remembers his infancy imperfectly, if at all. Another approach, and the one I have adopted, is to observe the infant's behavior, which is undoubtedly related to his inner experience, although not a transparent communication thereof. A substantial proportion of scientists now observing the infant's behavior in his earliest interactions are themselves psychoanalysts or are psycho-analytically oriented; I see very little difference between my approach and theirs. I have not attempted to draw any systematic parallels between my observations of infant behavior and a psychoanalytic interpretation of infantile experience. It is my belief that it would be very profitable to seek parallels. Such a search would both provide a necessary check on the thoughtful speculations and reconstructions of psychoanalytic theorists and enormously enrich the understandings that may be derived from purely behavioral studies—although it would take me too far afield to specify the ways in which enrichment could be expected.

The chief respect in which my present view departs from the main body of psychoanalytic theory is in regard to instinct theory. Freud talked of instincts or instinctual drives; I follow the ethologists (and Bowlby) in talking of instinctive behavior. The difference goes further than merely talking of different things. Drives are internal and are not directly observable; behavior is external and observable. Freud was a very wise man who had a long and productive life. He said many different things in his lifetime; sometimes the things he said revised things he had said earlier; and sometimes the things he said suggested new departures to which he did not later return for the follow-through. Therefore, one can usually speculate that some of his statements support the view that one wishes to advance. Nevertheless, the main body of subsequent Freudian theory[13] clearly favored the importance of drives in accounting for the development of the infant's attachment to his mother. The infant became attached to his mother because it was she who gratified his drives and fulfilled his needs. Drives and needs were primary and social behavior was a secondary, derived development. Not only psychoanalytic theory but psychological learning theory holds this view of the origin of attachment. The infant's physiological drives are primary; his need for his mother must be acquired and secondary.[14]

Recent research demands a change in our view of motivation. Drives have no simple locus in the body. We used to believe that hunger, for example, rested upon the perception of contractions of an empty stomach; we now know that hunger and feeding behavior are infinitely more complicated, involving intricate interactions between stimulus situation, nutritional state, behavior, and excitatory and inhibitory centers in the central nervous system, and that a feedback mechanism is crucial.[15] If central mechanisms and the interaction between environmental situation, inner state, and behavior are essential in

13 The relevant references to Freud's position and to the subsequent development of Freudian theory are much too numerous to cite in the context of the present argument. Let me, however, direct the reader to Anna Freud, *Normality and pathology in childhood* (New York: International Universities Press, 1965).

14 See, for example, J. Dollard and N. E. Miller, *Personality and psychotherapy* (New York: McGraw-Hill, 1950).

15 See E. Stellar, The physiology of motivation, *Psychol. Rev.*, 1954, *61*, 5–22, for A new theory of motivation, with a review of supporting evidence. See K. H. Pribram, A review of theory in physiological psychology, *Ann. Rev. Psychol.*, 1960, *11*, 1–40, for a neurophysiological description of the role of feedback mechanisms.

regulating hunger and feeding, it is likely that they are even more conspicuous as regulators of the various components of sexuality to which Freud rightly attributed great significance, and the extreme lability of which he stressed.[16] The biology upon which Freud based his view of motivation is outmoded. A revolution in motivational theory is not only overdue but underway. This revolution does not threaten the essentials of psychoanalytic theory, in my opinion, but it makes untenable what Bowlby terms the secondary drive theory of attachment.[17]

The view to which I adhere is that the child is born with a behavioral repertoire which includes responses already biased toward mediating social interaction—and that this is part of his built-in, species-specific equipment. In addition to actions which have a primarily social function, his repertoire includes some which have potential multiple function and can be turned to social ends. Thus the potential for attachment is part of the equipment of the newborn, although obviously attachment itself is only gradually acquired in the course of development—acquired in the course of interaction with his environment and the feedback he experiences as a consequence of his actions. His experience of having his needs for food and warmth met is important, but its significance is within the context of feedback. Fulfillment and gratification, as well as privation and frustration, are aspects of the feedback that the infant receives. Furthermore, it is obvious that the infant's survival is impossible if his basic requirements are not met at least minimally, and healthy development is hampered by too much privation or frustration. These things are true, and yet it is a gross oversimplification to focus on gratification and frustration while ignoring the role of organism-environment interaction and the fact that feedback refers to the consequence of the infant's own actions and not to need-gratification.

There is some evidence from the Ganda investigation to support the view that attachment does not rest on need-gratification. First, it is evident that babies become attached very early to people who have little or no responsibility for gratifying

16 Freud held that the infant has instinctual drives and certain innate channels for discharge of tension (aim of instinct) and that maturation provides some shift in these channels or aims. But the lability of the sexual drives he attributed to the lack of an innate connection between a drive and its object or gratifier. The belief that instinctual drives were initially objectless sometimes led psychoanalysts, particularly the earliest ones, to write as though the instinctual drives originated and developed in an environmental vacuum, relatively uninfluenced by organism-environment interaction. Nowadays, any analyst worth his salt operates professionally with full cognizance of organism-environment interaction. Nevertheless, much theoretical writing still gives too little attention to it. Prominent among those who must be excepted from this generalization are the so-called object-relations theorists, beginning with Melanie Klein, who held that instinctual drives were related to objects from the outset. Although in this regard object-relations theory is more akin to the position I espouse than Freudian theory, the fact that it is concerned to such an extent with inner life and fails to trace the parallels between inner life and behavior makes it extremely difficult to perceive similarities.

17 Bowlby, The nature of the child's tie to his mother.

their basic needs—to fathers and selected siblings. One child—Nora—showed signs of attachment to the father who came home on weekends and who merely responded to her advances and played with her, but she did not seem attached to the mother, who fed her, nor to the other wife in the family, who shared with the mother the task of gratifying her basic needs. Other babies, more fortunate than Nora, developed good relationships with their mothers but nevertheless became strongly attached almost simultaneously to other figures who could not have been selected on the basis of need-gratification. Secondly, the conspicuous characteristic shared by the mothers of the non-attached babies was not so much ineffectiveness in satisfying basic needs but failure in interaction— failure in responsiveness to signals, in timing of interventions, and in general accessibility. But let us not carry the argument further on the basis of the Ganda evidence. Harlow[18] has much more telling evidence from his study of infant monkeys, and Bowlby[19] has argued the theoretical points more cogently. All that I set out to do was to register one point of difference with widely held psychoanalytic theory, within the context of general compatibility with the psychoanalytic viewpoint, and to voice my hope that this point of difference—and perhaps others which I myself have not identified as difficulties—will not interfere with the highly desirable search for parallels between observable behavior and reconstructions of inner life. An understanding of child development is our mutual concern; our viewpoints are supplementary rather than contradictory.

Developmental studies of infant-mother interaction distinguish stages or phases of development.[20] Here I refer back to the sequence of phases of development described in Chapter 22. Let us review these.

During the first year attachment develops through the following phases: (1) an undiscriminating phase, during the first part of which the baby is relatively unresponsive to social advances, and during the second part of which he is responsive but in an undiscriminating way; (2) a phase of discrimination and differential responsiveness to a figure close at hand; (3) a phase of discrimination and differential responsiveness at some distance; (4) a phase of active initiative in making, sustaining and renewing contact and interaction; and (5) a phase of stranger anxiety. Although not identified and described in this study, probably because it is not clearly developed until well on into the second year of life or

18 Harlow stated that from his studies "there was no evidence that nursing, through the mechanism of secondary reinforcement, became an effectional variable of any real importance." Harlow, The development of affectional patterns in infant monkeys, *Determinants of infant behavior*, ed. Foss, 77.

19 Bowlby, The nature of the child's tie to his mother.

20 The stages of development of mother-interaction identified by Sander deserve special mention; they dovetail very closely with the stages of development of attachment outlined in this book. (L. W. Sander, Issues in early mother-child interaction, *J. Amer. Acad. Child Psychiat.*, 1962, *1*, 141–66.)

later, there is undoubtedly a further phase during which attachment becomes increasingly internalized and the child can begin to sustain his relationship with a beloved person through periods of absence, at first brief but becoming ever longer.

Even though there may be individual differences in the specific organization of the patterns of attachment behavior, and thus differences in the course of development of the particular patterns included within the organization, the phases of development described above may hold true in general. The first four phases represent epigenetic stages of development—that is, stages of development which each child must pass through on the way to a full-blown attachment, each stage depending on the one preceding it. It is well-known that a baby responds in an undiscriminating way before he responds discriminatingly. It seems reasonable that he learns to discriminate between figures close at hand before he can discriminate across even several yards of distance. I, myself, attach particular importance to the next phase of active initiative in making, sustaining, and renewing contact and interaction, although perhaps the special significance of this phase may not be immediately perceptible to others. I believe that there are threads of evidence testifying to the importance of the baby's own activity in becoming attached—and these I shall mention in another context later. I believe—as does Piaget—that the child learns largely through his own actions and his experience of their effects. Furthermore, attachment is more than a discrimination between people and implies something far more active—a literal or figurative seeking out, fastening on, holding to, and resisting the severance of the tie. If an attachment once formed is an active process, it is reasonable to suppose that at one phase in his development of attachment the child's own activity will be the conspicuous feature.

Although I am confident that the first four phases I have identified will stand up to the test of further research, I am less confident about the fifth phase of stranger anxiety. One of my misgivings is that stranger anxiety differs so greatly in intensity between children who appear to be equally attached and seems to depend both on accidents of individual experience and upon general insecurity level. I believe it to be likely that stranger anxiety is one aspect of a fifth phase which has other important features not yet adequately described and in terms of which the phase might be better characterized.

It will be recalled that the starting point of my search, which resulted in identification of patterns of attachment behavior and a delineation of phases of development, was an attempt to elucidate criteria in terms of which a child could be judged to be attached to his mother or not—or to what degree he was attached. In the literature most discussion has hinged on separation anxiety and stranger anxiety as indicators of attachment. Some hold that stranger anxiety is *the* criterion of attachment on the grounds that it is not clear that a child truly distinguishes his mother from other people until he makes this clear by showing fear of strangers.[21] Others hold that separation anxiety is the crucial criterion and that a child is not attached to his mother who does not manifest distress when separated from her or when such a separation is perceived as a threat.[22] According to this second view the essence of attachment is a drive for proximity to the mother, and the presence of the drive may best be perceived through the distress occasioned when it is frustrated. It should by now be evident that I believe that these two criteria comprise part of the truth about attachment but not the whole truth.

First let us consider stranger anxiety as a criterion of attachment. To be sure, fear of strangers proves that the child can discriminate his mother from strangers, but it has been seen that such discrimination has a long history before the emergence of clear-cut stranger anxiety. The early appearance of differential crying and differential smiling shows discrimination, and even before this there is undoubtedly differentiation in rooting, sucking, and postural adjustment.[23] Furthermore, the response to strangers may itself be seen to have a long history, with perception of a stranger as being new and different manifesting itself earlier and in much less dramatic ways than the terror of strangers that frequently emerges toward the end of the first year. A child of about nine months of age may suddenly show marked fear of strangers, and fear even of a relatively unfamiliar figure to whom he had previously been friendly. Whatever the explanation of this phenomenon may be—and it certainly deserves further study— it is not that the

21 Spitz has been influential in focusing attention on the significance of stranger anxiety, which he calls eight-month anxiety. He believes that the emergence of this anxiety "marks a distinct stage in the development of the psychic organization . . . the percept of the stranger's face . . . is confronted with the memory traces of the mother's face. It is found to be different and will therefore be rejected. We assume that this capacity of cathectic displacement on reliably stored memory traces in the eight-month-old child reflects the fact that he has now established a true object relation, and that the mother has become his libidinal object, his love object. Before this, we can hardly speak of love, for there is no love until the loved one can be distinguished from all others, and there is no libidinal object as long as it remains interchangeable." (R. A. Spitz, *The first year of life* [New York: International Universities Press, 1965], p. 156.) It is only fair to note that this statement, taken out of context, gives a somewhat distorted view of Spitz's position. Especially, it should be noted that he believes the dynamic basis for eight-month anxiety to be fear of loss of the object—his mother —and thus, in his view, stranger anxiety is a special case of separation anxiety. In this he follows Freud, who said that "missing someone who is loved and longed for" lay behind the manifestations of anxiety that occur "when a child is alone or in the dark, or when it finds itself with an unknown person instead of one to whom it is used—such as its mother." (*Inhibitions, symptoms and anxiety* [Standard ed.; London: Hogarth, 1959], XX, 136).

22 For example, H. R. Schaffer and Peggy E. Emerson, The development of social attachments in infancy, *Monog. Soc. Res. Child Develpmt.*, 1964, No. 3.

23 Both Spitz (*The first year of life*) and J. D. Benjamin (Further comments on some developmental aspects of anxiety, in H. S. Gaskill [ed.], *Counterpoint* [New York: International Universities Press, 1963], pp. 121–53.) acknowledge these early differentiations but judge them to be related to the "pre-object," not to the true love object.

child could not previously differentiate between his mother and strangers. Our findings strongly suggest that the baby who is afraid of strangers has previously shown clear signs of attachment to his mother; it was also found that babies who showed no such clear signs of attachment were not afraid of strangers.

Furthermore, our findings suggest that response to strangers is influenced by a number of variables which have little to do with the child's attachment to his mother. There is reason to believe that a baby who has had recurrent experiences with strangers—provided that they are not in themselves painful or frightening experiences—will be less afraid of them than a baby who has had little or no previous experience with strangers. The nature of the stranger himself is of significance—how similar to or different from the familiar figures in in the child's experience he may be.[24] Other significant variables are, however, related to infant-mother attachment. Under certain circumstances a baby, strongly attached to his mother, may show no fear of strangers, as though his mother gave him security to face the stranger, just as she can serve as a secure base from which he can explore the world.[25] On the whole it seems likely that babies who have an insecure attachment to the mother in general or who are currently experiencing separation anxiety will react more anxiously to strangers than those who are more secure. Therefore we must conclude that stranger anxiety, although undoubtedly related significantly to the growth of attachment, cannot serve as the sole criterion of attachment.

How about separation anxiety as a criterion? It is reasonable to describe a baby as attached to his mother if he shows distress when he sees her leave and is not easily comforted by anyone else. Indeed, the persistent distress of infants and young children separated from their mothers and the concomitant disturbances in development that may occur if there is no adequate substitute for her have given great impetus to empirical research into the nature of the infant's tie to his mother. Several studies now point to six or seven months of age as the time at which separation anxiety begins dependably to emerge with the great majority of infants; they emphasize that it is the disturbance of the relationship with the mother that is at the core of the distress rather than a strange or institutional environment. But these studies were of major separations—the baby who is sent away from his mother to hospital because he is ill,[26] the baby who remains in a familiar environment (even an institutional environment) but whose mother is

24 Benjamin (Further comments on some developmental aspects of anxiety, *Counterpoint*, ed. Gaskill) distinguishes fear of the strange from "infantile stranger anxiety proper." It can occur earlier than true stranger anxiety. But, he implies that it interacts with fear of object loss as the dynamic determinant of stranger anxiety.

25 Spitz (*The first year of life*) cautions those who wish to elicit "eight-month anxiety" not to try to do so in the presence of the mother, if the phenomenon is to be observed in unmistakable form.

26 For example, H. R. Schaffer, Objective observations of personality development in early infancy, *Brit. J. med. Psychol.*, 1958, *31*, 174–83.

sent away for several months,[27] or the baby sent to live with an adoptive mother after having become attached to a foster mother.[28] Separation experiences such as these are more disturbing than the minor separation experiences that occur in everyday home life, such as when the mother leaves the room, or goes out for the evening leaving the baby at home with a sitter. Distress upon being separated may, I am convinced, serve as a reliable criterion that infant-mother attachment has been formed, if the separation is a "major" one, either because of change of environment or because of the length of the separation, or both. Distress upon being separated briefly in one of the minor separation situations which recur frequently in everyday life is a less dependable criterion of attachment.

In particular, I do not believe that the degree of disturbance in minor separation situations may be used as an indication of how strong or intense the attachment is.[29] The seven Ganda babies whom I classified as insecure-attached seemed to be more intensely and more consistently disturbed by minor separation situations than the sixteen babies classified as secure-attached, but I do not believe that they were more strongly attached—merely more insecure. When ill, babies in the secure-attached group were "clingy" and behaved much like the insecure-attached. Were they more attached to the mother when ill or merely more insecure? Similarly, we may contrast preweaning and postweaning behavior. The demand-fed babies in particular showed more intense and consistent separation anxiety after weaning than before. They surely did not become more strongly attached to their mothers through having been weaned, but it is likely that they went through a period of being less secure in their attachment because of the weaning experience. Therefore we may conclude that separation anxiety, although significantly related to attachment, cannot serve as the sole criterion of attachment.

Considerations such as these lead me to believe that attachment should be assessed through observation of a variety of behavior patterns and that no single pattern should be taken as the sole criterion of attachment. Stranger anxiety and separation anxiety can have striking and conspicuous manifestations in behavior, but other less dramatic behavior is equally important to note—the orientation of the whole body silently but tensely toward the beloved one, the lifting of a hand in trustful anticipation that the mother's hand will come to meet it, the look of delight directed toward the mother as though inviting her to share a new

27 For example, R. A. Spitz and Katherine Wolff, Anaclitic depression, *Psychoanal. Study Child*, 1946, *2*, 313–42.

28 For example, L. J. Yarrow, Research in dimensions of early maternal care, *Merrill-Palmer Quart.*, 1963, *9*, 101–14.

29 I regret that I must disagree with H. R. Schaffer and Peggy E. Emerson (*The development of social attachments*) in their use of distress in minor separation situations as the criterion of the intensity of attachment; otherwise, and in more important respects, we have the pleasure of knowing that our views and findings coincide.

and interesting experience—all these and many others are the more subtle but, surely, equally valid manifestations of an infant's attachment.

To ask what constellation of patterns might serve as a criterion of attachment is misleading, for such a question implies that there is a sharp dividing line between attachment and non-attachment. It implies that up to a certain point in development a baby is not yet attached, but that after that point he is. On the contrary, the observations herein reported suggest that attachment comes about through a gradual process of development, beginning at or near the beginning of life, continuing throughout the first twelve or fifteen months that I observed, and undoubtedly continuing beyond it. I believe that the most meaningful assessments that can be made are age-relevant comparisons—and this has proved to be true for many other aspects of development, especially in the earliest years. I am not concerned with deciding whether a baby in phase three, who cries when his mother leaves the room, is attached to her or whether he is not really attached until phase five when he clings to her as a haven of safety when threatened by a stranger; I am concerned, however, with comparing his attachment behavior with that of other babies and judging whether he seems advanced, at age, or delayed in his development.

Deserving much more attention than they have received in the literature are the behavior patterns that emerge in the fourth phase of active initiative—e.g., following, approaching, and active greeting. Through these the baby is active in making, sustaining, and renewing contact and interaction. Not only does a baby through such behavior show that he is becoming attached, but, as implied earlier, it is through such behavior that he *becomes* attached. He becomes attached through following and approaching and greeting—and it seems likely also that he begins to become attached even earlier through smiling and crying and other behaviors that stem back to the earliest weeks of life.

Perhaps this statement is exaggerated; it is certainly incomplete. The child would not become attached through following or through smiling or through crying if nothing ever followed as a consequence of these activities—as a fairly stable and predictable consequence. But, in the usual home environment, something usually does happen when he takes the social initiative. Someone responds to him. If the response is consistent enough, and particularly if it is of such a nature as to encourage him to repeat or continue his social advances or demands, he comes to have some confidence that he, through his own actions, has some control over his world and the people in it. And he becomes attached to the person or persons over whom he feels he has some control. Thus attachment grows through feedback in response to active behavior.

I am sure that the average parent, if he has been able to travel with me this far, will want to raise two questions. First, he will want to protest that a baby who felt he could control his world through his parents would be a spoiled baby. Shouldn't he learn right away that he can't always have his own way, that he must consider other people, and that there are distinct limits to the extent to which he can control what happens to him? And then he might think to ask whether attachment is wholly a good thing. Can't a child be too attached to his mother? Sooner or later he must learn to be independent and to stand on his own feet. If one responds to him as a baby in a way that encourages the growth of attachment, would this not then discourage the growth of independence?

To reply to these questions I must go even further beyond the limits of what my observations of Ganda babies suggest, for, after all, I did not follow them through to a point that one could judge how they had "turned out." But my reply is part of the general viewpoint that I am here advancing. First of all, the child's development of attachment, and indeed all of his development, takes place in interaction with his environment and the people in it, and it proceeds gradually through a succession of phases. Just as infant behavior appropriate to one phase would be inappropriate to a later phase, parental behavior which is appropriate to and facilitates development in one phase might well be inappropriate to or hinder development in another phase. Later, I shall discuss parental behavior variables that seem to facilitate development in the first year. Here I merely wish to assert that there is a time to give a baby confidence in his control of his world and there is a time to demonstrate to him that there are limits to his control. There is a time to nurture a tender attachment and there is a time to encourage self-reliance. If you ask whether this or that practice is a good thing, I could answer only, "it depends." It depends on the stage of development the child has reached[30]—and on other things as well.

Let me return for a moment to the biological orientation. Students of mother-infant interaction in subhuman mammalian species, when discussing attachment or its animal equivalent, point out that the peak of mother-infant interdependence in behavior is followed by a stage of development in which independence emerges. The kitten, after having had his mother usually accessible to him, and after having been retrieved by her when he strayed, becomes more competent in looking after himself, and then finds his mother increasingly impatient with his demands and likely to go where he cannot reach her.[31] The infant monkey, after having clung to his mother most of the time during earliest infancy, and after having been pulled back by her long arm from any attempt to explore the world at a distance, finds that his mother both tolerates his expeditions away from her and pushes him off if he clings too long.[32] Just as there seems to be a biological

30 My view here is similar to that taken by J. McV. Hunt (*Intelligence and experience* [New York: Ronald Press, 1961], pp. 267–88) when he stresses the importance of matching environmental stimulation to the stage of cognitive development so far reached in the child.

31 Rosenblatt, Turkewitz and Schneirla, Early socialization in the domestic cat as based on feeding and other relationships between female and young, *Determinants of Infant Behaviour,* ed. Foss.

32 Harlow, in his paper The maternal affectional system (*Determinants of Infant Behaviour*, *II*, ed. Foss.) describes a phase of independence in the development of interaction between infant and

basis for the development of attachment, there seems to be a biological basis for the development of independence, although maternal behavior and the wider environmental context in which mother-infant interaction takes place may hasten or delay this development.

Throughout the animal series, as well as in the human, the development of independence has a dual basis—in the increasing competence of the infant and in the increasing encouragement of independence on the part of the mother. The human infant, like the baby monkey, is curious about his world, and as he becomes more and more competent he becomes increasingly eager to venture out to explore it. His mother may gradually release her control over him, or even push him away, but in the normal course of events he will himself initiate much of the growing away from her. There are overprotective monkey mothers, just as there are overprotective human mothers, who for reasons of their own keep pulling back the infant whose growing capabilities lead him to want to explore in ever-widening circles. But the point I want to make is that at the same time that the infant is becoming more and more attached to his mother, he is becoming both more competent and more interested in mastering the world on his own account. Instinct in lower animals may perhaps gear the mother's withdrawal more accurately to the level of actual competence of the infant, and certainly in other species the time span of helplessness is shorter than in the human; but, I believe, without undue "retrieval behavior" on the part of the mother, the developmental process of the human infant will make him gradually more independent and, no matter how lovingly attached he is to his mother, he will want to do things on his own.

This moving out and away may be observed quite clearly even during the first year of life. The behavior pattern to which I have referred as "using the mother as a secure base" highlights the fact that there can be a sound development of close attachment at the same time that there is increasing competence and independence. It is the insecure child who clings to his mother and refuses to leave her. The secure child, equally closely attached, moves away and shows his attachment by the fact that he wants to keep track of his mother's whereabouts, wants to return to her from time to time, and in his occasional glances back to her, or in his bringing things to show to her, he displays his desire to share with her his delight in exploring the wonders of the world. So in reply to one question from parents I reply that attachment does not normally or necessarily interfere

mother living under laboratory conditions. Perhaps even more relevant for our purposes is the description of infant-mother interaction living in larger social groups given by Thelma Rowell (The social development of some rhesus monkeys, *Determinants of Infant Behaviour, II*, ed. Foss) and R. A. Hinde (Rhesus monkey aunts, in B. M. Foss, [ed.], *Determinants of Infant Behaviour, III* [London: Methuen, 1965]).

with the development of competence and self-reliance but rather supports this development.

What about the question of control and omnipotence? This is a more difficult one, and I cannot find a clear parallel with kittens or monkeys. But I fall back again on Ecclesiastes—there is a time for omnipotence and there is a time when omnipotence should be discouraged. I believe that a baby gains his first firm sense of reality—what the real world is about—through discovering that his own actions alter and control what happens. At first he is so helpless that his own actions do not accomplish much of anything at all. Much of his gratification—and certainly his survival—depends on the intervention of parental figures. Whether they intend to do so or not—and certainly few parents are conscious of trying to stimulate a baby's development when they attend to his simple and immediate needs—parents give a baby a sense of control and competence and a growing sense of reality when they respond to him, and this in turn facilitates his actual development of control, competence, and reality.

There is a point, however, toward the end of the first year of life or early in the second year, when a baby's confidence in being able to control his world through his own actions is well enough established that parents can begin to show him the limits of his power.[33] Much of his assurance rests on his parents' cooperation. If they did not go along with him—acceding to his signals, demands, and requests—he would have little power or control. On the other hand, if they had not gone along with him this far, he could not have built up any kind of trust in himself, in them, or in the world. It may be difficult to judge when the time has come to begin to demonstrate to an infant the limits of his power, but sooner or later—yet not too soon—he must learn that he is not king and cannot control his parents at his whim. He must find out, perhaps largely through trial and error, just what he can control and what he cannot control, and what he can influence by the right techniques but cannot be sure of controlling. But before that time comes, the development of a sense of omnipotence is an inevitable concomitant of gaining feelings of efficacy and a sense of competence and control.[34]

I held out the hope to my Ganda participants that through studies such as this one, we might learn which of their customs and which of Western customs were better ways of rearing infants. Was this entirely a false hope? I think not, and yet my opinions again must be stated as conjectures rather than as

33 L. W. Sander (Issues in early mother-child interaction) describes a "monotropic" phase of infant-mother interaction occurring toward the end of the first year. If I understand him correctly, the issue which must be resolved before the infant proceeds to the next phase is that, having become monotropically attached to his mother, he must learn that his mother is not under his control and not an extension of his own will.

34 Throughout this discussion I have used the terms "efficacy" and "competence"; I mean to imply by them what White implies in his discussion of ego development. (R. W. White, *Ego and reality in psychoanalytic theory* [New York: International Universities Press, 1963].)

conclusions—conjectures which I hope to explore more fully in future research. My conjectures come from two sources. First, in Chapter 23 it was pointed out that individual differences in methods of infant care were related to differences in the babies' development of attachment. Secondly, a similar comparison may be made between the Ganda sample and Western infant-mother pairs, even though the latter must be confined to the few in my present study of American babies and the comparison must be impressionistic at this stage in the research.

In Chapter 23 it was found that three variables distinguished at a statistically significant level between the three groups of babies— secure-attached, insecure-attached, and not-yet-attached. The first of these significant intrasample comparisons suggested that babies who developed a secure attachment had mothers who gave more time, care, and attention to them than did the mothers of babies in the other two groups; that babies who had not yet developed an attachment had mothers who gave much less time, care, and attention than did the mothers of babies in the other two groups; and that the babies who developed an insecure attachment tended to have mothers intermediate between the other two groups in respect to amount of time, care, and attention. "Amount of time, care, and attention," as it was pointed out, however, is a rough approximation of several underlying variables which required further work to begin to sort out.

Here it is relevant to cite the interim results of some work still in progress with a sample of American babies.[35] At about one year of age those babies who had developed a secure attachment to their mothers, and who displayed it by being able to use their mothers as a secure base to explore a strange situation, differed both from babies who seemed relatively weakly attached to their mothers and pre-maturely independent and from babies who seemed attached but disturbed in their relationship to the mother in terms of the following variables. (1) They experienced frequent and sustained physical contact with their mothers, especially during the first six months of life. (2) Their mothers were able to soothe them effectively through physical contact when they were distressed. (3) Their mothers were sensitive to their signals and responsive to their demands. (4) Their mothers were able to time their caretaking interventions in harmony with the babies' rhythms. (5) The mother so regulated the baby's environment that he could derive a sense of the consequences of his own actions and come to feel that what he did could have some consistent and hence predictable effect on what happened to him; this feedback promoted feelings of efficacy.

It is believed that these five variables, and perhaps others not yet identified, lie behind the blanket variable "amount of time, care, and attention" that was found to be significant in the Ganda sample. It is acknowledged that a mother

35 Mary D. Salter Ainsworth and Barbara A. Wittig, Attachment and exploratory behavior of one-year-olds in a strange situation, in B. M. Foss (ed.), *Determinants of Infant Behaviour, IV* (in press).

may spend much time in the same house with a baby, and even in the same room, and still not give him adequate care and attention. It is also acknowledged that a mother may give care and attention adequate to look after a baby's basic needs for nourishment and protection and still not foster a secure attachment. It also seems reasonable to believe that if the mother cannot give full-time care and attention to her baby, he could thrive if one or two other persons shared in his care in a sensitive and responsive way. But, nevertheless, if a mother or a substitute mother does not spend enough time with a baby and does not give him enough of her attention, she cannot learn what his signals signify and what his rhythms are; she cannot therefore respond sensitively to his signals and time her interventions in harmony with his rhythms. Furthermore, if the mother shares her responsibility for the baby with others, it is difficult, although perhaps possible, for her to arrange an environment with a consistent and predictable feedback that gives the baby some sense of having an effect on what happens to him. On the other hand, if all caretakers stress physical contact and especially give physical contact when soothing, several caretakers could combine to give adequate care at least in this respect.

In regard to these five variables the mothers of the secure-attached Ganda babies—who were most numerous proportionally in the Ganda sample—receive high marks. The typical Ganda baby experiences much physical contact, especially during his early months before he can sit and crawl. He receives this chiefly from his mother, but also from other caretakers and visitors. His mother picks him up when he cries, and soothes him by holding him, and may also give him the breast as many other Ganda mothers do. The typical Ganda mother is sensitive to her baby's signals and responsive to his demands. Even though some of the secure-attached babies were schedule-fed, the tendency certainly was for their mothers to gear their interventions to the babies' rhythms. Finally, the typical Ganda baby—and here I refer to the secure-attached baby—does experience the kind of environment in which he can sense the consequences of his own actions, both because his caretakers are sensitive to his signals and because he is given so much occasion for social interaction and so much freedom to take initiative. Therefore, it appears that some central and crucial methods of Ganda infant care are good and can be endorsed. It is better for a baby to be held a lot, to be picked up when he cries, to be given what he wants when he wants it, and to be given much opportunity and freedom to interact than it is for a baby to be kept for long periods in his crib apart from other people, where his signals cannot be perceived and consequently where he cannot experience a sense of predictable consequence and control.

A second variable which emerged as significant in the Ganda sample in differentiating between the groups was the mother's excellence as an informant. It was suggested earlier that this reflected the mother's interest in the baby, but it also reflects the amount of time the mother spends with him; otherwise she could not have observed him enough to be able to describe his behavior in response to inquiries. A third variable which proved to be significant was the mother's enjoyment of breast feeding. Both of these variables seem to be related to one which emerged as important in the American study, in which the mother-infant interaction characteristic of the secure-attached babies was one of mutual delight. In the American sample this was manifested chiefly in mother-infant play situations, but it was also reflected in the mother's delight in informing the interviewer about her child. This delight on the mother's side tended to extend to all aspects of the infant's behavior, including the more negative aspects of protest and pouting. It seems reasonable to suppose that enjoyment of breast feeding may contribute to the mother's delight in her baby, although it is not essential to mutual delight—for, as the American sample bears witness, delight can occur when babies are bottle-fed.

Although we have been concerned primarily with the development of attachment, we have given attention also to sensorimotor development, in which the Ganda babies were found to be advanced beyond Western norms. My American sample was also advanced, but one of the interim impressions of that study has been that the babies who were most advanced were those who had been given freedom to explore and to learn, first in a visual-motor sense and later through locomotion. In other words, babies who were confined to crib or playpen after they were capable of locomotion tended to be slower in sensorimotor development than those who were given more freedom to explore, and babies who earlier were kept apart with little visual stimulation and who had their movements hampered so that they could not reach for what they saw were also slower in sensorimotor development. Again, the normative practices of the Ganda rate high. Although the four not-yet-attached babies were kept confined and isolated much of the time, the others were given much freedom to explore once locomotion had developed, and before that had experienced much stimulation through being so much a part of the social group. Furthermore, it is my hunch that physical contact facilitates sensorimotor development, especially in the earliest months. When a baby is held, he has to adjust his posture to the person who holds him, and since he tends to be shifted about he has to keep adjusting. It seems likely to me that these early, frequent postural adjustments facilitate early locomotor development in that they involve neck and trunk musculature. In contrast, the baby who is kept on his back in his crib most of the time—or even prone on his tummy—has much less occasion to strengthen neck and trunk musculature and to acquire the sensorimotor coordinations associated with postural adjustment. If he is laid in a prone position, he has some opportunity to reach for and perhaps to manipulate objects placed in his crib beside him, but if he is laid on his back he cannot reach much of anything, and thus eye-hand coordination is likely to be delayed.

To return for a moment to the issue of the dangers of an indulged first year, the Ganda provide a test case. The typical Ganda baby is indulged in the sense that he gets what he wants when he wants it and is frequently picked up and held. And yet the secure-attached group did not show signs of being spoiled. It was the insecure-attached group who seemed "spoiled," and their undesirable characteristics seemed attributable more to the factors making for their insecurity than to indulgence. Indeed, the caretaking practices which offered freedom to explore were seized upon with alacrity by the secure-attached babies, who consequently gained quite a substantial degree of competence and independence while still being closely attached.

Ganda babies, on the other hand, have perhaps a sharper push towards independence and a more abrupt cessation of indulgence than do those Western babies who enjoy an indulged infancy. Although it lay beyond the age limits of the Ganda study, and hence was not systematically observed, it seemed unmistakable that the birth of a new baby represented a greater and probably more traumatic change to the Ganda infant than to his Western counterpart. Since Ganda mothers typically devote so much time and attention to the baby, they have relatively little time for the toddler. If the timing is right, perhaps this is of no consequence, but if a new baby arrives when the child is still little more than an infant, it is difficult for him to cope with the shift from being indulged to being largely ignored. It seems to me that Western mothers tend, on the whole, to spread their concerns and attentions more evenly among their preschool children than do Ganda mothers, and although the baby may get less, the next-oldest gets more. In ancient days, when the baby was not weaned until he was two and a half or three years of age, perhaps he could cope with the withdrawal of his mother's focus of attention. But nowadays it is hard for Ganda babies of fifteen months or so to adjust to a new baby in the family.

So far I have said nothing about the relative virtues of breast feeding and bottle feeding, demand feeding and schedule feeding, and early versus late weaning. In respect to these aspects of infant care it is obvious that Ganda practices differ from contemporary middle-class American practices. Does this study of Ganda infants have any light to throw on the controversy which perennially rages over infant feeding practices?

Perhaps no other aspects of infant care have prompted more vociferous proponents of one extreme or the other. Few aspects of infant care have evoked more research. Opinions may be strongly stated, but research evidence is equivocal.[36] There are several good reasons why research has failed to yield clear-cut results. First, most investigators have relied on secondhand information rather than on firsthand observation, and only too often the information has been retrospective, having been obtained some years after the child has left

36 Of several reviews of the literature I recommend that by Bettye M.Caldwell, as most recent and most insightful. (The effects of infant care, in M. L. Hoffman and L. W. Hoffman [eds.], *Review of child development research, I*, 9–88 [New York: Russell Sage Foundation, 1964].)

infancy behind. Thus the information available about infant feeding practices is less reliable than in here-and-now research which uses direct observation. Secondly, until very recently investigators have tended to study one of these infant-care practices at a time and have neglected to take account of other infant-care practices which may interact with the one under investigation. Thus, for example, it seems unlikely that one can ascertain much about the effect of breast feeding if one does not at the same time consider age of weaning; surely, any real effects are obscured if the study lumps together all those who have ever been breast-fed—whether for a few weeks or for a year or more. Furthermore, interest has generally been directed toward long-term effects of infant-care practices, despite the fact that, important though infancy probably is, the ultimate outcome is undoubtedly very much influenced by life experiences during the intervening years.

I can scarcely offer definitive evidence in regard to these issues in view of the small sample of Ganda infants and an even smaller sample of American babies observed to date. On the other hand, the present data are not retrospective; they are based on firsthand observation as well as upon interview; they may be examined in the context of other possibly relevant infant-care practices; since we can be concerned only with short-term effects, we therefore may expect to find sharper contrasts than would be found some years from now, after important intervening experiences have blurred them.

Let us first consider breast versus bottle feeding. Should you ask me which is better for the Ganda at the present time, I would answer unequivocally—breast feeding. This answer is primarily practical. The techniques of bottle feeding are difficult to carry through in an undeveloped country—the measurement of the ingredients of a formula, the sterilization of bottles and nipples, the boiling of the component milk or water. In Buganda, cow's milk is difficult for most people to obtain, and imported commercial preparations are very expensive. The baby's best chance for good health and nutrition is through breast feeding. But in the psychological literature the issue pertains not to nutrition and health but to mother-infant interaction. In Western countries it is obviously quite feasible to nourish a baby well indeed through "artificial" feedings. But is the artificial feeding as good as breast feeding for emotional and interpersonal development?

Within the Ganda sample there was only one baby who was not breast-fed, but there is nevertheless pertinent evidence. The mothers who reported that they enjoyed breast feeding tended significantly to have babies who were attached and secure in their relationship with their mothers. In this country we have been told by experts that a bottle-fed baby can develop just as fine a relationship with his mother as a breast-fed baby, provided that his mother holds him during feeding and interacts with him—and I think there is much good sense in that pronouncement. Yet it may be that, other things being equal (which, of course, they rarely are), mothers who undertake breast feeding and enjoy it tend to have a closer, more sensitive, more delighted interaction with the baby than those who rely on the bottle. The Ganda sample, however, emphasizes the importance of the mother herself enjoying breast feeding. Not all mothers do, even in Buganda. And we have all heard horror stories about mothers who have suffered pain, humiliation, frustration, and guilt in regard to unsuccessful attempts to breast feed.

Even among the Ganda, where breast feeding is the norm, its course does not always run smoothly. There, perhaps, much of the difficulty comes about through the alternatives diffusing into Ganda culture from the West. Supplementary bottles are becoming increasingly common—and instinct is not sufficient to inform the mother that the supplementary bottle may decrease the stimulation of the breast through sucking, and thus decrease the milk secretion. But, whether or not supplementary bottles have been used, Ganda mothers, like Western mothers, may have anxieties about providing enough nourishment for the baby. The fact that there are alternatives now—bottle feeding and earlier introduction of solid foods—bring these anxieties to light whereas previously they were perhaps kept hidden.

Let us assume, as the Ganda evidence suggests, that mothers who wish to breast feed and who are predisposed to enjoy it may develop a better relationship with their babies than those who do not. Then, it seems to me, thay should receive every encouragement and assistance. But they do not in this country. They are advised by their obstetricians often enough—as well as by relatives and friends—not to be silly. If they persist despite discouragement from others, they are likely to run into many difficulties. Instinct may prompt a woman to want to breast feed, but instinct is too watered down in the human species to tell her how to go about it. In relatively undeveloped countries or communities experienced women may give good advice, but here, unforunately, bottle feeding has been too widespread for too long for even grandmothers to be able to help, and the medical professions have all too frequently little to offer. The obstetrical wards of most hospitals merely tolerate breast feeding, but do not help it along. Many pediatricians favor breast feeding and encourage mothers who wish to do so; but they do not instruct them how to accomplish this successfully or counsel them against practices which may defeat their efforts. By default, the field is open to non-medical societies whose exhortations include some nonsense as well as sound advice.

How about demand versus schedule feeding? The research literature is highly equivocal about this issue. I believe that the equivocal findings are due largely to the investigators' reliance on interview information. I found it very necessary in my Ganda study to inquire in detail about practices, and to check the information through firsthand observation. Some mothers who stated that they fed by schedule were obviously very flexible. Some who said they fed on demand—when the baby was hungry—seemed to schedule their perceptions of his hunger. In my work with American mothers I have found it even more important to observe directly than with the Ganda mothers. Some who claim to feed on demand manage to get their babies onto three meals a day within an astonishingly short time. Some who claim to adhere to a schedule introduce between-meal snacks which they do not count as feedings. I have no confidence in a mother's categorization of her method of feeding as "demand" or "schedule" without much detailed further information.

Sensitivity to signals and responsiveness to demands emerged as an important variable in the American sample and seemed to lie behind the significant differentiations in the Ganda sample. One of the chief ways in which a mother can be sensitive and responsive to a baby is in regard to signals of hunger and demands to be fed. Yet my intensive observations with American infant-mother pairs suggests that mothers may be differentially responsive to different kinds of signals and demands, and there is no one-to-one relationship between responsiveness to hunger signals and responsiveness to other signals. Indeed, some mothers, for reasons of their own which even they may not consciously understand, respond to signals of distress and social signals and ignore all but the most desperate hunger signals; yet they manage to establish a fairly good relationship with the baby. After all, time is on their side. Whereas at first hunger frequently overwhelms the baby, he becomes better and better able to sustain delays between feedings and becomes increasingly interested in social interchange. Nevertheless, because sensitivity to signals and responsiveness to demands seems to me to be such an important variable in maternal care, I am inclined to side with those who hold with demand feeding. Therefore, I attach importance to the fact that the Ganda mothers who fed "for comfort" tended to have secure-attached babies, even though the tendency was below the level of statistical significance.

On the other hand, as I pointed out earlier, the Ganda babies who were fed on demand tended to be more disturbed by weaning than those who were fed on schedule. The cases were too few for statistical significance, but the differences in behavior were sharp enough to suggest significance. I interpreted this finding to suggest that those fed on demand tended to have feeding behavior built into the attachment pattern whereas those fed on schedule did not. Here, I believe, we have the key to much that is bewildering in the psychological and psychoanalytic literature. We hear that weaning is the first major trauma that a baby experiences. And yet, we usually do not find babies in middle-class American society traumatized by weaning. Indeed, in this society we are not too sure how weaning should be defined. Is it when breast feeding stops and something else starts? Or when breast feeding is no longer the sole mode of nutrition, as when supplementary bottles or solids are first started? Or is it when sucking is no longer the major mode of nutrition, whether from breast or bottle, and is supplanted by taking food from spoon, cup, or fingers? In any event, despite the fact that weaning seemed to be traumatic in middle-class Vienna early in the century, just as it is now with Ganda babies fed truly on demand, it does not seem to be traumatic among middle-class American babies, whether breast- or bottle-fed, on demand or otherwise.

This discussion about weaning emphasizes the fact that one must evaluate an infant-care practice in its context. The context is at the intersection of two dimensions—one cross-sectional and the other historical. One must evaluate the infant-care practice in the context of the other practices pertinent to the infant in question, and one must recognize that both the practice and its context may undergo changes through time so substantial that it is no longer the same practice. This, I hold, is true of weaning in Western societies. What was implied by "weaning" in 1900 has nothing much to do with present-day weaning. The context has changed too much. Weaning nowadays among the Ganda seems comparable to Western weaning in 1900, but it is dissimilar to present-day Western weaning.

It has always seemed to me that a scientist—especially a behavioral scientist—must have a great tolerance of ambiguity and uncertainty if he is to keep his equilibrium in his vocation. It takes such a long time to find the clear and unambiguous answers that one can be sure that in one's lifetime most of the questions will remain unanswered. It is difficult to hold an open mind over an extended time —and yet, that is what is required of the scientist. It is required also, increasingly, of the ordinary citizen in this age. Science has been so successful that we have arrogant expectations of it; and yet the practical answers, especially, are slow to come. In matters such as rearing an infant—a matter which is of immediate and urgent concern to his parents—it would indeed be good if all the answers were known. They are not—and therefore parents also, and perhaps especially, must have tolerance of uncertainty and be content to do the best they can with the information they have available to them. And despite the alarming incidence of neurosis in this world, full as it is of uncertain or conflicting information, parents—both Ganda and non-Ganda—by and large do well.

REFERENCES

Ainsworth, Mary D. The effects of maternal deprivation: a review of findings and controversy in the context of research strategy. *Deprivation of maternal care: a reassessment of its effects* (Public Health Papers, No. 14 [Geneva: World Health Organization, 1962]), pp. 97–165.

——— The development of infant-mother interaction among the Ganda. *Determinants of infant behaviour. II* (B. M. Foss, ed.). London: Methuen, 1963, pp. 67–112.

——— Patterns of attachment behavior shown by the infant in interaction with his mother. *Merrill-Palmer Quart.*, 1964, *10*, 51–58.

———, and Wittig, Barbara A. Attachment and exploratory behavior of one-year-olds in a strange situation. *Determinants of infant behaviour. IV* (B. M. Foss, ed.). (In press.)

Albino, R. C., and Thompson, V. J. The effects of sudden weaning on Zulu children. *Brit. J. med. Psychol.*, 1956, *29*, 177–210.

Benjamin, J. D. Further comments on some developmental aspects of anxiety. *Counterpoint* (H. S. Gaskill, ed.). New York: International Universities Press, 1963, pp. 121–53.

Billington, W. R., *et al.* Custom, child health, pregnancy and child-birth. *Trop. Geogr. Med.*, 1963, *15*, 124–33.

Blauvelt, Helen, and McKenna, J. Mother-neonate interaction: capacity of the human newborn for orientation. *Determinants of infant behaviour* (B. M. Foss. ed.). London: Methuen, 1961, pp. 3–36.

Bowlby, J. *Maternal care and mental health* (2nd ed.) Geneva: World Health Organization, 1952.

——— Critical phases in the development of social responses in man. *New Biology, No. 14.* London: Penguin, 1953, pp. 25–32.

——— The nature of the child's tie to his mother. *Internat. J. Psychoanal.*, 1958, *39*, 1–34.

——— *Child care and the growth of love* (2nd ed.) London: Penguin, 1964.

Caldwell, Bettye M. The effects of infant care. *Preview of child development research. I* (M. L. Hoffman and Lois W. Hoffman, eds.). New York: Russell Sage Foundation, 1964, pp. 9–88.

David, Myriam, and Appell, Genevieve. A study of nursing care and nurse-infant interaction. *Determinants of infant behaviour* (B. M. Foss, ed.). London: Methuen, 1961, pp. 121–42.

DeVore, I. (ed.). Primate Behavior. New York: Holt, Reinhart and Winston, 1965.

Dollard, J., and Miller, N. E. *Personality and psychotherapy.* New York: McGraw-Hill, 1950.

Fallers, L. A. (ed.). *The King's men: leadership and status in modern Buganda on the eve of Independence.* London: Oxford University Press. 1964.

———, assisted by F. K. Kamoga and S. B. K. Musoke. Social stratification in modern Buganda. *The King's men: leadership and status in modern Buganda on the eve of Independence.* (L. A. Fallers, ed.). London: Oxford University Press, 1964, pp. 64–116.

Flavell, J. H. *The developmental psychology of Jean Piaget.* Princeton, N. J.: Van Nostrand, 1963.

Foss, B. M. (ed.). *Determinants of infant behaviour*. London: Methuen, 1961.

——— *Determinants of infant behaviour. II*. London, Methuen, 1963.

——— *Determinants of infant behaviour. III*. London: Methuen, 1965.

——— *Determinants on infant behaviour. IV*. (In preparation.)

Fraiberg, Selma H. *The magic years.* New York: Scribners, 1959.

Freud, Anna. *Normality and pathology in childhood.* New York: International Universities Press, 1965.

Freud. S. Inhibitions, symptoms and anxiety (1926). *Standard edition,* XX. London: Hogarth, 1959.

Géber, Marcelle. Développement psychomoteur de l'enfant africain. *Courrier*, 1956, *6*, 17–29.

——— L'enfant africain occidentalisé et de niveau social supérieur en Uganda. *Courrier*, 1958, *8*, 517–23.

——— Problèmes posés par le développement du jeune enfant africain en fonction de son milieu social. *Le Travail Humain,* 1960, *23*, 97–111.

———, and Dean R. F. A. The psychological changes accompanying kwashiorkor. *Courrier*, 1956, *6*, 1–14.

———, and ——— Gesell tests on African children. *Pediatrics.* 1957, *6*, 1055–65.

———, and ——— The state of development of newborn African children. *Lancet,* 1957, *I*, 1216–19.

Gesell, A., and Amatruda, Catherine S. *Developmental diagnosis.* (2nd ed.) New York: Harper, 1947.

Griffiths, Ruth. *The abilities of babies.* London: University of London Press, 1954.

Gunther, Mavis. Instinct and the nursing couple. *Lancet,* 1955, *I, 575–78.*

Harlow, H. F. The development of affectional patterns in infant monkeys. *Determinants of infant behaviour* (B. M. Foss, ed.). London: Methuen, 1961, 51–74.

——— The maternal affectional system. *Determinants of infant behaviour. II* (B. M. Foss, ed.). London: Methuen, 1963, pp. 3–34.

Hinde, R. A. Rhesus monkey aunts. *Determinants of infant behaviour. III* (B. M. Foss, ed.). London: Methuen, 1965, pp. 67—76.

——— *Animal behavior: a synthesis of ethology and comparative psychology.* New York: McGraw-Hill, 1966.

Hunt, J. McV. *Intelligence and experience.* New York: Ronald, 1961.

Lorenz, K. Companionship in bird life. *Instinctive behavior* (Claire H. Schiller, ed.). New York: International Universities Press, 1957, pp. 83–116.

Low, D. A., and Pratt, R. C. *Buganda and British overrule, 1900–1955.* London: Oxford University Press, 1960.

Mair, Lucy B. *An African people in the twentieth century.* London: Routledge, 1934.

Mead, Margaret, and Gorer, G. *Tentative questionnaire for handbook of psychological leads for ethnological field workers: life cycle* (rev. by E. Sapir *et al.).* Issued by the Committee on Culture and Personality of the National Research Council. Mimeographed.

Mead, Margaret. A cultural anthropologist's approach to maternal deprivation. *Deprivation of maternal care: a reassessment of its effects* (Public Health Papers No. 14 [Geneva: World Health Organization, 1962]), pp. 45–62.

Medical Research Council Infantile Malnutrition Group. *Lactation enquiry.* Mimeographed.

Miller, G. A., Galanter, E., and Pribram, K. H. *Plans and the structure of behavior.* New York: Holt, Rinehart and Winston, 1960.

Piaget, J. *The origins of intelligence in children.* New York: International Universities Press, 1952.

——— *The construction of reality in the child.* New York: Basic Books, 1954.

Pratt, R. C. The crisis of 1953–55. *Buganda and British overrule, 1900–1955.* D. A. Low and R. C. Pratt. London: Oxford University Press, 1960, pp. 317–49.

Pribram, K. H. A review of theory in physiological psychology. *Ann. Rev. Psychol.*, 1960, *11*, 1–40.

Read, Margaret. *Children of their fathers.* New Haven: Yale University Press, 1960.

Richards, Audrey I. Authority patterns in traditional Buganda. *The King's men: leadership and status in modern Buganda on the eve of Independence* (L. A. Fallers, ed.). London: Oxford University Press, 1964, pp. 256–93.

——— Traditional values and current political behavior. *The King's men: leadership and status in modern Buganda on the eve of Independence* (L. A. Fallers, ed.). London: Oxford University Press, 1964, pp. 294–335.

Roscoe, J. *The Baganda.* London: Macmillan, 1911.

Rosenblatt, J. S. The basis of synchrony in the behavioral interaction between the mother and her offspring in the laboratory rat. *Determinants of infant behaviour. III* (B. M. Foss, ed.). London: Methuen, 1965, pp. 3–46.

———, Turkewitz, G., and Schneirla, T. C. Early socialization in the domestic cat as based on feeding and other relationships between female and young. *Determinants of infant behaviour* (B. M. Foss, ed.). London: Methuen, 1961, pp. 51–74.

Rowell, Thelma. The social development of some rhesus monkeys. *Determinants of infant behaviour. II* (B. M. Foss, ed.). London: Methuen, 1963, pp. 35–52.

Sander, L. W. Issues in early mother-child interaction. *J. Amer. Acad. Child Psychiat.*, 1962, 7, 141–66.

Schaffer, H. R. Objective observations of personality development in early infancy. *Brit. J. med. Psychol.*, 1958, *31*, 174–83.

———, and Emerson, Peggy E. *The development of social attachments in infancy.* Monog. Soc. Res. Child Develpmt., 1964, No. 3.

Sluckin, W. *Imprinting and early learning.* London: Methuen, 1964.

Spitz, R. A. *The first year of life.* New York: International Universities Press, 1965.

———, and Wolff, Katherine. Anaclitic depression. *The Psychoanalytic Study of the Child,* 1946, *2,* 313–42.

Stellar, E. The physiology of motivation. *Psychol. Rev.*, 1954, *61*, 5–22.

Tennes, Katherine H., and Lampl, E. Esther. Stranger and separation anxiety in infancy. *J. nerv. ment. Dis.*, 1964, *139*, 247–54.

Welbourn, Hebe F. The danger period during weaning: a study of Baganda children. *J. trop. Pediat.*, 1955, *1*, 34–46.

——— Bottle feeding: a problem of modern civilization. *J. trop. Pediat.*, 1958, *3,* 157–66.

——— Weaning among the Baganda. *J. trop. Pediat.*, 1963, *9*, 14–24.

——— *Baganda Childhood.* (In preparation.)

White, R. W. *Ego and reality in psychoanalytic theory.* New York: International Universities Press, 1963.

Whiting, J. W. M. *et al. Field guide for a study of socialization in five societies.* Mimeographed.

Yarrow, L. J. Maternal deprivation: toward an empirical and conceptual re-evaluation. *Psychol. Bull.*, 1961, *58*, 459–90.

——— Research in dimensions of early maternal care. *Merrill-Palmer Quart.*, 1963, *9*, 101–14.

——— Separation from parents during early childhood. *Review of child development research. I* (M. L. Hoffman and Lois W. Hoffman, eds.). New York: Russell Sage Foundation, 1964, pp. 89–136.

INDEX

For Product Safety Concerns and Information please contact our EU representative GPSR@taylorandfrancis.com Taylor & Francis Verlag GmbH, Kaufingerstraße 24, 80331 München, Germany

Batch number: 10830924

Printed by Printforce, the Netherlands